Care of People with Diabetes:

A Manual of Nursing Practice

Trisha Dunning
RN, MEd, PhD, CDE, FRCNA
Professor Director Endocrinology and Diabetes Nursing Research
and Clinical Nurse Consultant Diabetes Education
St Vincent's Hospital and University of Melbourne
Melbourne, Australia

Editorial offices:
Blackwell Publishing Ltd, 9600 Garsington Road, Oxford OX4 2DQ, UK
Tel: +44 (0)1865 776868
Blackwell Publishing Inc., 350 Main Street, Malden, MA 02148-5020, USA
Tel: +1 781 388 8250
Blackwell Publishing Asia Pty, 550 Swanston Street, Carlton, Victoria 3053, Australia
Tel: +61 (0)3 8359 1011

First edition published 1994
Second edition published 2003
Reprinted 2005

Library of Congress Cataloging-in-Publication Data
Dunning, Trisha.
Care of people with diabetes: a manual of nursing practice / Trisha Dunning.—2nd ed.
p. cm.
Includes bibliographical references and index.
ISBN 1-4051-0111-3 (alk. paper)
1. Diabetes—Nursing—Handbooks, manuals, etc. I. Title.
[DNLM: 1. Diabetes Mellitus—nursing—Handbooks. WY 49 D924c 2003]
RC660.D785 2003
610.73'69–dc21

ISBN-10: 1-4051-0111-3
ISBN-13: 978-14051-0111-0

A catalogue record for this title is available from the British Library

Set in 10/11.5 Souvenir
by DP Photosetting, Aylesbury, Bucks
Printed and bound in Great Britain
by TJ International Ltd, Padstow, Cornwall

The publisher's policy is to use permanent paper from mills that operate a sustainable forestry policy, and which has been manufactured from pulp processed using acid-free and elementary chlorine-free practices. Furthermore, the publisher ensures that the text paper and cover board used have met acceptable environmental accreditation standards.

For further information on Blackwell Publishing, visit our website:
www.blackwellpublishing.com

Dedication

This book is dedicated to all people with diabetes who may one day need nursing care, and to all nurses who care for them.

Contents

List of Figures xvii
List of Tables xviii
Example Forms and Instruction Sheets xx
Foreword xxi
Preface xxiii
Acknowledgements xxvi
List of Abbreviations and Symbols xxvii

1 Diagnosis and Classification of Diabetes 1

1.1 Key points 1
1.2 What is diabetes mellitus? 1
1.3 Classification of diabetes 1
1.4 Type 1 and Type 2 diabetes 2
1.5 Diagnosis of diabetes 8
1.6 Oral glucose tolerance test (OGTT) 9
Example Instruction Sheet 1: Preparation for an oral glucose tolerance test 10
1.7 Screening for diabetes 11
1.8 Management of diabetes mellitus 11
1.9 Diabetes education 16
1.10 Complications of diabetes 17
1.11 Cost of diabetes 18
1.12 Aim and objectives of nursing care of people with diabetes 19
References 21

2 Assessment and Nursing Diagnosis 22

2.1 Key points 22
Rationale 22
2.2 Characteristics of the nursing history 22
2.3 Nursing history 23
Example of an assessment chart 24

3 Documenting and Charting Patient Care 29

3.1 Documenting in the medical record 29
3.2 Nursing responsibilities 33

3.3 Documentation by people with diabetes 33
References 33

4 Monitoring Diabetes Mellitus **34**

Rationale 34
4.1 Introduction 34
Monitoring 1: blood glucose **35**
4.2 Key points 35
4.3 The role of blood glucose monitoring in the care of diabetes 35
4.4 Guidelines for the frequency of blood glucose monitoring 36
4.5 Blood glucose meters 38
4.6 Reasons for inaccurate blood glucose results 39
4.7 Non-invasive/minimally invasive blood glucose testing 39
4.8 Monitoring blood ketones 40
Blood glucose testing checklist **41**
Monitoring 2: urine glucose/ketones and blood ketones **44**
4.9 Key points 44
4.10 Introduction 44
4.11 Limitations of urine glucose testing 44
4.12 Indications for urine glucose tests 45
4.13 Monitoring ketones 45
4.14 Urine tests of kidney function 46
4.15 Micral-test 46
Monitoring 3: additional assessment **47**
4.16 Nursing responsibilities 47
4.17 Blood glucose 48
4.18 Glycosylated haemoglobin (HbA1c) 48
4.19 Fructosamines 48
4.20 Serum lipids 49
4.21 C-peptide 49
4.22 Islet cell antibodies 50
4.23 Creatinine clearance and urea 50
4.24 Oral glucose tolerance test (OGTT) 50
References 51

5 Nutritional Aspects of Caring for People with Diabetes **52**

5.1 Key points 52
Rationale 52
5.2 Role of the nurse 52
5.3 Obesity 53
5.4 Method of screening for dietary characteristics and problems 54
5.5 Principles of dietary management for people with diabetes 55
5.6 'Sugar-free' foods 56
5.7 Non-nutritive sweeteners 57
5.8 Carbohydrate modified foods 57
5.9 Dietetic foods 57
5.10 Alcohol 57
5.11 'Exchanges' and 'portions' 58
5.12 Glycaemic index 58

5.13 Exercise/activity 58
5.14 Example questions to ask when taking a diet history 58
References 59

6 Oral Hypoglycaemia and Lipid Lowering Agents 60

6.1 Key points 60
Rationale 60
6.2 Introduction 60
6.3 Sulphonylureas 61
6.4 Biguanides 61
6.5 Glitinides 63
6.6 Thiazolidinediones 63
6.7 Alpha-glucosidase inhibitors 63
6.8 Drug interactions 66
6.9 Combining OHAs 67
6.10 Combining OHAs and insulin 67
6.11 Lipid lowering agents 68
References 69

7 Insulin Therapy 71

7.1 Key points 71
Rationale 71
7.2 Basic insulin action 71
7.3 Objectives of insulin therapy 72
7.4 Types of insulin available 72
7.5 Storage of insulin 74
7.6 Injection site and administration 74
7.7 Mixing short- and long-acting insulins 77
7.8 Common insulin regimes 77
7.9 Continuous subcutaneous insulin infusion (CSII) 84
7.10 Sliding scale and top-up regimes 86
7.11 Intravenous insulin infusions 87
7.12 Uses of insulin infusions 88
7.13 Risks associated with insulin infusions 89
7.14 Factors affecting insulin delivery via infusion 90
7.15 Mistakes associated with insulin infusions 90
7.16 Inhaled insulin 91
7.17 Insulin allergy 91
7.18 Pancreas transplants 92
References 92

8 Hypoglycaemia 94

8.1 Key points 94
Rationale 94
8.2 Introduction 94
8.3 Definition of hypoglycaemia 94
8.4 Recognising hypoglycaemia 95
8.5 Counter-regulatory hormonal response to hypoglycaemia 96

8.6 Objectives of care 96
8.7 Treatment 96
8.8 Nocturnal hypoglycaemia 98
8.9 Chronic hypoglycaemia 99
8.10 Relative hypoglycaemia 99
8.11 Drug interactions 99
8.12 Patients most at risk of hypoglycaemia 100
8.13 Psychological effects of hypoglycaemia 100
8.14 Guidelines for the administration of glucagon 101
8.15 Adverse reactions 102
References 102

9 Stabilisation of Diabetes **103**

9.1 Key points 103
Rationale 103
9.2 Stabilisation of diabetes in hospital 104
9.3 Outpatient stabilisation 104
References 107
Example protocol for outpatient stabilisation onto insulin **108**

10 Hyperglycaemia, Diabetic Ketoacidosis (DKA), Hyperosmolar Coma and Lactic Acidosis **110**

10.1 Key points 110
Rationale 110
10.2 Hyperglycaemia 110
10.3 Diabetic ketoacidosis (DKA) 110
10.4 Hyperosmolar non-ketotic coma (HONK) 117
10.5 Prevention 119
10.6 Euglycaemic DKA 119
10.7 Lactic acidosis 119
References 120

11 Cardiovascular Disease and Diabetes **121**

11.1 Key points 121
Rationale 121
11.2 Objectives of care 123
11.3 Nursing responsibilities 123
11.4 Medical tests/procedures 125
11.5 Rehabilitation 125
11.6 Modification of risk factors associated with the development of cardiac disease 126
11.7 Coaching 126
11.8 Cerebrovascular disease 126
References 127

12 Management During Surgical Procedures **128**

12.1 Key points 128
Rationale 128

12.2 Introduction 128
12.3 Aims of management 129
12.4 Preoperative nursing care 130
12.5 Major procedures 131
12.6 Postoperative nursing responsibilities 132
12.7 Minor procedures 132
12.8 Emergency procedures 134
References 134

Example Instruction Sheet 2(a): Instructions for diabetic patients on oral hypoglycaemic agents having procedures as outpatients under sedation or general anaesthesia 135

Example Instruction Sheet 2(b): Instructions for diabetic patients on insulin having procedures as outpatients under sedation or general anaesthesia 136

13 Care During Investigative Procedures 137

13.1 Key points 137
Rationale 137
13.2 The objectives of care 137
13.3 General nursing management 138
13.4 Colonoscopy 138
13.5 Eye procedures 138
13.6 Care of the patient having radiocontrast media injected 140

14 Special Situations and Unusual Conditions Related to Diabetes 142

Introduction 142

14a Enteral and parenteral nutrition 143
14.1 Key points 143
14.2 Aims of therapy 143
14.3 Routes of administration 144
14.4 Choice of formula 145
14.5 Nursing responsibilities 145
References 147

14b Diabetes and cancer 148
14.6 Key points 148
14.7 Objectives of care 148
14.8 Nursing responsibilities 149
References 150

14c Autonomic neuropathy 151
14.9 Key points 151
Rationale 151
14.10 Introduction 151
14.11 Diagnosis and management 152
14.12 Nursing care 154
References 155

14d Diabetes and corticosteroid medications 156
14.13 Key points 156

	Rationale	156
14.14	Introduction	156
14.15	Effect on blood glucose	156
14.16	Predisposing factors	157
14.17	Management	157
	References	158
14e	**Brittle diabetes**	**159**
14.18	Key points	159
	Rationale	159
14.19	Introduction	159
14.20	Management	159
	Reference	160
14f	**Teeth, gums and diabetes**	**161**
14.21	Key points	161
14.22	Introduction	161
14.23	Causal mechanisms	162
14.24	Management	162
	References	162
14g	**Haemochromatosis and hepatic iron overload**	**163**
14.25	Key points	163
14.26	Haemochromatosis	163
14.27	Iron overload	163
14.28	Management	163
	References	164
14h	**Diabetic mastopathy**	**165**
14.29	Key points	165
14.30	Diabetic mastopathy	165
14.31	Diagnosis	165
14.32	Management	165
	Reference	165
15	**Diabetes and Eye Disease**	**166**
15.1	Key points	166
	Rationale	166
15.2	Introduction	166
15.3	Risk factors for retinopathy	167
15.4	Eye problems associated with diabetes	167
15.5	Resources for people with visual impairment	168
15.6	Aids for people with low vision	169
15.7	Nursing care of visually impaired patients	169
	References	170
16	**Diabetes and Renal Disease**	**171**
16.1	Key points	171
16.2	Introduction	171
16.3	Risk factors for renal disease	171
16.4	Renal failure	172

16.5 Renal disease and anaemia 172
16.6 Diet and renal disease 173
16.7 Renal disease and the elderly patient 173
16.8 Kidney biopsy 174
16.9 Renal dialysis 174
16.10 Objectives of care 175
16.11 Nursing responsibilities 176
16.12 Commencing CAPD in patients on insulin 176
16.13 Protocol for insulin administration in people with diabetes on CAPD – based on four bag changes each day 177
16.14 Education of patient about CAPD 177
16.15 Renal disease and herbal medicine 178
References 179

17 Diabetes and Sexual Health 180

17.1 Key points 180
Rationale 180
17.2 Sexual health 180
17.3 Sexual development 181
17.4 Sexual problems 181
17.5 Possible causes of sexual difficulties and dysfunction 182
17.6 Sexuality and the elderly 183
17.7 Women 183
17.8 Men 184
17.9 Investigation and management 185
17.10 Sexual counselling 186
17.11 The PLISSIT model 187
17.12 Role of the nurse 187
References 188

18 Diabetes in the Older Person 189

18.1 Key points 189
Rationale 189
18.2 Introduction 189
18.3 Metabolic changes 192
18.4 Aims of treatment 193
18.5 Education approaches 193
18.6 Access and equity to diabetes services 194
18.7 Factors that can affect metabolic control 194
18.8 Infection 195
18.9 Quality of life 195
18.10 Safety 196
18.11 Medications 196
18.12 Nutrition 198
18.13 Hypoglycaemia 199
18.14 Diabetes and falls 200
18.15 Nursing care 201
References 201

19 Foot Care **203**

19.1 Key points 203
Rationale 203
19.2 Vascular changes 204
19.3 Infection 204
19.4 Neuropathy 205
19.5 Objectives of care 207
19.6 Nursing responsibilities 207
19.7 Classification of foot ulcers 209
19.8 Wound management 209
19.9 Rehabilitation 211
References 211

20 Diabetes in Children and Adolescents **213**

20.1 Key points 213
Rationale 213
20.2 Introduction 213
20.3 Diabetes in children and adolescents 214
20.4 Strategies to enhance compliance in adolscence 215
20.5 Ketoacidosis in children 216
References 217

21 Diabetes in Pregnancy and Gestational Diabetes **218**

21.1 Key points 218
Rationale 218
21.2 Introduction 218
References 220

22 Psychological and Quality of Life Issues Related to Having Diabetes **221**

22.1 Key points 221
Rationale 221
22.2 Introduction 221
22.3 Depression 224
22.4 Type 1 diabetes 224
22.5 Type 2 diabetes 225
22.6 Compliance/non-compliance 226
22.7 Quality of life 227
References 228

23 Diabetes Education **230**

23.1 Key points 230
Rationale 230
23.2 Introduction 230
Sample diabetes education record chart **232**
23.3 Empowerment 234
23.4 Special issues 235
23.5 The role of the bedside nurse in diabetes education 235

23.6 Insulin administration 237
23.7 Guidelines for instructing patients about insulin delivery systems 237
Example Instruction Sheet 3: How to draw up insulin – one bottle only 239
Example Instruction Sheet 4: How to draw up insulin – two bottles 240
Example Instruction Sheet 5: How to give an insulin injection 241
Example Instruction Sheet 6a: Managing your diabetes when you are ill: patients with Type 1 diabetes 242
Example Instruction Sheet 6b: Managing your diabetes when you are ill: patients with Type 2 diabetes 245
References 248

24 Discharge Planning 249

24.1 Key points 249
24.2 On day of discharge 249

25 District Nursing and Home-based Care 251

25.1 Key points 251
25.2 Introduction 251
25.3 How to obtain help 252
25.4 General points 252
25.5 Diabetic problems nurses commonly encounter in the home 252
25.6 Nursing actions 252
25.7 Interpreting the blood glucose level 253
25.8 Hypoglycaemia 253
25.9 Hyperglycaemia 254
25.10 The patient with chest pain 255
25.11 The patient who has not taken their insulin or diabetes tablets and it is 11 AM or later 255
25.12 Managing diabetic foot ulcers at home 256
25.13 The patient who does not follow the management plan 257
25.14 Disposal of sharps in the home situation 258
25.15 Storage of insulin 258
25.16 Guidelines for premixing and storing insulin doses for home and district nursing services 259
References 260

26 Complementary Therapies and Diabetes 261

26.1 Key points 261
Rationale 261
26.2 Introduction 261
26.3 Complementary therapy philosophy 263
26.4 Integrating complementary and conventional care 263
26.5 Can complementary therapies benefit people with diabetes? 264
26.6 How can complementary therapies be used safely? 269
26.7 Nursing responsibilities 270
References 271

27 Nursing Care in the Emergency and Outpatient Departments **273**

Rationale 273
27.1 The emergency department 273
27.2 The outpatient department 275

***Appendix A:* Associations Providing Services for People with Diabetes** **276**

A.1 Diabetic associations 276
A.2 Professional diabetes associations 277
A.3 International Diabetes Federation (IDF) 277
A.4 Other professional associations 277
A.5 Pharmaceutical companies 278

***Appendix B:* Diabetes Reference Material for Nursing Staff** **279**

B.1 Reference texts 279
B.2 Practical texts 279
B.3 Recommended journals 279

***Appendix C:* Reading Material for People with Diabetes** **280**

Index **281**

List of Figures

1.1 Schematic representation of the slow progressive loss of beta cell mass following the initial trigger event in Type 1 diabetes 3
1.2 Consequences of the insulin resistance syndrome 4
1.3 Diagrammatic representation of insulin binding, insulin signalling, translocation of GLUT-4 and glucose entry into the cell 5
1.4 Example of a screening and preventative model of health care 12
1.5 Suggested diabetes management model. Most diabetes management occurs in primary care settings in collaboration with secondary and tertiary care services 14
1.6 Normal energy sources during exercise 15
3.1 Example of a combination genomap and ecomap of a 50-year-old woman with Type 2 diabetes and a history of childhood molestation and sexual abuse. It shows a great deal of conflict within and outside the family and identifies where her support base is 30
3.2 Sample diabetes record charts for (a) 2-T hourly testing (e.g. when using an insulin infusion); (b) 4-hourly or less frequent testing 32
4.1 An example quality control flow chart for checking blood glucose meters 40
7.1 Range of Lilly insulins, their presentation and schematic action profiles 78
7.2 (a) Range of Novo Nordisk insulins with their time action characteristics and insulin profiles and (b) the delivery systems available within each insulin 80
7.3 Diagrammatic representation of insulin action showing different regimes: (a) daily, (b) twice daily, (c) basal bolus using short-acting insulins and (d) basal bolus using rapid-acting insulins 85
7.4 Possible results of blocking of the IV cannula and three-way adaptor during the concurrent administration of insulin and dextrose/saline 91
10.1 An outline of the physiology, signs and symptoms and biochemical changes occurring in the development of diabetic ketoacidosis (DKA) 112
10.2 An outline of the development of hyperosmolar coma 118
19.1 Diagrammatic representation of the factors leading to foot problems in people with diabetes 206
22.1 Model of the diabetic grief cycle 223

List of Tables

1.1	Characteristics of Type 1 and Type 2 diabetes mellitus	6
1.2	Diagnostic criteria for diabetes based on the World Health Organisation guidelines. Fasting plasma glucose is the preferred test for diagnosis, but any of the three tests are acceptable	8
1.3	Guidelines for assessment of control of diabetes	13
4.1	Blood ketone levels and potential management	42
4.2	Currently available urine test strips	45
4.3	Non-glycaemic factors affecting results of glycosylated haemoglobin assays	49
5.1	Drugs whose absorption can be modified by food	56
6.1	Oral hypoglycaemic agents, dose range and frequency, possible side effects, the duration of action and main site of metabolism	64
6.2	Potential drug interactions between oral hypoglycaemic agents and other drugs (based on Shenfield 2001)	67
6.3	Lipid lowering agents	69
7.1	Readily available insulin devices and some of the issues to be aware of with each device	75
7.2	Some commonly encountered factors that affect insulin absorption	86
8.1	Signs and symptoms of hypoglycaemia	95
8.2	The counter-regulatory hormonal response to hypoglycaemia	96
8.3	Commonly prescribed drugs which can increase the hypoglycaemic effect of sulphonylurea drugs	99
10.1	Signs, symptoms and precipitating factors in diabetic ketoacidosis (DKA)	111
10.2	The metabolic consequences of diabetic ketoacidosis and associated risks	113
11.1	Diabetes-specific cardiovascular abnormalities that predispose an individual to heart disease	122
12.1	Hormonal, metabolic and long-term effects of surgery	129
14.1	Organs commonly affected by diabetes autonomic neuropathy and the resultant clinical features	153
18.1	Particular problems encountered in the elderly person with diabetes and the resultant risks associated with the problem	190
18.2	Factors that can affect diabetes control and management in elderly patients	195
18.3	Risk factors for inadequate nutrition and malnutrition in the elderly	198
19.1	Changes in the feet due to normal ageing	206
19.2	Risk factors for the development of foot problems in people with diabetes	207
19.3	Management of specific foot problems while the person is in hospital	210
23.1	Factors which influence teaching and learning	236

26.1 Commonly used complementary therapies 262
26.2 Commonly used herbs and supplements, their potential interactions, reported adverse events and some management strategies to use should an adverse event occur 267

Example Forms and Instruction Sheets

Forms

Example of an assessment chart, formulated for people with diabetes 24
Blood glucose testing checklist 41
Example protocol for outpatient stabilisation onto insulin 108
Sample diabetes education record chart 232

Example Instruction Sheets

1 Preparation for an oral glucose tolerance test 10
2a Instructions for diabetic patients on oral hypoglycaemic agents having procedures as outpatients under sedation or general anaesthesia 135
2b Instructions for diabetic patients on insulin having procedures as outpatients under sedation or general anaesthesia 136
3 How to draw up insulin – one bottle only 239
4 How to draw up insulin – two bottles 240
5 How to give an insulin injection 241
6a Managing your diabetes when you are ill: patients with Type 1 diabetes 242
6b Managing your diabetes when you are ill: patients with Type 2 diabetes 245

Foreword

Worldwide, the prevalence of diabetes is increasing at an alarming rate and much of the care previously considered the domain of the medical practitioner will now need to be undertaken by nursing staff. Hence, it is essential that nurses, whatever the context of their working environment, develop a sound clinical understanding of diabetes management.

This remarkably comprehensive book reflects the depth of knowledge and experience of its author and will assist nurses in the process of diabetes management. The text encompasses many areas of diabetic care and bridges the gap between traditional nursing texts and diabetes medical textbooks. It will be valuable to nurses working on the periphery of diabetes in a hospital or community environment as well as to nurses who have developed a career in diabetes care. The author provides carefully detailed aspects of clinical care such as the caution required when using radio-contrast medium in people with diabetes and renal impairment while also including information about the use of complementary therapies for diabetes management.

The diagnosis of diabetes, whether it is type 1 or type 2, has a significant impact on the life of the person and their family. Living with diabetes is not easy and requires considerable dedication and commitment to adapt to the life-long regimen imposed by this chronic disease. While it is inevitable that nurses will take on an increased clinical role, it is also important that they do not forget the fundamental purpose of nursing which is to care for patients. Nursing staff must recognise not only the medical aspects of diabetes but also its psychosocial impact and thus not be judgemental when caring for the patient with diabetes. This book emphasises the need for a holistic approach and provides insight into the many physiological and psychological facets of diabetes care.

It is with much delight that I write the foreword to this excellent textbook written by my friend and colleague Dr Trisha Dunning. Her vast experience in diabetes education, clinical management and research is obvious. I wholeheartedly recommend this text to all health professionals whether working directly in, or on, the fringe of diabetes. This textbook should be considered essential reading for diabetes management.

Marg McGill MSc (Med)
Chair, International Diabetes Federation Consultative Section on Diabetes Education

Preface

Background to the second edition

It has been 30 years since I trained as a nurse in the days of Fehling's solution to test for urine glucose and glass reusable insulin syringes. My first exposure to diabetes was the complete devastation of a school friend who developed diabetes during her first pregnancy. I had no intuitive flash to become a diabetes nurse specialist/diabetes educator – they did not exist. Diabetes itself was hardly considered. Today diabetes is the focus of my working and a great deal of my personal life.

Diabetes has come a long way too, since it was first described as *diabetes maigre* (bad prognosis) and *diabetes gros* (big diabetes). Science and technology have made major contributions to our understanding of the pathophysiology of diabetes and its complications, and to our management options, and have enabled people with diabetes to have autonomy over their disease.

The incidence of diabetes is increasing, particularly in the elderly. People are living longer and there is an increasing incidence of Type 2 diabetes in developing countries and depressed populations. There truly is a diabetes epidemic. The information presented in this Manual offers suggestions for the nursing management of people with diabetes. Where references exist, they are included to support the nursing care recommendations and as a framework for continuing education. A number of guidelines for managing diabetes exist, but most refer to medical management and primary and outpatient care, rather than nursing care in acute settings.

The nursing care described in this Manual has been partly extrapolated from these documents and is based on the clinical experience and knowledge gleaned over 17 years of practice in diabetes education and care and discussion with nursing colleagues.

The book was written to fill the gap between academia and clinical practice by providing easy-to-access information that can be directly applied in busy clinical situations. The purpose is to guide the practice of diabetes nursing and assist nurses to provide consistent care and achieve better outcomes for their patients with diabetes. The first edition was successful in meeting these goals.

A number of changes have occurred since the Manual was first published that require the information to be revised and updated. They include improvements in diabetes technology, understanding of the disease process and its complications and shifting the focus to empowering people with diabetes.

In particular, the results of the Diabetes Control and Complications Trial (DCCT 1993) and the United Kingdom Prospective Diabetes Study (UKPDS 1998) have had a significant impact on current diabetes management. In addition, the Australian *National Diabetes Strategy* (NDS) (Colagiuri *et al.* 1998) and the British *Diabetes National*

Service Framework: Standards for Diabetes Services (Department of Health 2001) define the standards of care in those countries. The NDS does not address nursing care or management in the acute setting. The British National Service Framework consists of 12 standards in nine areas due to come into operation in 2003. One standard refers to care of people with diabetes during a hospital admission.

For the past six years I have been privileged to be a member of the Victorian Nurses Care Awards, a committee that receives nominations from patients of nurses they consider to have demonstrated excellence in nursing practice. These nominations demonstrate that people value the 'art', or caring aspects of nursing practice, but also expect to be cared for by competent, knowledgeable nurses.

Almost all countries, especially the UK and Australia, are moving towards managing diabetes in primary care settings with integrated care programmes. This means that people with diabetes in hospital are likely to be sicker and require skilled nursing care. Because the incidence and prevalence of diabetes is increasing worldwide, most nurses can expect to care for a person with diabetes at some stage of their nursing career.

In order to address these issues, some chapters have required extensive revision, others very little. New chapters have been added, for example, on care of the elderly, to increase the relevance of the Manual to aged and community settings, and on complementary therapies, to reflect the increasing use of these therapies by the general public and nurses. References have been included that serve as the evidence base for the recommendations.

There is a growing trend to prefer the term 'people with diabetes' rather than 'diabetics' or 'patients'. The terms 'people with diabetes' and 'patients' are used interchangeably throughout the Manual, as appropriate to the particular reference. Most people, including people with diabetes, still regard people in hospital as patients.

A trend in some parts of the world, including Australia and the UK, is the development of the nurse practitioner role. Diabetes nurse specialists/diabetes educators will be one category of nurse practitioner. The nurse practitioner is an experienced advanced clinical nurse with an extended scope of practice that includes medication management, one component of which is prescribing. Diabetes educator nurse practitioners are likely to play a major role in diabetes care in the future and will be in an ideal position to support ward nurses.

It is my hope that the revised edition of the Manual will continue to contribute to the body of nursing knowledge about diabetes, and that it will be of assistance to nurses (and other health professionals) involved in the care of people with diabetes. I have endeavoured to make the information general and applicable to all nurses; I hope each person who reads the Manual will find something of value.

Using the Manual

> The nurse, more than any other member of the health team, is the person who interprets to the patient the care he must take of himself and his family. Her belief in the comprehensiveness of adequate care will influence the scope of her care beyond the treatment prescribed by the physician.
>
> (Henderson 1966)

In spite of the age, and sexism, of this reference, the philosophy is still relevant today, especially given the rise of the nurse practitioner role and advanced nursing practice. Nursing is both an art and a science whose essence is caring. Nurses have a responsibility, with other health professionals, for planning, implementing and evaluating the care given to patients under their care. Nurses function in a variety of settings and the components of the nurse's role varies according to the setting (hospital, community health centres, city or remote areas).

Nursing care is distinct from medical care, but nursing and medical care complement each other. Some nursing actions occur as a result of the medical orders, others are the basis on which the medical orders are formulated. It is of the utmost importance, then, that nurses have adequate knowledge about disease processes and their effect on individuals in order to provide optimal care.

People who have had diabetes for some time are often aware of omissions and poorly performed procedures relating to their care in hospital. In the case of people with diabetes, this is particularly true of blood glucose testing, and hypoglycaemia, management. A lack of trust in the staff, considerable anxiety and confusion about the correct method can result if nursing practice is not consistent with the teaching of the diabetes education team.

This Manual has been designed as a quick reference source for specific nursing actions needed in the care of people with diabetes mellitus to allow nursing care plans to be formulated quickly in busy situations and to provide references where more information can be found. A list of key points is given at the beginning of most chapters. Important information is referenced throughout the text. In addition, practice points based on research findings, and clinical observations based on personal experience are included.

Chapters are cross-referenced where appropriate. The pathophysiology and medical management of diabetes is discussed only briefly because it is more than adequately covered in other publications, see Appendix B.

The care outlined in this Manual does not negatve the provision of basic general nursing care as indicated by the presenting condition, but focuses on the specific and extra needs of people with diabetes. The presence of diabetes will have physiological effects on the presenting condition if diabetes is not adequately controlled. A careful assessment of individual physical, psychological and spiritual needs should form the basis of all nursing care.

Practice point

The procedure and policies of the employing institution should be followed. This Manual does not replace these documents.

References

Colagiuri, S., Colagiuri, R. & Ward, J. (1998) *National Diabetes Strategy and Implementation Plan*. Diabetes Australia, Canberra.

DCCT (Diabetes Control and Complications Trial Research Group) (1993) The effect of intensive treatment of diabetes on the development and progression of long term complications in insulin dependent diabetes. *New England Journal of Medicine*, **329**, 977–986.

Department of Health (2001) *Diabetes National Service Framework: Standards for Diabetes Services*. Department of Health, London.

Henderson, V. (1966) *The Nature of Nursing*. Macmillan, New York.

United Kingdom Prospective Diabetes Study (UKPDS) (1998) Intensive blood glucose control with sulphonylureas or insulin compared with conventional treatment and risk of complications in patients with Type 2 diabetes (UKPDS 33). *Lancet*, **352**, 837–853.

Acknowledgements

I would especially like to thank Blackwell Publishing for promoting the book and for supporting a second edition.

I work in a supportive team of doctors and nurses and to that team I say a special thank you, in particular, to doctors Frank Alford and Glenn Ward, and my colleagues Linda Jackson, Linda Stevenson, Bridget Wilkes, Rachel Miller and Louise O'Brien. To the nurses on the wards who reviewed the first edition and made helpful suggestions about the proposed revisions, I am truly grateful. Their input enhances the applicability of the information to all nurses who will use the Manual.

I am in debt to the librarians of St Vincent's Hospital, Sandra, Lorraine and Hilary, who are always interested in what I am doing, ask after progress, track down references for me and look forward to having a copy of the new edition in the library.

To Michelle Robins from Melbourne Extended Care and Rehabilitation Service who advised about the chapter on the care of the elderly, Dr Richard Gilbert for his helpful advice about renal disease, Dr Frank Alford for reviewing the medication chapters, and Meredith Plummer and the renal nursing team from St Vincent's Hospital Renal Unit for their helpful comments about renal nursing, my sincere thanks.

My thanks go to Louise McLaren, Product Manager, Novo Nordisk Australia and Jehangir Sidhwa, National Sales Manager, Eli Lilly Australia for permission to use their respective insulin charts in Chapter 7.

Elisabeth Davies deciphered my hand-drawn figures and turned them into works of art. Thank you, Liz.

I have learned a great deal about diabetes from the people with diabetes I teach and care for and their families. I thank them for the privilege of caring for them.

To my editor Eleanor Rivers thank you for your skill and patience – I know how much work is involved in turning a manuscript into a book.

The support and understanding of my family continue to be invaluable. My especial thanks and love go to my husband, John, who is still 'the wind beneath my wings'.

List of Abbreviations and Symbols

↑	Increased
↓	Decreased
$<$	Less than
$\geq$	Equal to, or greater than
$>$	Greater than
BG	Blood glucose
BMI	Body mass index
BP	Blood pressure
BUN	Blood urea nitrogen
CAPD	Continuous ambulatory peritoneal dialysis
CCF	Congestive cardiac failure
CCU	Coronary care unit
CSII	Continuous subcutaneous insulin infusion
DA	Diabetes Australia
DKA	Diabetic ketoacidosis
ECG	Electrocardiogram
EN	Enteral nutrition
FFA	Free fatty acids
HbA1c	Glycosylated haemoglobin
HM	Human insulin
HONK	Hyperosmolar non-ketotic coma
ICU	Intensive care unit
IV	Intravenous therapy lines
LFT	Liver function test
MODY	Maturity onset diabetes in the young
NDSS	National Diabetes Supply Scheme
OGTT	Oral glucose tolerance test
OHA	Oral hypoglycaemic agent
TPN	Total parenteral nutrition
TPR	Temperature, pulse and respiration
WHO	World Health Organisation

The words are used in full the first time they appear in the text. All abbreviations are widely accepted and recognised.

Chapter 1
Diagnosis and Classification of Diabetes

1.1 Key points

- Diabetes represents a considerable economic and social burden for the person with diabetes and the health system.
- The classification of diabetes was revised by the American Diabetes Association in 1997 and adopted by the World Health Organisation in 1998. It was adopted in Australia and by Diabetes UK in 1999.
- Type 2 diabetes is a progressive disease and complications are often present at diagnosis.

1.2 What is diabetes mellitus?

Diabetes mellitus is a metabolic disorder in which the body's capacity to utilise glucose, fat and protein is disturbed due to insulin deficiency or insulin resistance. Both states lead to an elevated blood glucose concentration and glycosuria.

The body is unable to utilise glucose in the absence of insulin and draws on fats and proteins in an effort to supply fuel for energy. Carbohydrate is necessary for the complete metabolism of fats, however, and when carbohydrate metabolism is disordered fat metabolism is incomplete and intermediate products (ketone bodies) can accumulate in the blood leading to ketosis, especially in Type 1 diabetes. The protein breakdown in this situation leads to weight loss and weakness and contributes to the development of hyperglycaemia and lethargy.

There are different types of diabetes which have different underlying causal mechanisms and clinical presentation. In general, young people are insulin-deficient (Type 1 diabetes), while older people may have sufficient insulin secretion and plasma insulin levels but demonstrate resistance to its action (Type 2 diabetes). Type 2 diabetes is the most common, accounting for 85% of diagnosed cases; Type 1 accounts for 15% of diagnosed cases. N.B. Type 2 diabetes occurs in children and Type 1 diabetes occurs in the elderly.

1.3 Classification of diabetes

The American Diabetes Association (ADA) announced a revised diabetes classification system and diagnostic criteria in 1997. These revised data were a joint activity between the ADA and the World Health Organisation (WHO). As part of the new classification the terms insulin-dependent diabetes (IDDM) and non-insulin-dependent diabetes (NIDDM) were replaced with Type 1 and Type 2 diabetes (Expert Committee on the Diagnosis and Classification of Diabetes Mellitus 1997).

- Type 1 diabetes has two forms:
  - Immune-mediated diabetes mellitus, which results from autoimmune destruction of the pancreatic beta cells;
  - Idiopathic diabetes mellitus refers to forms of the disease that have no known aetiologies.
- Type 2 diabetes mellitus refers to diseases associated with relative insulin deficiency and insulin resistance.
- Impaired glucose homeostasis, which is an intermediate metabolic stage between normal glucose homeostasis and diabetes. It is a significant risk factor for cardiovascular disease. There are two forms:
  - Impaired fasting glucose, where the fasting plasma glucose is higher than normal but lower than the diagnostic criteria;
  - Impaired glucose tolerance, where the plasma glucose is higher than normal and lower than the diagnostic criteria after a 75 gram glucose tolerance test, see 1.6.
- Gestational diabetes mellitus, diabetes occurring in pregnancy.
- Other specific types, which include diabetes caused by other identifiable disease processes:
  - Genetic defects of beta cell function such as MODY;
  - Genetic defects of insulin action;
  - Diseases of the exocrine pancreas such as cancer and pancreatitis;
  - Endocrine disorders such as Cushing's disease, and Acromegaly;
  - Drug or chemical induced diabetes.

Diabetes affects approximately 0.5 to > 10% of the population depending on the type of diabetes, age group and ethnic group. The incidence of diabetes is increasing, particularly in the older age group and in developing countries.

A recent study in Australia (Dunstan *et al.* 2000), indicates that 7.5% of people over 25 years and 16.8% of people over 65 have diabetes and a further 16.1% have impaired glucose tolerance. In the UK, an estimated 1.4 million people have diabetes (Audit Commission 2000). In both countries Type 2 is the most common type, accounting for 80–90% of cases.

1.4 Type 1 and Type 2 diabetes

1.4.1 Type 1 diabetes

Type 1 diabetes is a disease of absolute insulin deficiency that usually affects children and young adults but can occur in older people. It often presents with the so-called classic symptoms of diabetes mellitus:

- Polyuria
- Polydipsia
- Lethargy
- Weight loss.

These symptoms usually occur over a short space of time (two to three weeks) as a result of destruction of the beta cells of the pancreas. The precipitating event may have occurred many years prior to the development of the symptoms. Type 1 diabetes can be due to an autoimmune or idiopathic process. It classically presents with elevated blood glucose and urinary glucose and ketosis. In severe cases the patient will present with diabetic ketoacidosis (DKA) (see Chapter 9).

Figure 1.1 is a schematic representation of the progression of Type 1 diabetes. It shows the progressive relentless destruction of the beta cells from the time of the initial triggering event. Three per cent of first-degree relatives of people with Type 1 diabetes have beta cell antibodies, usually with normal glucose tolerance and some progress to diabetes. Immunosuppression with Azathioprine or Cyclosporin and immunomodulation using Nicotinamide, to prevent further beta cell destruction have been used in newly diagnosed or pre-Type 1 diabetes but are not common. These drugs are potent immunosuppressive agents and their use cannot be warranted in the long term. Insulin has also been used in an attempt to stimulate immune tolerance, but not successfully.

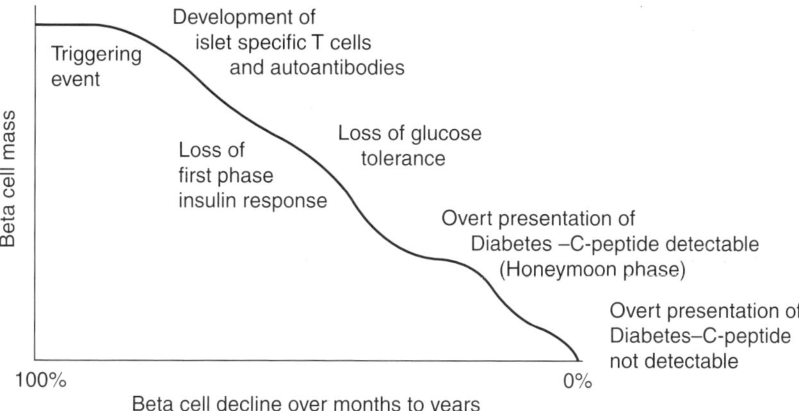

Figure 1.1 Schematic representation of the slow progressive loss of beta cell mass following the initial trigger event in Type 1 diabetes.

1.4.2 Type 2 diabetes

Type 2 diabetes is not 'just a touch of sugar' or 'mild diabetes'. It is an insidious progressive disease that is often diagnosed late when complications are present. Type 2 diabetes often presents with an established long-term complication of diabetes such as neuropathy, cardiovascular disease or retinopathy. Alternatively, diabetes may be diagnosed during another illness or on routine screening. The classic symptoms described above are often less obvious and occur over a longer period of time. Once treatment is instituted people often recognise that they have more energy and are less thirsty. Insulin resistance often precedes Type 2 diabetes.

Insulin resistance is the term given to an impaired biological response to both endogenous and exogenous insulin that can be improved with weight loss. Insulin resistance is a stage in the development of impaired glucose tolerance, which precedes the onset of Type 2 diabetes. When insulin resistance is present, insulin production is increased (hyperinsulinaemia) to sustain normal glucose tolerance; however, the hepatic glucose output is not suppressed and fasting hyperglycaemia and decreased postprandial glucose utilisation results.

Insulin resistance is a result of a primary genetic defect and secondary environmental factors (Turner & Clapham 1998). When intracellular glucose is high, free fatty acids (FFAs) are stored. When it is low FFAs enter the circulation as substrates for glucose production. Insulin normally promotes tryglyceride synthesis and inhibits postprandial lypolysis. Glucose uptake into adipocytes is impaired in Type 2 diabetes and circulating FFAs have a harmful effect on hepatic glucose production and insulin sensitivity. Increasing blood glucose also plays a role. Eventually the beta cells do not respond to glucose and this is referred to as glucose toxicity. Loss of beta cell function is present in over 50% of people with Type 2 diabetes at diagnosis. Figure 1.2 depicts the consequences of the insulin resistance syndrome.

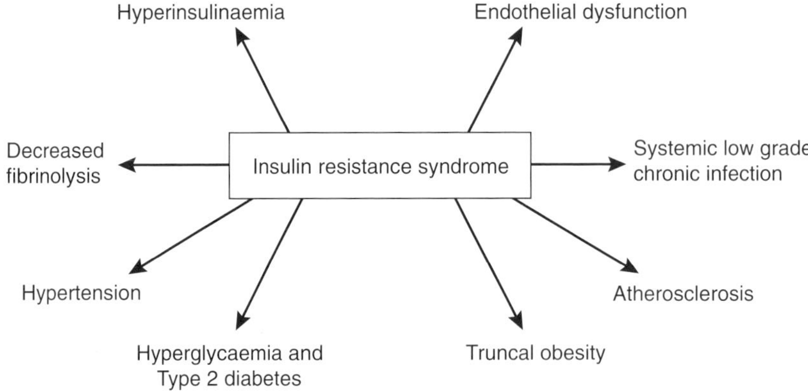

Figure 1.2 **Consequences of the insulin resistance syndrome.**

Insulin is secreted in phases and the early phase is considered important. People with Type 2 diabetes show a loss of the early phase insulin response (Dornhorst 2001). Interestingly, the beta cells do respond to other secretagogues, in particular sulphonylurea drugs.

The net effects of these abnormalities is sustained hyperglycaemia as a result of:

- impaired glucose utilisation
- decreased glucose storage as glycogen
- impaired suppression of glucose-mediated hepatic glucose production
- increased fasting glucose
- decreased postprandial glucose utilisation.

People most at risk of developing Type 2 diabetes:

- have insulin resistance syndrome,
- are overweight, i.e., truncal obesity, increased body mass index (BMI), and high waist:hip ratio (> 1.0 in men and > 0.7 in women). The increased level of FFAs inhibit insulin signalling and decrease glucose transport (see Figure 1.3) and are a source of metabolic fuel for the heart and liver. Binge eating precedes Type 2 diabetes in many

people and could be one of the causes of obesity; however, the prevalence of eating disorders is similar in Type 1 and Type 2 diabetes (Herpertz *et al.* 1998),

- are over 40 years of age,
- are closely related to people with diabetes,
- are women who have had gestational diabetes or who had large babies.

There is also an increasing incidence noticed in young people.

The characteristics of Type 1 and Type 2 diabetes are shown in Table 1.1.

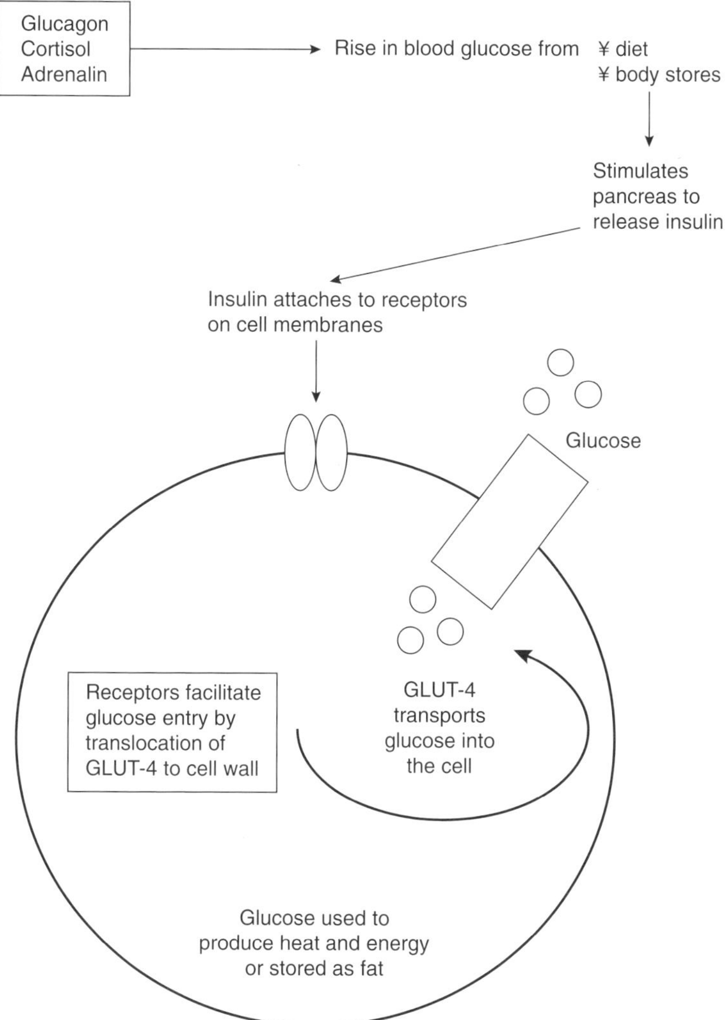

Figure 1.3 Diagrammatic representation of insulin binding, insulin signalling, translocation of GLUT-4 and glucose entry into the cell. GLUT-4 is a glucose transporter contained in vesicles in the cell cytoplasm. Once insulin binds to an insulin receptor GLUT-4 moves to the cell membrane and transports glucose into the cell. During fasting GLUT-4 is low and increases in response to the increase in insulin. Failure of GLUT-4 translocation could explain some of the insulin resistance associated with Type 2 diabetes.

Table 1.1 Characteristics of Type 1 and Type 2 diabetes mellitus.

	Type 1	*Type 2*
Age at onset	Usually <30 years	Usually >40 years
Speed on onset	Usually rapid	Usually gradual
Body weight	Normal or underweight; often recent weight loss	80% are overweight
Heredity	Associated with specific human leukocyte antigen (HLA)	No HLA association
	Autoimmune disease	
	Viral infection possible trigger	No evidence for viral trigger
Insulin	Early insulin secretion Impaired later; may be totally absent	Insulin deficiency or resistance to insulin action
Ketosis	Common	Rare
Frequency	15% of diagnosed cases	85% of diagnosed cases
Complications	Common	Common often present at diagnosis
Treatment	Insulin, diet, exercise	Diet, OHA, exercise, insulin

The majority of people with Type 2 diabetes require multiple therapies to attain acceptable blood glucose targets over the first nine years after diagnosis (UKPDS 1998). Between 50 and 70% require insulin that is often used in combination with OHAs. This means that diabetes management is more complicated for people with Type 2 diabetes, which increases the likelihood of non-compliance and increases the costs of managing the disease for both the patient and the health system.

1.4.3 Gestational diabetes

Gestational diabetes is defined as carbohydrate intolerance generally indicated by fasting blood glucose >6 mmol/L of variable severity which is first recognised during pregnancy. It affects about 3% of all pregnant women. The exact cause of gestational diabetes is unknown, but several factors have been identified including insulin resistance and hyperglycaemia as a result of the hormones produced by the placenta.

It is recommended that all pregnant women be screened for diabetes between 24 and 28 weeks gestation, the time the placenta begins to produce large quantities of hormones. If the screening test is abnormal an OGTT is performed.

Usually the blood glucose returns to normal after delivery of the baby. However, approximately 40% of women with gestational diabetes will develop diabetes in later life. In most cases the OGTT is repeated 6–8 weeks after delivery.

Who is at risk from gestational diabetes?

Gestational diabetes can occur in any pregnancy; however, those women at highest risk may be categorised as:

- Older.
- Overweight.
- Having a family history of diabetes or previous gestational diabetes or having had a large baby previously.
- Belonging to a race with an increased risk, e.g. Vietnamese.
- With maternal obesity > 12% of ideal bodyweight.

If the blood glucose cannot be controlled by diet, insulin will be required during pregnancy. Oral hypoglycaemic agents (OHAs) are contraindicated because they cross the placenta and cause neonatal hypoglycaemia. The aim of treatment is to keep blood glucose within the normal range (3–7 mmol), ensure the diet is appropriate and provide good obstetric care.

1.4.5 Malnutrition-related (tropical) diabetes

Childhood malnutrition, genetic predisposition and environmental factors are implicated in the development of diabetes in people living in tropical countries. It is not included as a specific category in the revised classification but could fit into the 'other' category. 'Tropical diabetes' or malnutrition-related diabetes differs from Type 1 diabetes because ketoacidosis is rare, and from Type 2 diabetes because it often occurs in young, thin people with no family history of diabetes. However, researchers have not yet agreed about the underlying causal mechanisms.

1.4.6 Maturity onset diabetes of the young (MODY)

Maturity onset diabetes of the young is a rare subgroup of Type 2 diabetes, formerly also called Mason-type diabetes and non-insulin-dependent diabetes of the young (NIDDY). It usually occurs in people younger than 25 years of age. It occurs in 1–2% of people with diabetes and there is considerable genetic heterogenicity between different races. MODY can be distinguished from Type 1 diabetes by the absence of ketosis. Treatment is with oral hypoglycaemic agents, diet and exercise, although insulin may eventually be required.

Recognition can be difficult and the diagnosis missed (Appleton & Hattersley 1996). This can have implications for the individual and their family in commencing appropriate treatment for the specific type of MODY and genetic counselling. The key features of MODY are:

- Autosomal dominant characteristic passed from one affected generation to the next generation.
- Young age of onset – usually before age 25.
- Type 2 diabetes, i.e. C-peptide present in the blood indicating endogenous insulin production and/or able to be treated without insulin for $\geq$ 5 years.

Practice points

(1) MODY is a different disease process from Type 2 diabetes that occurs in young people and which has a different genetic and inheritance pattern. Type 2 diabetes in children is a disease associated with obesity and insulin resistance (Sinha *et al.* 2002).

(2) MODY has been misdiagnosed as Type 1 diabetes and insulin commenced unnecessarily because of the young age at presentation. MODY has also been diagnosed instead of Type 1 diabetes in the UK (Health Service Ombudsman 2000).

These points demonstrate the importance of taking a careful clinical history and undertaking appropriate diagnostic investigations.

1.5 Diagnosis of diabetes

Urine tests alone should not be used to make a diagnosis of diabetes; if glycosuria is detected the blood glucose should be tested. When symptoms of diabetes are present an elevated blood glucose alone will usually confirm the diagnosis. See Table 1.2 for diagnostic criteria.

If the person is asymptomatic, abnormal fasting blood glucose values of >7 mmol/L should be demonstrated on at least two occasions before the diagnosis is made. A random plasma glucose of >11.1 mmol/L and symptoms are diagnostic of diabetes. An oral glucose tolerance test (OGTT) using a 75 g glucose load may be indicated to determine the presence of glucose intolerance if results are borderline. The criteria for diagnosing diabetes according to the World Health Organisation are shown in Table 1.2. For performance of test and patient preparation for an OGTT see section 1.6.

An abnormal plasma glucose identifies a subgroup of people at risk of diabetes-related complications. The risk data for these complications is based on the 2-hour OGTT plasma glucose level. However, the fasting glucose of 7.8 mmol/L does not equate with the 2-hour level that is used to diagnose diabetes. Recently the ADA and the WHO lowered the fasting level to 7.0 mmol/L to more closely align it to the 2-hour level.

The WHO continues to advocate a routine use of the OGTT to maximise early identification of people at risk of complications in order for early treatment to be instituted. The ADA does not advocate routine use of the OGTT because it believes that the revised fasting level is sensitive enough to detect most people at risk. Therefore, there could be

Table 1.2 Diagnostic criteria for diabetes based on the World Health Organisation guidelines. Fasting plasma glucose is the preferred test for diagnosis, but any of the three tests are acceptable.

Stage	*Fasting plasma glucose*	*Random plasma glucose*	*Oral glucose tolerance test (OGTT)*
Normal	<6.1 mmol/L		2 hour plasma glucose <7.8 mmol/L
Impaired glucose tolerance	Impaired fasting glucose – fasting glucose ≥6.1 and <7.0 mmol/L		Impaired glucose tolerance – 2 hour plasma glucose ≥7.8 and <11.1 mmol/L
Diabetes	≥7.0 mmol/L	≥11.1 mmol/L and symptoms	2 hour plasma glucose >11.1 mmol/L

In this table venous plasma glucose values are shown. Glucose in capillary blood is about 10–15% higher than venous blood.

differences internationally about the routine use of the OGTT. The ADA and the WHO do agree on how the test should be performed. Australia supports the continued use of the OGTT (Hilton *et al*. 2002).

1.6 Oral glucose tolerance test (OGTT)

An OGTT is used to diagnose diabetes:

- When fasting and random blood glucose results are equivocal.
- When there is a strong family history of diabetes, especially during pregnancy.
- If the suspicion of diabetes is high but blood and urine glucose tests are normal.

An OGTT should not be performed when the patient:

- Is febrile.
- Is acutely ill, e.g. postoperatively, or if uraemic.
- Has been immobilised for more than 48 hours.
- Has symptoms of diabetes or an elevated blood glucose before commencement of the test.

Rationale for OGTT
Early diagnosis and treatment of diabetes reduces the morbidity and mortality associated with the disease.

1.6.1 Preparing the patient for an OGTT

(1) Give specific oral and written instructions to the patient. A sample is given in Example Instruction Sheet 1 overleaf.
(2) Ensure the diet contains at least 200 g/day carbohydrate for at least 3 to 5 days before the test.
(3) If possible stop drugs which can influence the blood glucose levels 3 days before the test:
    - thiazide diuretics
    - antihypertensive drugs
    - analgesic and anti-inflammatory drugs
    - antineoplastic drugs
    - steroids.
(4) Fast from 12 midnight the night before the test.
(5) Avoid physical/psychological stress for 1 hour prior to, and during, the test.
(6) Avoid smoking for at least 1 hour prior to the test.
(7) Allow the patient to relax 30 minutes before beginning the test.

1.6.2 Test protocol

(1) The person should rest during the test to avoid dislodging the cannula.
(2) A cannula is inserted into a suitable vein for blood sampling.
(3) The blood glucose should be tested before commencing the test. If elevated clarify with the doctor ordering the test before proceeding. Two millimetres of blood are collected in fluoride oxalate tubes for laboratory analysis.

Example Instruction Sheet 1: Preparation for an oral glucose tolerance test

PATIENT INSTRUCTIONS FOR ORAL
GLUCOSE TOLERANCE TEST

Date of test: **Name:**

Time: **I.D. label**

Location where test will take place:

---

(1) Please ensure that you eat high carbohydrate meals each day for 3 days before the test. Carbohydrate foods are: breads, cereals, spaghetti, noodles, rice, dried beans and pulses, vegetables, fruit. These foods should constitute the major part of your diet for the 3 days.
(2) Have nothing to eat or drink after 12 midnight on the night prior to the test day, except water.
(3) Bring a list of all the tablets you are taking with you when you come for the test.
(4) Do not smoke at least one hour before the test.

The Test

The test is performed in the morning. You are required to rest during the test, which will take approximately 3 hours to complete. A small needle will be inserted into an arm vein for blood sampling. The needle will stay in place until the test is completed. You will be given 300 ml of glucose to drink. This is very sweet but it is important to drink it all over the 5 minutes, so that the results of the test can be interpreted correctly. Water is permitted.

You will be given a drink and something to eat when the test is finished. The doctor will discuss the results with you.

(4) The cannula is flushed with saline or heparinised saline between samples to prevent clotting. One to two milliletres of blood should be withdrawn and discarded before collecting each sample to avoid contaminating the sample.
(5) Blood samples are collected at:

minutes: −10
0
⇨ 75 g glucose, consumed over 5 minutes Water can be given after the glucose. It is very sweet and some people find it difficult to drink.
+ 30
+ 60
+ 120

The glucose used for an OGTT is prepacked in 300 ml bottles containing exactly 75 g of glucose.

(6) Ensure the person has a follow-up appointment with the referring doctor whose responsibility it is to explain the test results and commence appropriate management and education.
(7) In some cases only two venous samples will be collected. A fasting sample at the beginning of the test (time zero) and a second sample after two hours (the two-hour sample).

1.7 Screening for diabetes

Because of the insidious nature and increasing incidence and prevalence of Type 2 diabetes, many countries have instituted screening or case detection programmes in at-risk populations. Fasting plasma glucose tests are preferred to capillary (fingerpick) tests to identify the presence of diabetes, see Table 1.2 for the diagnostic criteria. Some programmes also involve checking for obesity and cardiovascular risk factors. At-risk groups include:

- age >55 years;
- high-risk ethnic groups;
- polycystic disease of the ovary;
- previous gestational diabetes;
- family history of diabetes;
- people with symptoms – often absent in Type 2 diabetes;
- the elderly;
- those with known diabetes complications such as cardiovascular and renal disease.

Screening for Type 1 diabetes is not usually necessary because it presents differently and has a more rapid onset and symptoms are usually present. First-degree relatives of people with diabetes can be tested for risk markers for diabetes but the preventative strategies applicable to Type 2 diabetes do not apply.

An example of a screening and preventative model of care is shown in Figure 1.4.

1.8 Management of diabetes mellitus

1.8.1 The diabetes team

Effective management of diabetes requires team care. The person with diabetes is a key player in the team. Good communication between team members is important and information given to the patient must be consistent between, and within, departments. The team usually consists of some or all of the following:

- Diabetologist
- Diabetes nurse specialist/diabetes educator
- Dietitian
- Podiatrist
- Social worker
- Psychologist
- General practitioner.

Other professionals who contribute regularly to the management of the patient are:

- Opthalmologist
- Renal physician
- Pharmacist
- Vascular and orthopaedic surgeons.

The ward staff who care for the patient in hospital also become team members:

- Doctors
- Nurses
- Physiotherapists
- Occupational therapists.

The management of diabetes consists of dietary modification, regular exercise/activity and in some cases insulin or OHAs. Diabetes education and regular medical assessment of diabetic control and complication status is essential.

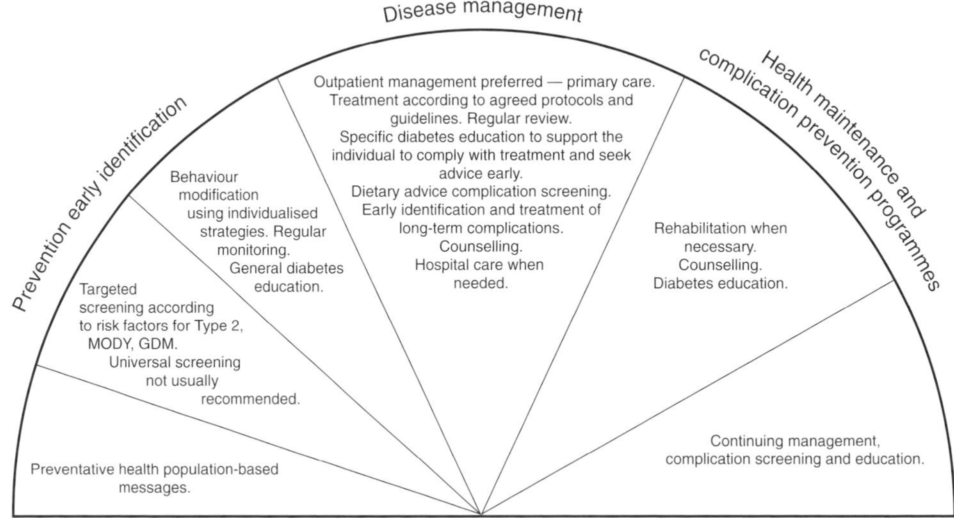

Figure 1.4 Example of a screening and preventative model of health care.

1.8.2 Aim of management

Management aims for Australia are defined in the National Diabetes Strategy and a number of other specific guidelines such as those described in the Australian Diabetes Society Position Statements and Clinical Management Guidelines for Diabetes in General Practice. The UK also has a number of specific guidelines including the newly released *Diabetes National Service Framework: Standards*, a ten-year implementation plan published in July 2001.

The aim of diabetes management is to maintain quality of life and keep the person free from the symptoms of diabetes, and the blood glucose in an acceptable range. The range is determined on an individual basis, usually between 4 and 9 mmol/L for 90% of tests, especially in young people and during pregnancy. The aim is to obtain results as near as possible to normal blood glucose but there must be a balance between the food plan, medication (insulin/OHAs) and exercise/activity. The regime should restrict lifestyle as little as possible, although some modification is usually necessary. Type 1 (insulin-dependent) people require insulin in order to survive. Type 2 (non-insulin-dependent) obese patients can be treated effectively with a combination of diet and exercise. In many people with Type 2 diabetes, OHAs will also be required, and often eventually insulin.

Practice point

In the current empowerment model of diabetes care the person with diabetes is the pivotal person. Forming a care partnership with the individual and accepting their choices is seen as essential to achieving optimal outcomes, see Chapters 22 and 23.

These are general recommendations only. Individual needs must be taken into consideration. For example, normoglycaemia achieved using insulin or OHAs in an elderly person could be dangerous, see Chapter 8.

Clinical observation

Diabetes is a balancing act. The individual's physical, psychological, spiritual and social life needs to be balanced in order to achieve good metabolic control. In fact the emphasis should be on balance rather than control.

Management involves educating the person with diabetes and other family members in order to help them:

- Obtain and maintain an acceptable weight.
- Achieve acceptable blood glucose levels.
- Achieve a normal blood lipid profile.
- Relieve symptoms of diabetes (polyuria, polydipsia and lethargy).
- Prevent complications of diabetes and of treatment.
- Maintain a healthy, independent lifestyle where the person is able to manage the necessary self-care tasks to achieve acceptable glycaemic control and have a good quality of life.

Some guidelines for assessing diabetic control are shown in Table 1.3.

A suggested model for the management of diabetes is shown in Figure 1.5. The model is divided into phases and indicates that management, education and counselling are required for life.

Table 1.3 Guidelines for assessment of control of diabetes.

% haemoglobin A1c	*Glucose (mmol/L)*		*Control*
	Fasting	*2 hours after food*	
4.0–6.0	4	7	Excellent or 'too good'*
6.0–7.4	7	9	Upper limit of normal
7.5–9.4	10	14.5	Unacceptable
>9.5	14	20	Unacceptable

* Risk of hypoglycaemia.

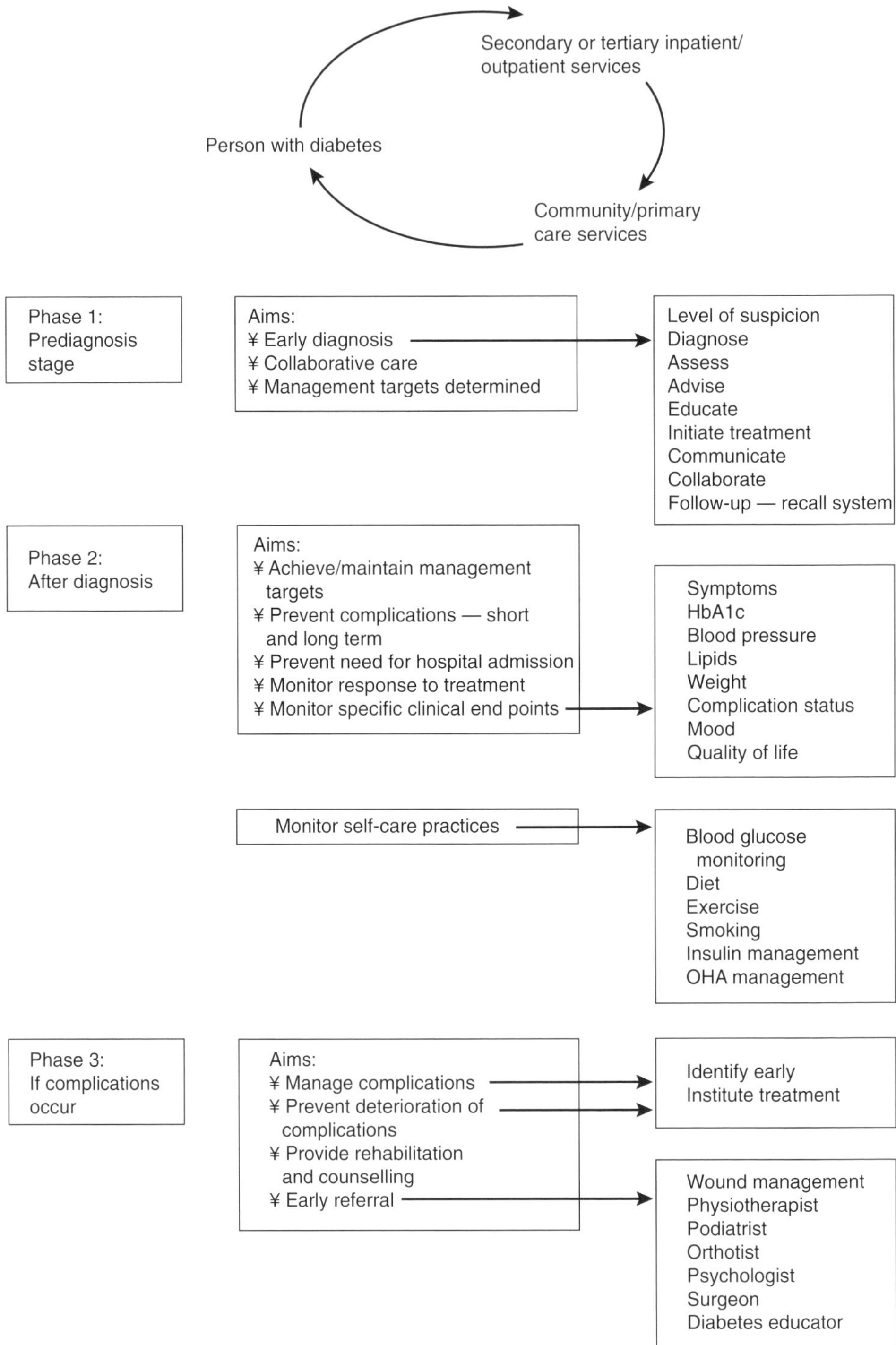

Figure 1.5 Suggested diabetes management model. Most diabetes management occurs in primary care settings in collaboration with secondary and tertiary care services.

1.8.3 Exercise/activity

Exercise plays a key role in the management of both Type 1 and Type 2 diabetes. It increases tissue sensitivity to insulin aiding in the uptake and utilisation of glucose during exercise and for several hours afterwards. The energy sources during exercise are depicted in Figure 1.6.

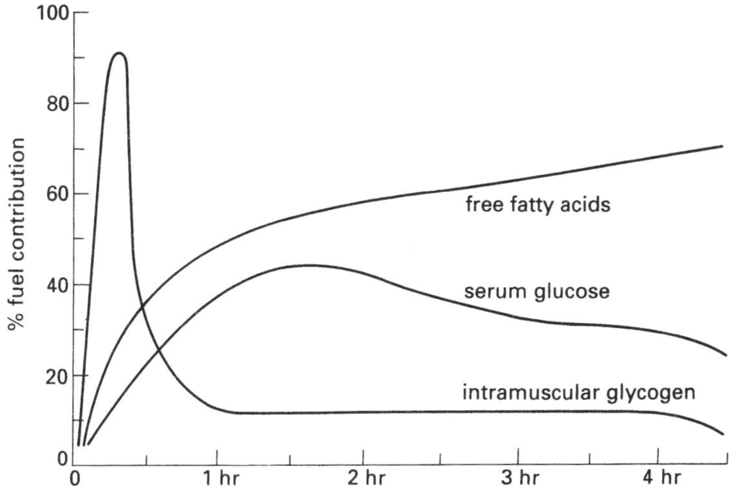

Figure 1.6 Normal energy sources during exercise.

Note: At rest free fatty acids are the major energy source. As exercise begins muscle glycogen is utilised as the predominant energy source. As exercise continues the blood glucose is utilised, reverting to free fatty acids as the major energy source if exercise is prolonged. Blood glucose is maintained by hormonal regulation of hepatic glucose output and lipolysis.

In addition, regular exercise may have beneficial effects on the risk factors that contribute to the development of diabetes complications (Boule *et al.* 2001). Exercise:

- Increases cardiovascular efficiency.
- Decreases blood pressure.
- Reduces stress.
- Aids in weight reduction and appetite control.
- Promotes a sense of wellbeing.
- Aids in blood glucose control.

All of these factors also decrease the risk of developing the long-term complications of diabetes. People are advised to have a thorough physical check-up before commencing an exercise programme; in particular, the cardiovascular system, eyes, nerves and feet should be examined. Food, fluid and clothing should be suitable for the type of exercise and the weather.

Insulin/OHAs might need to be decreased. Where the duration of the exercise is <30 minutes adjustments are generally not required. Adjustments are often necessary where the duration of the exercise exceeds 30 minutes (Perlstein *et al.* 1997). The exercise chosen should be suited to the person's physical condition. It is advisable to test the blood glucose before and after exercising and to have some carbohydrate available during exercise in case of hypoglycaemia. Infrequent exercise is not advisable; the aim should be to begin with 10–15 minutes exercise and progress to 30–60 minutes of moderate intensity three to five times per week, daily if possible. Footwear should be appropriate to the type of exercise and the feet inspected after exercising. Exercise is not recommended in extremes of temperatures, or at periods of poor diabetic control, especially if ketones are present in the urine. People should discuss their exercise plans with the diabetes team in order to plan an appropriate routine, adequate carbohydrate intake, and appropriate medication dose. Ensure adequate fluid intake to replace water loss especially in hot weather.

Practice point

Hypoglycaemia can occur several hours after vigorous or prolonged exercise due to continuing glucose uptake by muscles.

In general, anaerobic exercise (e.g. weight lifting) does not use glucose as a fuel. This type of exercise builds muscle mass, but does not improve the cardiovascular system. Anaerobic exercise is likely to cause an increase in blood glucose. Aerobic exercise (running, cycling, swimming) uses glucose as the major fuel source and a decrease in blood glucose can occur. It also confers cardiovascular benefits.

Specific advice about medications and food intake needs to be tailored to the individual. The relationship between hypoglycaemia and exercise is generally well recognised. Hyperglycaemia can also occur if insulin levels are low when excercising. In this situation the counter-regulatory hormones predominate and increase the blood glucose.

1.8.4 Exercise for the patient in hospital

(1) Encourage as much mobility/activity as the person's condition allows.
(2) Increase movement and activity gradually after a period of being confined to bed.
(3) Consider postural hypotension and differentiate it from hypoglycaemia to ensure correct management is instituted.
(4) Consult the physiotherapy department for assistance with mobility, chair or hydrotherapy exercises.

Practice point

Be aware that resuming normal activity after a period of prolonged inactivity, e.g. in rehabilitation settings, constitutes unaccustomed exercise and can result in hypoglycaemia, especially if the person is on insulin/OHAs and is not eating well. Exercise/activity increases the basal energy requirement by 20%.

1.9 Diabetes education

Diabetes education is an integral part of diabetes management. Regular support and contact with the diabetes care team assists people to manage their diabetes by providing advice and support when necessary. For more details see Chapter 23.

Practice points

(1) People with Type 2 diabetes *do not* become Type 1 when insulin is needed to control blood glucose. The correct term is insulin-treated or insulin-requiring diabetes. The basic underlying pathophysiology does not change and usually enough endogenous insulin is produced to prevent ketosis except in severe intercurrent illness.
(2) Type 2 diabetes is characterised by progressive beta cell destruction and insulin is eventually required by >50% of people (UKPDS 1998).

1.10 Complications of diabetes

Many people with diabetes are admitted to hospital because they have an active diabetes complication. The presence of a diabetic complication can affect the duration of the admission and the patient's ability to care for themself. Hence diabetic complications contribute to the overall cost of health care for these patients. In addition, they represent significant lifestyle costs to the person with diabetes.

Complications can be classified as acute or long term. Acute complications can occur during temporary excursions in blood glucose levels. Long-term complications occur with long duration of diabetes and persistent hyperglycaemia, especially in the presence of other risk factors. In Type 2 diabetes long-term complications are frequently present at diagnosis. Often there are few symptoms and both the diagnosis of diabetes and the coexisting complication/s can be overlooked.

1.10.1 Acute complications

(1) Hypoglycaemia (refer to Chapter 8).
(2) Hyperglycaemia:
    - diabetic ketoacidosis (refer to Chapter 10)
    - hyperosmolar coma (refer to Chapter 10).
(3) Infections can occur if blood glucose control is not optimal. Common infections include candidiasis and urinary tract infections.
(4) Fat atrophy/hypertrophy and insulin allergy occur very rarely with modern highly purified insulins and correct injection site rotation.

1.10.2 Long-term complications

Two important studies, the DCCT in 1993 and the UKPDS in 1998, demonstrated the relationship between the development and progression of the long-term complications of Type 1 and Type 2 diabetes, respectively. In addition, the UKPDS demonstrated the importance of controlling blood pressure to reduce the risk of cardiovascular disease. Since the publication of these findings, diabetes management guidelines and metabolic targets have been revised and efforts to achieve normoglycaemia increased.

(1) Macrovascular disease or disease of the major blood vessels, e.g.:
    - myocardial infarction
    - cerebrovascular accident
    - intermittent claudication.

(2) Microvascular disease or disease of the small blood vessels associated with thickening of the basement membranes of the small blood vessels, e.g.:
   - retinopathy
   - nephropathy.
(3) Neuropathy: diabetes can also cause damage to the central and peripheral nerves:
   - peripheral: decreased sensation in hands and particularly the feet, which can lead to ulcers, Charcot's arthropathy and amputation
   - autonomic: erectile dysfunction, atonic bladder, gastroparesis, mononeuropathies.
(4) Complications of pregnancy: diabetes during pregnancy carries risks for both mother and baby:
   - mother: toxaemia, polyhydramnous intrauterine death, caesarian section
   - baby: congenital malformations, prematurity, respiratory distress, hypoglycaemia at birth.

A number of other factors might play a role in the development of diabetic complications. For example, studies are under way to determine the role of free radicals, advanced glycated end products (AGE), changes in cellular signalling and endothelial humoral components that determine coagulation status and the tendency to form microthrombi. A list of recommended reading which deals with this subject has been included in Appendix B.

It is the responsibility of the nurse to assess the patient adequately for the presence of complications in order to determine self-care potential and devise an appropriate nursing care plan, and to be involved in preventative teaching about reducing risk factors for the development of diabetic complications.

1.11 Cost of diabetes

The Australian Institute of Health in 1991 estimated the cost of diabetes in Australia to be $7000 million per year. The cost of diabetes in the UK was recently estimated to be 10% of health service resources, nearly £5 billion per annum. These costs are increasing, especially for older people. In addition, the length of stay in hospital is longer for people with diabetes. Many of the hospitalisations are a result of diabetic complications which should be largely preventable.

Sixty per cent of the costs associated with diabetes are direct costs of providing service and medical supplies. The indirect costs (40%) are more difficult to assess; they include psychological costs to the person with diabetes, life years lost and loss of quality of life. There are also costs to the caregivers (relatives and family) which are difficult to estimate and which probably reduce direct health costs.

Diabetes is the fourth major cause of death after cardiovascular disease, cancer and musculo-skeletal disease, distributed across all age groups. Cardiovascular disease is a major complication of diabetes. Therefore it is not unreasonable to conclude that a person with diabetes will require at least one hospital contact/admission during their lifetime. It is documented that the need for hospital admission and the length of stay in hospital can be improved by diabetes education, and appropriate medical and nursing care. It is envisaged that this Manual will contribute to the provision of that care.

Practice points

(1) Hyperglycaemia and insulin resistance are commonly seen in critically ill patients, even those who do not have diabetes (Van den Berghe *et al.* 2001).
(2) It is important to control these states in people with diabetes during illness because of the extra stress of the illness and/or surgery, and their compromised insulin response. Elevated blood glucose in these situations in people without diabetes will require decisions about the presence of diabetes once the acute episode resolves.

1.12 Aim and objectives of nursing care of people with diabetes

1.12.1 Hospitalisation

Being hospitalised is more common for people with diabetes than those without, and they are more like to stay longer. Current diabetes management guidelines are heavily weighted towards screening and primary care management. Good evidence for acute care is more difficult to locate. The care suggested in this Manual is extrapolated from the research quoted, discussion with nurse experts in particular areas and the extensive clinical nursing experience of the author.

1.12.2 Metabolic factors that complicate illness

- Potentially erratic insulin absorption, especially in Type 1.
- Haemodynamic changes in blood flow.
- Counter-regulatory stress response to illness, hospitalisation, treatment, pain, psychological stress and fear.
- Timing of meals and snacks.
- Length of time between insulin administration and meals.
- Effect of medications on the gut, especially narcotics for pain relief. Glucose requirements may need to be increased to compensate for slow transit times, to supply sufficient energy and prevent hypoglycaemia.
- Increased white cell count and impaired leukocyte function as a result of hyperglycaemia.
- Decreased wound healing and strength of healing tissue.
- Increased risk of thrombosis.
- Risk of ketoacidosis in Type 1, and hyperosmolar coma in Type 2, if hyperglycaemia is not restrained, see Chapter 10.
- Impaired cognitive function and decreased mood can make learning difficult.

Clinical observations – patients' stories

(1) People with diabetes fear staff will make mistakes, especially with their medication doses and administration times and management of hypoglycaemia.
(2) They dislike being made to feel incompetent and not trusted by staff who take over the self-care tasks they usually perform for themselves, and who do not believe what they say.
(3) Some prefer the nurses to take on these tasks because it is an opportunity to 'let go' the responsibility for a short time.

(4) They find judgemental attitudes over eating sweet things demeaning, especially when they are accused of dietary indiscretion when their blood glucose is high.
(5) They dislike being labelled non-compliant, or uncooperative, if they have difficulty learning and remembering information.

1.12.1 Aims

To formulate an individual nursing management plan so that the person recovers by primary intention, maintains independence and quality of life as far as possible and does not develop any complications of treatment.

Recognise the importance of support from the family to the individual's wellbeing, self-care capacity and ability to take responsibility for their disease.

Rationale

Early diagnosis of diabetes and monitoring for short- and long-term complications enables early treatment and improved outcomes. The nurse's understanding of the pathophysiology and classification of diabetes will improve the care they provide.

1.12.2 Objectives

(1) To assess the person's:
- physical, mental and social status
- usual diabetic control
- ability to care for themselves
- knowledge about diabetes and its management
- the presence of any diabetes-related complications
- acceptance of the diagnosis of diabetes
- presence of concomitant disease processes.

(2) To encourage independence as far as the physical condition allows in hospital (test own blood glucose, administer own insulin, select own meals).
(3) To obtain and maintain an acceptable blood glucose range, thereby preventing hypoglycaemia or hyperglycaemia so that the person is free from distressing symptoms and fluctuating blood glucose levels.
(4) To prevent complications occurring as a result of hospitalisation (e.g. falls associated with hypoglycaemia).
(5) To observe an appropriate nursing care plan in order to achieve these objectives.
(6) To inform appropriate health professionals promptly of the patient's admission, e.g. diabetes nurse specialist/diabetes educator, dietitian, podiatrist.
(7) To ensure patient has the opportunity to learn about diabetes and its management, particularly self-management.
(8) To plan appropriately for discharge.
(9) To prevent further hospitalisations as a result of diabetes.

In the longer term, especially for diabetes nurse specialist/diabetes educators, who often see the patient regularly over many years, establishing a therapeutic relationship based on respect, equality and trust. The value of a therapeutic relationship has been recognised from the time of Hippocrates as being essential to healing.

References

Appleton, M. & Hattersley, A. (1996) Maturity onset diabetes of the young: a missed diagnosis. *Diabetic Medicine*, Suppl 2, AP3.

Audit Commission (2000) *Testing Times: a Review of Diabetes Mellitus Services in England and Wales*. Audit Commission, London.

Australian Diabetes Society (1990–1996) *Position Statements*. Australian Diabetes Society, Canberra.

Boule, N., Haddard, E., Kenny, G., Wells, G. & Sigal, R. (2001) Effects of exercise on glycaemic control and body mass index in Type 2 diabetes mellitus: a metanalysis of controlled clinical trials. *Journal of the American Medical Association*, **286**, 1218–1227.

Diabetes and Control and Complications Trial Research Group (1993) The effect of intensive insulin treatment on the development and progression of long term complications of insulin dependant diabetes. *New England Journal of Medicine*, **329**, 977–986.

Dornhorst, A. (2001) Insulinotrophic meglitinide analogues. *Lancet*, **358** (9294) 1709–1716.

Dunstan, D., Zimmet, P. & Welborn, T. (2000) On behalf of the AusDiab Steering Committee, Diabesity and associated disorders in Australia 200: the accelerating epidemic. *Australian Diabetes, Obesity and Lifestyle Report*. International Diabetes Institute, Melbourne.

Expert Committee on the Diagnosis and Classification of Diabetes Mellitus (1997) *Diabetes Care*, **20**, 1183–1197.

Health Service Ombudsman (2000) *Errors in the care and treatment of a young woman with diabetes*. The Stationary Office, London.

Herpertz, S., Albus, C. & Wagener, R. (1998) Cormorbidity of eating disorders. Does diabetes control reflect disturbed eating behaviour? *Diabetes Care*, **21** (7), 1110–1116.

Hilton, D., O'Rourke, P., Welbourn, T. & Reid, C. (2002) Diabetes detection in Australian general practice: a comparison of diagnostic criteria. *Medical Journal of Australia*, **176**, 104–107.

MacKinnon, M. (1998) *Providing Diabetes Care in General Practice. A Practical Guide for the Primary Care Team*. Class publishing, London.

National Divisions Diabetes Programs (1998) Commonwealth Department of Health and Family Services, Canberra.

Perlstein, R., McConnell, K. & Hagger, V. (1997) *Off to a Flying Start*. International Diabetes Institute, Melbourne.

Oakley, C. (1992) Care of gestational diabetes mellitus. *Diabetes Care*, **1**, 6–8.

Sinha, R., Fisch, G., Teague, B. *et al.* (2002) Prevalence of inpaired glucose tolerance among children and adolescents with marked obesity. *New England Journal of Medicine*, **346** (11), 802–810.

Smith, M. (2001) Pathogenesis of Type 2 diabetes and effect of lifestyle changes. *Journal of Diabetes Nursing*, **5** (4), 123–127.

Turner, N. & Clapham, C. (1998) Insulin resistance, impaired glucose tolerance and non-insulin-dependant diabetes pathologic mechanisms and treatment: current status and therapeutic possibilities. *Progress in Drug Research*, **51**, 33–94.

UKPDS (United Kingdom Prospective Diabetes Study) (1998) Intensive blood glucose control with sulphonylureas or insulin compared with conventional treatment and risk of complications in patients with Type 2 diabetes (UKPDS 33). *Lancet*, **352**, 837–53.

Van den Berghe, G., Wouters, P., Weekers, F. *et al.* (2001) Intensive insulin therapy in critically ill patients. *New England Journal of Medicine*, **345** (19), 1359–1367.

Chapter 2
Assessment and Nursing Diagnosis

2.1 Key points

- Assess general nursing needs.
- Incorporate specific diabetes assessment.
- Formulate individual care plans.
- Evaluate treatment outcomes.
- Discharge planning should be part of the care plan.

Rationale

Careful assessment enables physical, psychological, spiritual and social issues that impact on care to be identified and incorporated into nursing management and discharge plans.

2.2 Characteristics of the nursing history

The nursing history:

- Begins with demographic data (age, sex, social situation).
- Collects units of information to permit individual care plans to be formulated considering the person's goals and expectations.
- Obtains baseline information about a person's physical and mental status and presenting complaint.
- Should be concise to allow information to be collected in a short time.
- Assists in maintaining the person's independence while they are in hospital (e.g. allowing them to perform their own blood glucose tests).

The findings should be documented in the patient record and communicated to the appropriate caregivers. Consideration should be given to the privacy and confidentiality of all personal information and appropriate communication, access and storage mechanisms should be maintained.

Note: A guideline for obtaining a comprehensive nursing history follows. It is important, however, to listen to the patient and not be locked into 'ticking boxes', so that vital and valuable information is not overlooked.

Most of the information is general in nature, but some will be specifically relevant to diabetes (e.g. blood glucose testing and eating patterns). The clinical assessment in this example is particularly aimed at obtaining information about metabolic status.

Assessment of the person with diabetes does not differ from the assessment performed for any other disease process. Assessment should take into account social, physical and psychological factors in order to prepare an appropriate nursing care plan, including a plan for discharge.

Any physical disability the patient has will affect their ability to manage their diabetes (inject insulin, inspect feet, test blood glucose). Impaired hearing may preclude group education programmes. Management and educational expectations may need to be modified to take any disability into account.

If the person has diabetes, however, metabolic derangements may be present at admission, or could develop as a consequence of hospitalisation. Therefore careful assessment allows potential problems to be identified, a coordinated nursing care plan to be developed and appropriate referral to other health professionals (podiatrist, diabetes nurse specialist/diabetes educator, dietitian) to take place. A nursing problem list, ranking problems in order of priority, can also assist in planning individualised care that addresses immediate and future treatment goals. The first step in patient assessment is to document a nursing history.

Consider the font size, colour and language level of any written material provided, especially instructions for procedures and appointments and health professional contact details.

2.3 Nursing history

A nursing history is a written record of specific information about a patient. The data collected allows the nurse to plan appropriate nursing actions and to incorporate patient needs. A good patient care plan will allow consistency of treatment expectations within, and between, departments. An example patient assessment chart is shown in the sample Assessment Chart overleaf.

Example of an assessment chart, formulated for people with diabetes

EXAMPLE ASSESSMENT CHART

Formulated for People with Diabetes

A. GUIDELINES FOR OBTAINING A NURSING HISTORY

Name: ....

Age: .... Sex: ❑ Male ❑ Female

Type of diabetes: ❑ Type 1 ❑ Type 2 ❑ Other

Duration of diabetes .... years

Social

Language spoken: ....

Command of English: ❑ Written ❑ Spoken

Marital status: ....

Living arrangements: ❑ With partner ❑ Alone ❑ Other

Support systems: ....

Work type: ....

Hobbies ....

Meals

Regular meals: ❑ Yes ❑ No

Who does the cooking: ....

Eating out: ....

Alcohol consumption: ❑ Yes ❑ No How much: ....

How often: ....

Assessment chart *cont'd*

Smoking

❑ Yes ❑ No Cigarettes/pipe: . . . .

How many per day: . . . . Marijuana: . . . .

Current Medications

General: . . . .

Diabetic: . . . .

Self-prescribed: . . . .

Complementary therapies: . . . .

Usual Activity Level

Sports: . . . .

Gardening: . . . .

Walking: . . . .

Other: . . . .

Disabilities

What activities are limited: . . . .

To what degree: . . . .

(1) General: . . . .

(2) Hearing: . . . .

(3) Related to diabetic complications:

Decreased vision: ❑ glasses ❑ contact lenses ❑ registered blind

Neuropathy: (a) Peripheral: . . . .

(b) Autonomic: . . . .

Vascular: (a) Cardiac: . . . .

(b) Legs and feet: . . . .

Kidney function: . . . .

Sexuality: (a) Erectile dysfunction: . . . .

(4) Mobility: . . . .

(5) Dexterity (fine motor skills): . . . .

Assessment chart *cont'd*

Self-Monitoring of Diabetes Control (Testing Methods)

Urine test: ❑ Glucose ❑ Ketones Strips used: . . . .

Tests own blood glucose: ❑ Yes ❑ No Blood ketones ❑

Testing frequency: . . . .

System used:

(1) Visual, strip type . . . .

(2) Blood Glucose Meter Type: . . . .

Testing accuracy: . . . .

Insulin delivery system used . . . .

Insulin technique/accuracy: . . . .

Preparing injection using usual system: . . . .

Administration: . . . .

Type of insulin: . . . .

Patient can name type of insulin: ❑ Yes ❑ No

Frequency of dose: . . . .

Psychological Adjustment to Diabetes

❑ Anxiety ❑ Denial ❑ Depression ❑ Well adjusted

Mental state: . . . .

Diabetes Knowledge Assessment

Previous diabetes education: ❑ Yes ❑ No How long ago: . . . .

Attendance at education support groups: ❑ Yes ❑ No

Name of group: . . . .

Assessment chart *cont'd*

Patient's Stated Reason for Being in Hospital

. . . .

. . . .

B. CLINICAL EXAMINATION

A detailed physical examination of the patient is carried out by the medical staff; however, there is also a place for clinical examination of the patient by the nursing staff. Particular attention should be paid to the following areas.

(1) General Inspection

- Conscious state
- Temperature, pulse and respiration
- Blood pressure lying and standing; note any postural drop
- Height
- Weight and history of weight gain/loss; BMI
- Hydration status, skin turgor
- Presence of diabetic symptoms, thirst, polyuria, polydipsia, lethargy
- Full urinalysis
- Blood glucose
- Presence of ketones blood ❑ urine ❑

(2) Skin

- Pigmentation
- Skin tone/turgor, colour
- Presence of lesions, rashes, wounds, ulcers
- Inspect injection sites, including abdomen; note any thickening, lumps, bruises

Assessment chart *cont'd*

(3) Mouth

- Mucous membranes (dry/moist)
- Lips
- Infection, halitosis
- Teeth: evidence of dental caries, loose teeth, red gums, incorrectly fitting dentures

(4) Feet and Legs

- Temperature of feet and legs, noting any changes between legs and parts of the feet and legs.
- The skin of the feet and legs may be hairless and shiny due to poor circulation
- Muscle wasting
- Ulcers or pressure areas on soles of feet and toes, including old scars
- Loss of pain sensation that may be due to nerve damage; estimate the size and depth of any ulcers using a template filed in the medical record, note their location and how long they have been present
- Presence of oedema
- Infection including fungal infection; inspect between the toes
- Condition of nails and general cleanliness of feet
- Type of footwear
- Record podiatry contact or referral, if any

Chapter 3
Documenting and Charting Patient Care

3.1 Documenting in the medical record

Documentation is an essential part of health management. Alternative methods of documenting care are emerging, for example charting by exception, where only events outside the normal expected progress are recorded. This form of charting requires supportive documentation in the form of flow charts, care plans and care maps. They can avoid duplication and streamline documentation. The use of care pathways is becoming increasingly common in Australia and in the UK (O'Brien 2000).

Other ways of documenting holistic care incorporate genomaps and ecomaps (see Figure 3.1), which can effectively convey a great deal of information about the social, relationship and support base aspects of an individual's life (Cluning 1997). They are particularly useful for long-term chronic diseases such as diabetes, where these factors affect management outcomes, see Chapter 17. They also record information that is often passed on anecdotally during handover or in the corridor. This means that vital information that could assist in planning care is not available or is misinterpreted.

Genograms illustrate how the individual relates to other people in the family and ecomaps place the family in the context of the wider social situation in which they live. Ecograms and ecomaps can be simple or convey complex and detailed information. Together they give a great deal of information about:

- the individual's family structure
- family and extended support
- family health history
- family functioning
- health service utilisation
- social orientation.

3.1.1 Nursing care plans

The employing institution's policy regarding the method of documentation should be followed. Good nursing documentation allows communication of the care required, to all staff. In the future changes will occur to the methods of documenting care; for example narrative notes may be replaced by focus charting and flow charts. Flow charts are designed to enable all healthcare providers to document care on a single care plan. Much of the current duplication can thus be avoided.

Standardised care plans of common medical and nursing diagnosis are being developed to serve as blueprints and may reduce the time spent on documentation. There is a

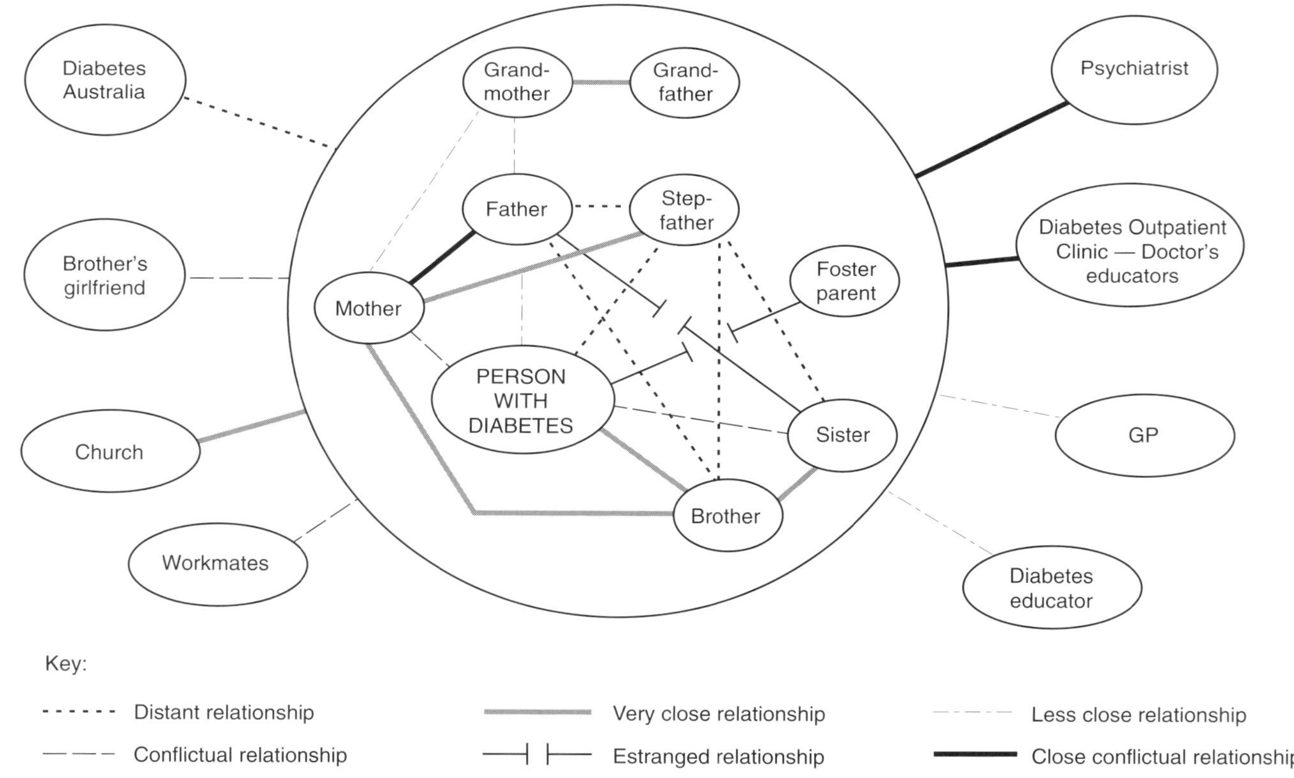

Figure 3.1 Example of a combination of a genomap (information inside the circle) and an ecomap (information outside the circle) of a 50-year-old woman with Type 2 diabetes and a history of childhood molestation and sexual abuse. It shows a great deal of conflict within and outside the family and identifies where her support base is.

move towards computerised or 'paperless' documentation. Where this form of documentation is used, due consideration of the security of the information is essential. Confidential information should be labelled as such in the record. Extra care is required with mobile technology such as laptops and palm pilots to ensure patient confidentiality is protected.

3.1.2 Nursing notes

Due consideration needs to be given to standard policies for good documentation and the laws governing privacy and confidentiality and people's right to access their medical records. Nursing notes are a record of the patient's hospital admission, healthcare and response to treatment, and act as a guide for discharge planning. They should be written legibly and objectively. They are not legal documents but may be subpoenaed for a court hearing.

Documentation should contain the following:

- The condition of the patient recorded objectively; for example, describe wounds in terms of size and depth.
- Qualification of the patient's condition, recording swelling, oedema, temperature, pulse and respiration (TPR) and blood pressure (BP).
- All teaching the patient receives.
- The patient's response to treatment.
- All medications received.
- Removal of all invasive medical devices (e.g. packs, drains, IV lines).
- Psychological and social factors.

Clinical observation

In some cases it is possible to refer to standard protocols in medical records if there is a set procedure documented and regularly revised, e.g. there is a standard procedure for performing an oral glucose tolerance test. The documentation could note relevant details such as the time, date and person's name and then state 'OGGT performed according to the standard protocol'. Where any deviation from the protocol occurred it should be recorded. If required, the standard protocol could be produced.

3.1.3 Diabetes documentation

The purposes of the chart are:

- To provide a record of blood and urinary glucose measurements.
- To record ketones in urine or blood.
- To provide a record of the amount and time of administration of insulin/oral hypoglycaemic agent doses.
- To record episodes of hyper or hypoglycaemia.
- To provide a basis for the adjustment of insulin/oral hypoglycaemic agents.

Frequency of blood and urine testing is dependent on the patient's status and the treatment being given (see Chapter 4).

DIABETIC FREQUENT MONITORING

IDENTIFICATION

DATE	TIME	INSULIN		BLOOD SUGAR	URINE								NURSING COMMENTS E.g. Adverse reactions or food omission
		TYPE	DOSE		GLUCOSE						ACETONE	PROTEIN	
					0 %	1/10 %	1/4 %	1/2 %	1 %	2 %			

(a)

INSTRUCTIONS
TYPE OF INSULIN, BLOOD GLUCOSE AND URINE TESTS MUST BE RECORDED IN FULL.

IDENTIFICATION

Date		0700	1100	1600	2100	COMMENTS
	Insulin type					
	Dose					
	Blood glucose mmols/l					
	Urine glucose					
	Ketones					
	Insulin type					
	Dose					
	Blood glucose mmols/l					
	Urine glucose					
	Ketones					

(b)

Figure 3.2 Sample diabetes record charts for (a) 2-hourly testing (e.g. when using an insulin infusion); (b) 4-hourly or less frequent testing.

Practice point

A common error is that medication doses are not recorded and it can be difficult to interpret the blood glucose profile without the medication information.

3.2 Nursing responsibilities

(1) Write legibly.
(2) Record all medication doses accurately in the correct column.
(3) Record hypoglycaemic episodes (symptoms, treatment, time, activity and food omission) in the appropriate column. Hypoglycaemia should also be documented in the patient's unit record.
(4) Do not add unnecessary details.
(5) Sign and include the date and time of all entries.

Figure 3.2 depicts example charts for (a) frequent testing and (b) testing 4-hourly or less often.

3.3 Documentation by people with diabetes

People with diabetes also document a great deal of information about their disease. They use a variety of record-keeping methods including blood glucose monitoring diaries, complication screening records and other management information such as medication doses and the results of investigative procedures. These records are a vital part of the documentation process. They not only supply written information, but can also give a great deal of information about an individual's self-care ability, e.g. a blood glucose diary covered with blood smears could mean the person is having difficulty placing the blood on the strip. Discussion with the patient might reveal that they often get the shakes and their vision is blurred due to hypoglycaemia. It is important, however, that all such assumptions are checked out.

References

Cluning, T. (1997) Social assessment documentation: genomaps and ecomaps, Chapter 7 in J. Richmond (ed.) *Nursing Documentation: Writing What We Do*. Ausmed Publications, Melbourne.

O'Brien, S. & Hardy, K. (2000) Impact of a care pathway driven diabetes education programme. *Journal of Diabetes Nursing*, **4**(5), 147–150.

Chapter 4
Monitoring Diabetes Mellitus

Rationale

Blood glucose monitoring allows a profile to be identified and treatment appropriately tailored to the individual. The accuracy of the testing technique and appropriate maintenance of equipment ensure treatment decisions are based on correct data. Self-monitoring allows people with diabetes to identify the effects of treatment, diet, exercise and other factors, on their blood glucose levels and gives them greater insight into their disease.

4.1 Introduction

Monitoring blood glucose is an important part of diabetes management. The results obtained form the basis for adjusting medication, food intake and activity levels. Urine glucose is now rarely used to assess metabolic control, but might still be useful for some people, provided the renal threshold for glucose has been established.

People with diabetes are expected to monitor their diabetes at home. They should be encouraged to continue to self-monitor in hospital if they are well enough to do so. Always inform the patient of the result of their blood glucose test. This time can be used as teaching time.

The results of blood and urine tests are useful only if tests are accurately performed.

Section 1 of this chapter explores monitoring blood glucose (see over).

Monitoring 1: blood glucose

4.2 Key points

- Follow correct procedure when performing tests.
- Perform control and calibration tests regularly.
- Clean and maintain equipment regularly.
- Calibrate and clean meter regularly.
- Record and interpret results.

4.3 The role of blood glucose monitoring in the care of diabetes

Blood glucose monitoring provides insight into the effectiveness of the diabetes management plan. It allows direct feedback to the patient about their blood glucose.

Clinical observation

In the home situation it allows the person with diabetes more responsibility for, and control over, their disease and is a tool they can use to maintain their quality of life. It is *not* a means of control by health professionals and is only one aspect of an holistic, individualised assessment.

Blood glucose testing is performed to:

- Monitor the effectiveness of diabetes therapy and guide adjustments to food plan, OHAs/insulin dose, exercise/activity.
- Detect lack of control as indicated by elevated glycosylated haemoglobin (HbA1c) levels.
- Achieve better control and acceptable blood glucose levels which have a role in preventing or delaying the onset of diabetes-related complications.
- Diagnose hypoglycaemia, including nocturnal hypoglycaemia, which can present as sleep disturbances, snoring, restlessness or bad dreams.
- Establish the renal threshold and therefore the reliability of urine testing in those rare cases where people still test their urine glucose.
- Achieve 'tight' control in pregnancy and thereby reduce the risks to both mother and baby.
- Provide continuity of care following hospitalisation.

Blood glucose monitoring is of particular use in:

- Frequent hypoglycaemic episodes.
- Unstable or 'brittle' diabetes.
- Management of illnesses at home, and in those recovering from an illness.
- Pregnancy.
- Establishing a new treatment regime.
- People whose urine tests are unreliable.

- Stabilisation onto insulin.
- Patients with renal failure, autonomic neuropathy, cardiovascular or cerebrovascular insufficiency where hypoglycaemic signs can be masked or not recognised.
- Detecting actual or potential drug/drug or drug/herb interactions.

The target blood glucose range and frequency of testing should be assessed individually.

4.3.1 Factors which influence blood glucose levels

(1) Food: times of last food intake, quantity and type of carbohydrate/fibre consumed.
(2) Exercise: timing with respect to food, medication and insulin doses, injection site, type of exercise and blood glucose level when commencing exercise.
(3) Intercurrent illness, e.g. influenza, urinary tract infection.
(4) Medications used for diabetes control: oral agents, insulin.
(5) Other drugs, e.g. steroids, oral contraceptives, beta blockers, including non-prescription medications that contain glucose, ephedrine, pseudoephedrine or alcohol, e.g. cold remedies.
(6) Alcohol: type, relationship to food intake, amount consumed.
(7) Insulin type, injection site, injection technique.
(8) Complementary therapies, e.g. herbs, stress management techniques.
(9) Emotional and physical stress – not only stress itself but medications used to treat stress.
(10) Accuracy of monitoring technique, including not handwashing before testing if sweet substances have been handled.
(11) Pregnancy in people with diabetes and gestational diabetes.
(12) Childhood: erratic swings in blood glucose levels are common.
(13) Adolescence: hormonal factors during adolescence can make control difficult.
(14) Renal, liver and pancreatic disease.
(15) Other endocrine disorders, e.g. thyroid disease, Cushing's disease.
(16) Parenteral nutrition.

Clinical observation

Insulin absorption can be delayed if injected into an oedemateous or ascitic abdomen. The delayed absorption can affect blood glucose control. The thigh or upper arm may be a preferable site in this instance.

4.4 Guidelines for the frequency of blood glucose monitoring

(1) Capillary blood glucose tests should be performed only by adequately qualified health professionals.
(2) Medical staff are usually responsible for interpreting the results and adjusting diabetes management.

The following recommendations are guidelines only; the policy and procedure manual of the employing institution should be followed.

Clinical observation

The diabetes educator–nurse practitioner role is emerging on both Australia and the UK and these practitioners may take on more responsibility for initiating and adjusting the treatment regime in the future.

4.4.1 Suggested protocol

Blood glucose and urinalysis are performed before meals and before bed (standard times are 7 AM, 11 AM, 4 PM and 9 PM), in order to obtain a profile of the effectiveness of diabetes therapy and to establish the renal threshold. Some practitioners prefer to test 2 hours after food, especially in Type 2 diabetes, to provide information about glucose clearance from the blood stream after a glucose load. Results should usually be <10 mmol/L. Tests may be performed at 2 AM or 3 AM for two to three days to ascertain if nocturnal hypoglycaemia is occurring.

Urine ketones should be monitored in all patients with Type 1 diabetes and in some Type 2 people during severe stress, e.g. surgery, infection, myocardial infarction if blood glucose tests are elevated. Each person's needs should be assessed individually and the testing schedule tailored to individual requirements where work routines and staffing levels allow. One way to achieve an individualised monitoring regime is to allow the patient to perform their own blood glucose tests where their condition permits them to do so.

4.4.2 Regime for patients on insulin

Initially, for 48 hours, monitor at 7 AM, 11 AM, 4 PM and 9 PM to assess the effectiveness of current insulin therapy. Review after 48 hours and alter test frequency if indicated. If the insulin regime is altered, review again after 48 hours.

N.B. The timing of blood glucose monitoring depends on the insulin regime and the type of insulin used.

4.4.3 Patients on oral hypoglycaemic agents

Initial monitoring as for insulin treated patients. Review after 48 hours and reduce monitoring frequency to twice daily, daily or once every second or third day, alternating the times of testing, as indicated by the level of control and the general medical condition of the patient.

4.4.4 Patients controlled by diet

Initially, twice daily monitoring, decreasing to daily or once every second or third day, unless the patient is having total parenteral nutrition (TPN), diagnostic procedures, is undergoing surgery or is actually ill.

In the acute care setting, patients are usually ill and require at least 4-hourly monitoring. The frequency can often be reduced in rehabilitation, mental health and care facilities for the elderly.

4.4.5 Special circumstances

These might require a prescription from the medical staff. They include:

(1) Insulin infusion: tests are usually performed every 2 hours during the infusion and reviewed every 2 hours. Reduce to 3–4 hourly when blood glucose levels are stable (see Chapter 7).
(2) People on steroid therapy:
 (a) non-diabetic patients: alternate weeks to screen for hyperglycaemia, unless results are abnormal when more frequent testing is required.
 (b) people with diabetes: see protocols in sections 4.4.2, 4.4.3 or 4.4.4.
(3) TPN guidelines suggest:
 (a) routine blood glucose testing for the first 48 hours, 7 AM, 11 AM, 4 PM and 9 PM, until the patient is stable on TPN, then revert to protocol in section 4.4.2 or 4.4.3;
 (b) monitor urine and blood for ketones, 7 AM, 11 AM, 4 PM and 9 PM.

Practice point

Never prick the feet of an adult because it causes trauma and increases the risk of infection. Heel pricks can be performed on babies.

4.5 Blood glucose meters

Blood glucose meters are devices used to monitor blood glucose in the home or at the bedside in hospital. Technology of both meters and strips is changing rapidly. Staff should become familiar with the system in use in their place of employment. Consult the diabetes educator/specialist team or manufacturer for specific advice.

Where meters are used, a blood glucose meter quality management programme with a centralised coordinator is desirable. As part of such a programme it is recommended that:

- Individual nurses demonstrate competence to use the system in operation.
- Meters are subject to regular control testing (at least daily), are calibrated as required, usually when a new pack of strips is opened, are appropriately cleaned and maintained and that these processes are documented.
- A procedure for dealing with inaccurate results and meter malfunction is in place.

There are two main types of meter, light reflectance meters and electronic devices. Electronic devices are more accurate than light reflectance meters and are superseding them. Examples of electronic devices are Medisense PC and Precision PCx (Australia) and the Boehringer Advantage (Australia and the UK). Electronic devices are preferred in acute care settings because they are less subject to technique errors and are therefore more accurate.

Practice points

(1) Incorrect operator technique and inadequate quality control testing are the major causes of inaccurate results using blood glucose meters.
(2) Some people still use visual comparison methods but they are not reliable and will gradually be phased out.

4.6 Reasons for inaccurate blood glucose results

Inaccurate blood glucose readings can occur for the following reasons:

(1) Meters
- using the incorrect strip for the meter
- using the incorrect calibration or code
- using an unclean meter
- low or flat battery
- inserting the strip incorrectly or facing the wrong way
- insufficient blood on the strip will give a false low reading
- quality control tests/calibration are not performed.

(2) Light reflectance meters and visual comparison methods
- blood wiped from the strip too soon can give low readings
- blood left on the strip too long can give high readings
- incomplete removal of blood from the strip makes interpretation difficult
- touching the pad of the finger onto some test strips leads to patchy colour development and difficulty in interpreting colours
- strips used after expiry date may not be accurate
- failure to wash hands before testing, especially if sweet substances have been handled
- humidity and high temperatures affect some testing systems.

If in doubt, repeat the test or confirm biochemically.

Figure 4.1 outlines the steps to be taken when performing quality control testing of blood glucose monitoring equipment.

4.7 Non-invasive/minimally invasive blood glucose testing

In 2001 a non-invasive blood glucose monitoring method was released. It is not widely used at present and may not be appropriate in acute illness. It is called the Glucowatch, and is a watch-sized device that automatically monitors blood glucose as often as every 20 minutes through the skin.

The device works by reverse iontophoreses and uses an electric current that stimulates sweat production. Glucose is absorbed from the sweat by an autosensor, a small disposable pad, on the back of the device. The autosensor transforms the electrical signal to a glucose reading that can be displayed by pressing a button. The autosensor must be changed every 24 hours.

An alarm sounds if the blood glucose goes too low or too high, but is not as effective in the low range. The Glucowatch holds up to 4000 tests in the memory and is only approved for adult use at present.

Practice points

(1) It is not necessary to swab the finger with alcohol prior to testing because it can dry the skin. Alcohol swabbing does not alter the blood glucose results (Dunning *et al.* 1994).

(2) The hands should be washed in soap and water and dried carefully before testing, especially if the person has been handling glucose, e.g. in an accident and emergency department/casualty, where the person presents with hypoglycaemia.

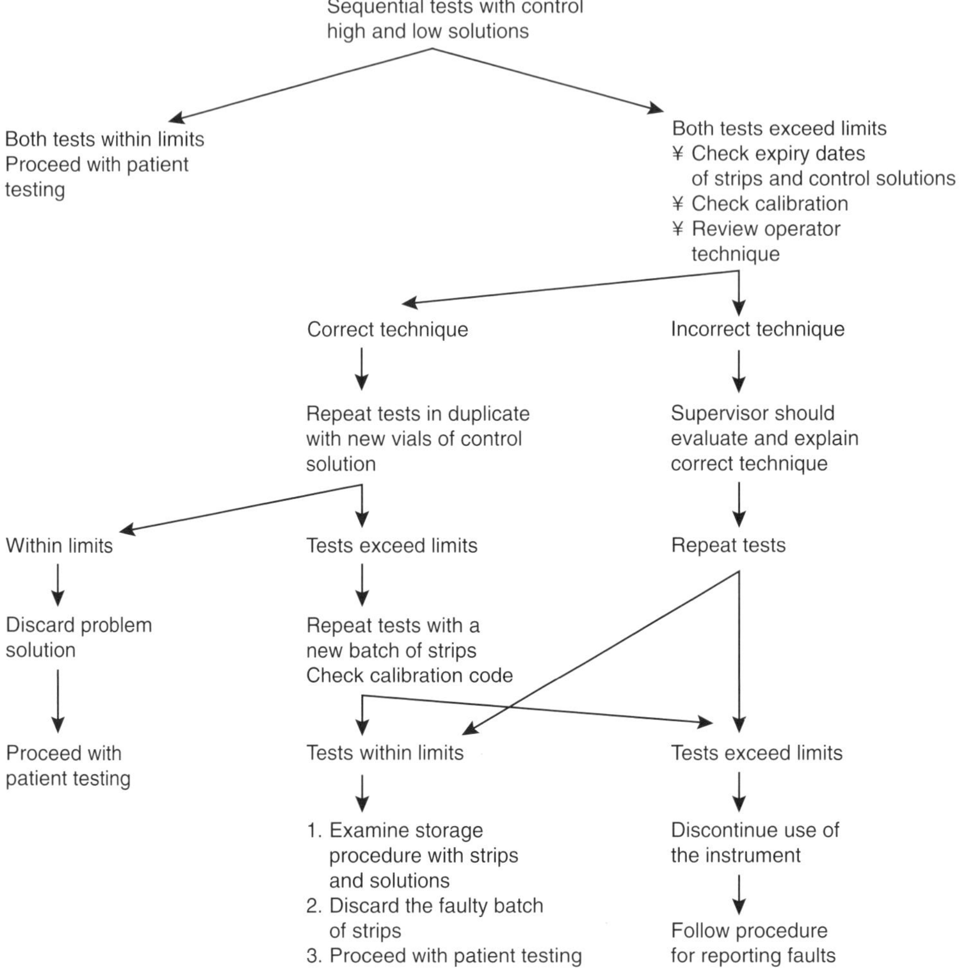

Figure 4.1 An example quality control flow chart for checking blood glucose meters.

4.8 Monitoring blood ketones

A 30-second capillary blood ketone testing hand-held meter was launched in 2001. It will be a useful adjunct to blood glucose testing for people with Type 1 diabetes during illness by allowing them to distinguish between hyperglycaemia and ketosis and to institute early treatment of hyperglycaemia and prevent ketoacidosis. It could also be useful in the clinical setting for the same reasons as well as giving an indication of the adequacy of the treatment (Wallace *et al.* 2001).

The meter measures capillary betahydroxybuterate (B-OHB). Levels >1 mmol/L require further action, e.g. extra insulin, levels >3 mmol/L require medical assessment. Ketones are formed in the liver from free fatty acids as a source of energy during fasting, exercise and insulin deficient states such as illness in Type 1 diabetes. Ketoacidosis can develop if the formation of ketones is not restrained, see Chapter 10.

Blood glucose testing checklist

BLOOD GLUCOSE TESTING CHECKLIST

Nursing Actions

(1) Assemble materials and prepare environment according to hospital policy and testing system used:
- test strip removed from vial and cap replaced immediately or open foil package;
- dry cotton or rayon ball or tissue if required;
- disposable fingerpricking device or a device with disposable end cap to avoid the possibility of cross-infection from blood left on the device.

(2) Explain procedure to patient.

Obtaining a Drop of Blood

(1) Wash patient's hands with soap and warm water, dry carefully.

(2) Choose a site on any finger, near the side or tip. Avoid using the pad of the finger where nerves and arteries are concentrated: it is more painful.

(3) Prick finger firmly, using a fingerprick device.

(4) Squeeze finger, milking along the length of the finger to well up blood at the puncture site.

(5) Allow the drop of blood to fall onto the strip or be drawn up by capillary action depending on the type of meter and strips in use.

Documenting the Results

(1) Record test results on diabetes chart and in any other pertinent record.

(2) Communicate results to appropriate person, e.g. doctor and the patient.

(3) Dispose of sharps into appropriate sharps container.

Tips

(a) Warm hands bleed more readily.

(b) If peripheral circulation is deficient, obtaining blood can be difficult. Trap blood in fingertip with one hand, by milking the length of the finger and applying pressure with finger before pricking.

(c) Excess squeezing can dilute the red cells with plasma and lead to inaccurate results.

(d) Check with biochemistry result.

The main ketone bodies are:

- Acetoacetate, which is an end product of fatty acid metabolism.
- Acetone, which is formed from spontaneous decarboxylation of acetoacetate. Acetone is volatile and expelled in expired air. It is the ketone responsible for the acetone smell of ketoacidosis.
- Betahydroxybuterate (B-OHB), which is a reduced form of acetoacetate and the major ketone formed in acidosis.

People with Type 1 diabetes are advised to test for ketones during illness, hyperglycaemia, pregnancy, if polyuria, polydipsia and lethargy are present and if they have abdominal pain. Abdominal pain is common in ketoacidosis and usually resolves as the ketosis clears. If it persists it could indicate an abdominal emergency. Blood ketone testing for B-OHB is more reliable than urine ketone testing (Fineberg *et al.* 2000). Currently available urine ketone test strips do not measure B-OHB and laboratory ketone testing often does not do so either unless it is specifically requested. The meter has not yet been tested in acute care settings and its use in acute care is still to be determined. Type 1 patients with hyperglycaemia and HbA1c > 8.5%, in association with B-OHB, are insulin deficient and at risk of ketosis. Normal blood B-OHB is 0–0.5 mmol/L. Table 4.1 depicts normal and abnormal ketone levels and suggests the management required.

Table 4.1 Blood ketone levels and potential management.

Blood ketone level (B-OHB)	*Potential management*
Normal <0.5 mmol/L	
Elevated 0.5–1.5 mmol/L and blood glucose ≥16 mmol/L	Ketosis risk/impending ketosis Insulin dose may need to be increased Food intake might be low due to fasting, poor intake or anorexia
Acidosis >1.5 mmol/L and blood glucose >16 mmol	Ketones established and ketoacidosis risk Medical review required Insulin required, possibly as an IV infusion Infection could be present

It should be noted that these levels are an indication and are not evidence based (Laffel & Kettyle 2000).

Clinical observation

Lower than actual blood glucose levels can occur on capillary testing with some commonly used blood glucose meters in the presence of moderate to heavy ketosis. The reason for this finding is not clear. It can lead to an underestimation of the severity of the hyperglycaemia, miss developing ketoacidosis and delay appropriate treatment.

Practice points

(1) Ketones are present in non-diabetic individuals during fasting and can be detected in 30% of first voided morning urine specimens of pregnant women.

(2) Ketone test strips using nitroprusside reagents (used on urine test strips) give false positive ketone results in the presence of sulphydryl drugs such as captopril.
(3) As insulin replacement corrects the acidosis B-OHB is converted to acetoacetate, meaning the ketosis is resolving but the urine ketone test can indicate that the ketones are still high.
(4) Urine ketone test strips give false negative results when they have been exposed to the air for some time, have passed their expiry date and if the urine is highly acidic such as in a person taking large doses of vitamin C.

The rate of fall of B-OHB using the new blood ketone strips can potentially avoid these situations and improve self-care and allow early intervention for people with diabetes.

Blood ketone strips can be used as an indicator of the adequacy of the treatment in acute care settings.

Section 2 explores monitoring urine glucose/ketones and blood ketones (see over).

Monitoring 2: urine glucose/ketones and blood ketones

4.9 Key points

Urine glucose testing is not recommended. If it is used:

- Establish renal threshold to determine reliability of urine tests.
- Hydration status affects results.
- Renal status affects the results.
- Double voiding is unnecessary.
- Test for ketones if blood glucose is elevated, especially in people with Type 1 diabetes.
- In future blood ketone testing will be the preferred method.
- Perform a full ward urine test on admission.

4.10 Introduction

In the presence of normal kidney function glycosuria is correlated to the blood glucose concentration. Glycosuria occurs when the tubular maximum reabsorption has been exceeded, usually around 8–10 mmol/L blood glucose. The test reflects the average glucose during the interval since the person last voided, rather than the level at the time the test is performed. This is called the renal threshold for glucose and varies within and between individuals. The renal threshold may be changed by:

- Increasing age
- Renal disease
- Long-standing diabetes.

Therefore:

- The blood glucose can be elevated without glycosuria being present.
- Traces of glucose in the urine can indicate loss of control.
- The renal threshold can be low in children and glycosuria present when blood glucose is normal.

It is important to establish the renal threshold at a period of good control by simultaneously testing blood and urine glucose.

Practice point

Urine glucose monitoring does not give warning of impending hypoglycaemia and a negative urine glucose finding does not indicate hypoglycaemia.

4.11 Limitations of urine glucose testing

(1) Fluid intake hydration status and urine concentration influence the glucose concentration.

(2) The time since voiding influences the result.
(3) Urine glucose is a limited predictor of blood glucose.

4.12 Indications for urine glucose tests

(1) If a person refuses to monitor their blood glucose.
(2) Very well controlled stable patients with Type 2 diabetes.
(3) When the aim is to avoid glycosuria.

Double voiding prior to testing is no longer considered necessary.

The currently available urine test strips are listed in Table 4.2. Moderate to heavy ketones in the urine can depress the colour reaction for glucose on Diastix and Ketodiastix. Blood glucose tests should be performed if ketones are present in the urine.

Table 4.2 Currently available urine test strips.

Trade name	*Manufacturer*	*Uses*
Clinistix Bottles of 100 strips	Ames–Bayer	Test for urine glucose
Diastix Bottles of 100 strips	Ames–Bayer	Test for urine glucose
Keto-diabur-Test 5000	Boehringer Mannheim	Test for both glucose and ketones
Ketodiastix Bottles of 100 strips	Ames–Bayer	Test for both glucose and ketones
Ketostix Bottles of 100 strips	Ames–Bayer	Test only for ketones

All urine test strips have a graded colour scale on the label to estimate the amount of glucose/ketones in the urine.

4.13 Monitoring ketones

Urine ketone testing is still important at the time of writing. In time capillary blood ketone monitoring will supersede it. Testing for ketones is important during illness in:

- All people with Type 1 diabetes.
- People with Type 2 who are severely ill.

Ketonuria can be a consequence of:

- Insulin deficiency.
- Starvation.
- After-severe hypoglycaemia.

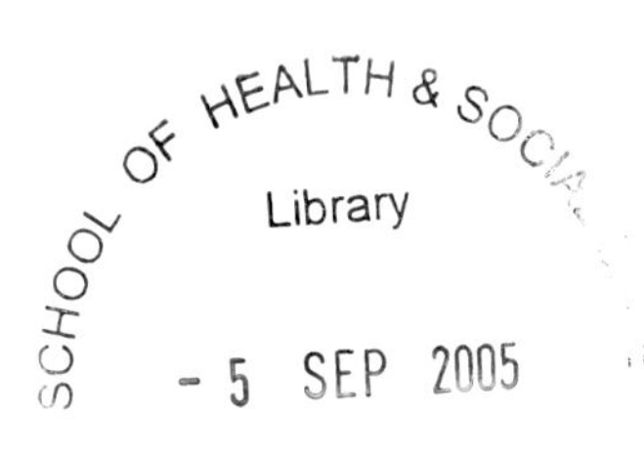
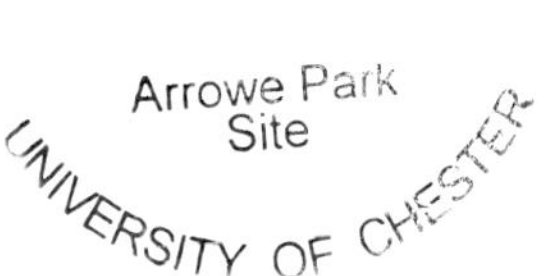

- Severe stress.
- TPN feeds high in glucose or lipids.

4.14 Urine tests of kidney function

Twelve- and 24-hour urine collections are used to monitor kidney function and detect early kidney damage by monitoring creatinine clearance rates and microalbumin excretion rates. Microalbuminuria is the earliest marker of the onset of kidney and cardiovascular damage and 30% of people with Type 1 diabetes develop nephropathy. Early diagnosis and treatment can delay the onset by 24 years and decrease the need for dialysis and increase life expectancy (Borch-Johnsen *et al.* 1993). Seventeen per cent of people with essential hypertension develop proteinuria despite satisfactory treatment (Ruilope *et al.* 1990). Therefore, nurses have a role in screening and detecting declining renal function and educating the person about appropriate preventative measures. The procedure for collecting the urine should be explained to the patient carefully. Written instructions should be supplied if the collection is to be performed at home. Collections are best obtained at a period of good control and normal activity, not during illness or menstruation; therefore the urine is often collected on an outpatient basis.

The opportunity can be taken during a hospital admission to collect 12- or 24-hour timed urine collections when people repeatedly fail to collect them as outpatients. In some cases the first early morning voided specimen will be collected – 50 ml.

Ensure the correct containers are used for the collection. Ensure correct labelling of the specimen. The urine is tested for the presence of microalbuminuria, which is a predictor of kidney damage before overt proteinuria is detected by Multistix or Albustix.

Two new dipstick tests have recently become available for testing for microalbuminuria, and can be used in the ward situation. These are the:

- Micral-test and Micral-test II
- Microbumin test.

4.15 Micral-test

Microalbuminuria can also be detected via an optically read immunoassay used in Micral-test and Micral-test II strips. These strips are packaged in lots of 12 and 30. The test is performed by dipping the reagent end into fresh urine. The strip is read within five minutes by comparing the colour change with the microalbuminuria calibrator and ranges from negative, 20, 50 and 100 mg/L.

Section 3 explores additional assessment (see over).

Monitoring 3: additional assessment

In addition to blood and urine testing, diabetic control is assessed by:

(1) Regular weight checks.
(2) Regular physical examination, especially of:
- blood pressure (lying and standing to detect any postural drop that could indicate the presence of autonomic neuropathy)
- eyes (retina) and visual acuity
- cardiac status
- feet
- kidney function.

(3) Regular education about:
- diet
- self-monitoring techniques
- injection sites
- general diabetic knowledge
- changes to diabetes care as a result of research.

In addition, special blood tests may be requested by the medical staff.

Practice point

Normal ranges for the tests described will differ between laboratories depending on the assay method used.

4.16 Nursing responsibilities

(1) To have a basic knowledge of the tests in order to be able to explain them to the patient.
(2) Ensure patients who are required to fast are given appropriate *written* instructions before the test about their medications and any other preparation required.
(3) To ensure the correct collection technique, appropriate amount of blood and correct tubes are used.
(4) Mix the sample by inverting the tube two or three times if an anticoagulant tube is required. Vigorous shaking causes haemolysis of red blood cells.
(5) To ensure the specimen reaches the laboratory in the appropriate time span.
(6) To ensure results are available for medical evaluation.
(7) To know the effects of illness and stress on the results of the test.
(8) To ensure appropriate sterile blood collection technique is used.
(9) To ensure appropriate disposal of used equipment.
(10) To ensure patients are given their medication and something to eat after completing the test.

4.17 Blood glucose

Venous glucose is measured to:

- Screen for and diagnose diabetes.
- Monitor effectiveness of diabetic medication.
- Determine medication requirements.
- Evaluate diabetic control.
- Confirm high/low capillary glucose result.

Specimens should reach the laboratory within 30 minutes of collection or be refrigerated to prevent glycolysis occurring and consequent deterioration of the sample.

4.18 Glycosylated haemoglobin (HbA1c)

Circulating blood glucose attaches to the haemoglobin in the red blood cells and undergoes a chemical reaction (Amadori) whereby the glucose becomes permanently fixed to the haemoglobin (glycosylation). The glycosylated haemoglobin (HbA1c) can be measured and quantified to give an indication of metabolic control, in particular the average blood glucose concentration over the preceding 3 months.

It should be noted that:

- The rate of glycosylation of haemoglobin is influenced by chronic hyperglycaemia.
- HbA1c complements capillary blood glucose tests and the clinical assessment of the patient.
- Fasting prior to obtaining the blood sample for HbA1c is not necessary.
- Tests are usually performed at least three months apart but can be done sooner to gauge the effect of a treatment modification.

Practice points

(1) People who experience frequent hypoglycaemic episodes may have satisfactory HbA1c results.
(2) HbA1c results should be evaluated as part of the total clinical picture and not viewed in isolation.
(3) HbA1c does not represent the blood glucose profile, but gives an average level. Considered to be the 'gold standard' for monitoring metabolic control.

There are several assay methods available for the determination of HbA1c values. Table 4.3 lists some factors which may affect HbA1c results.

4.19 Fructosamines

The fructosamines are a group of glycosylated blood and tissue proteins.

(1) They are dependent on blood glucose levels.
(2) They reflect average blood glucose levels within the preceding 3 weeks.

(3) They are useful for monitoring:
- diabetes during pregnancy
- initial response to diabetes medication
- patients with chronic anaemia
- patients with haemoglobinopathies.

Fructosamine results can be lower in patients with low serum albumin, cirrhosis of the liver or haemoglobinopathies. Fructosamine estimations are not performed very often.

Table 4.3 Non-glycaemic factors affecting results of glycosylated haemoglobin assays.

False high	*False low*
Chronic alcohol abuse	Anaemia
Fetal Hb	Abnormal haemoglobins
Hyperlipidaemia	such as HbS, HbC, HbD found in some
Hyperbilirubinaemia	ethnic groups
Renal failure	Chronic blood loss
Splenectomy	Haemolysis
	Haemorrhage

4.20 Serum lipids

Serum lipids are usually elevated if the blood glucose is elevated. Three classes of lipids are measured:

(1) Cholesterol
(2) Triglycerides
(3) Lipoproteins:
- very low density lipoprotein (VLDL)
- low density lipoprotein (LDL)
- high density lipoprotein (HDL).

Fasting blood samples are most useful. Alcohol should not be consumed for 24 hours before the blood sample for serum lipid measurements is taken.

High lipids, especially elevated triglycerides and LDL and low HDL, are risk factors for cardiovascular disease. This is a common lipid profile in people with poorly controlled Type 2 diabetes and may be secondary to hyperglycaemia. It is another reason to strive for normoglycaemia. Elevated triglycerides can make it difficult to achieve good control and medications such as fibrates, fish oil concentrates or nicotinic acid may be required depending on the type of lipid abnormality present, see Chapter 6.

4.21 C-peptide

C-peptide is the connecting peptide which determines the folding of the two insulin chains during insulin production and storage in the pancreas. It splits off in the final stages and can be measured in the blood. It is used to measure endogenous insulin production, to distinguish the type of diabetes if this is not clear in the clinical presentation. C-peptide is present in normal or elevated amounts in Type 2 diabetes, indicating that insulin is being produced and that diet and/or OHAs with exercise could achieve acceptable control.

- C-peptide will be absent or low in people with Type 1 diabetes and can be a useful indicator in slow onset Type 1 diabetes occurring in adults (Cohen 1996).
- It is not changed by injections of insulin.
- Fasting results are most useful.

4.22 Islet cell antibodies

Islet cell antibodies (ICA) are found in most newly diagnosed people with Type 1 diabetes, indicating that diabetes is an autoimmune disease. The beta cells of the pancreas are the specific target in diabetes and other pancreatic functions are not affected. In the laboratory, impaired insulin release can be demonstrated when ICA are present but the clinical implication is still unclear.

ICA are present in the prediabetic state before the disease is clinically obvious. They can also be present in close relatives who are at high risk of developing diabetes if they have ICA.

GAD antibodies are also present in 80% of people with Type 1 diabetes and enable it to be distinguished from Type 2 diabetes (Cohen 1996).

4.23 Creatinine clearance and urea

These are used to estimate renal function and nutritional status in relation to protein, especially during TPN and continuous ambulatory peritoneal dialysis (CAPD). An increase in the blood urea nitrogen (BUN) may indicate impaired renal function, however the BUN can also be increased if the patient is dehydrated, has internal bleeding or is on steroids. Anorexia, a low protein diet and fasting can lead to a decrease in urea.

Creatinine is a more sensitive marker of renal function. The serum creatinine is compared with the urine creatinine clearance rate over the same period of time. An increased serum creatinine indicates renal impairment. A significant rise may only occur when up to 50% of kidney function is lost. Creatinine is measured regularly to note *any* increase in the creatinine level.

4.24 Oral glucose tolerance Test (OGTT) (see section 1.6)

OGTT is used to confirm diabetes when fasting and random blood glucose results are equivocal, and:

- When there is a strong family history, especially during pregnancy.
- In the presence of the symptoms of diabetes, when all blood and urine glucose tests are normal.
- When the fasting and random blood glucose results are slightly elevated.

References

Borch-Johnsen, K., Wenzel, H., Vibert, G. & Mogensen, C. (1993) Is screening and intervention for microalbuminuria worthwhile in patients with IDDM? *British Medical Journal*, **306**, 1722–1725.

Cohen, M. (1996) *Diabetes: A Handbook of Management*. International Diabetes Institute, Melbourne.

Dunning, T., Rantzau, C. & Ward, G. (1994) Effect of alcohol swabbing on capillary blood glucose. *Practical Diabetes*, **11** (4), 251–254.

Fineberg, S. (2000) Comparison of blood beta-hydroxybutyrate and urine ketones in 4 weeks of home monitoring by insulin-requiring children and adults. American Diabetes Association Scientific Meeting, USA, June.

Laffel, L. & Kettyle, W. (2000) Frequency of elevations in blood b-hydroxybutyrate (B-OHB) during home monitoring and association with glycaemia in insulin-treated children and adults. *Proceedings*, ADA Scientific Meeting, USA.

Ruilope, L., Alcazar, J., Hernandez, E. & Rodico, J. (1990) Does an adequate control of blood pressure protect the kidney in essential hypertension? *Journal of Hypertension*, **8**, 525–531.

Wallace, T., Meston, N., Gardnert, S. & Matthews, D. (2001) The hospital and home use of a 30-second hand-held blood ketone meter: guidelines for clinical practice. *Diabetic Medicine*, **18** (8), 640–645.

Chapter 5
Nutritional Aspects of Caring for People with Diabetes

5.1 Key points

- Everybody, not just people with diabetes, should eat a balanced diet. A balanced diet, not a 'diabetic diet' is required.
- Good nutrition is important. The diet should contain essential vitamins and minerals as well as foods from the five food groups and at least 6–8 glasses of water each day.
- The amount of fat should be decreased.
- Complex carbohydrate should be evenly spread throughout the day.
- The amount of salt should be decreased.
- Alcohol should be limited.
- Meals should be regular.
- Eating is an enjoyable social activity.

Rationale

Good nutrition is vital to the wellbeing of everybody and is an essential basis of diabetes management. Nutritional monitoring is important to ensure the optimal health of people with diabetes.

Practice point

Labels on the bed that state *Diabetic diet* are demeaning and unnecessary.

5.2 Role of the nurse

Good nutrition is essential to health. Inadequate nutrition leads to many diseases and affects the primary condition and response to treatment (Sydney-Smith 2000). Sixty per cent of deaths are related to nutritional factors, e.g. diabetes-associated cardiovascular disease (Middleton *et al*. 2001). In particular, micronutrients and protein intake are often inadequate and mineral deficiencies are common in Australia, especially in people living in poverty.

Tiredness, fatigue and obesity can indicate inadequate protein intake which can be calculated by comparing the blood urea nitrogen (BUN) with the serum creatinine. If the creatinine is low, protein intake is low. If both BUN and creatinine are low it could suggest that a state of tissue catabolism exists, such as hyperglycaemia. Increased free fatty acids are common, but total fat intake is not a determinant of blood fats.

Diets low in vitamins and minerals are also deficient in antioxidants that prevent oxidative tissue damage. Oxidative tissue damage is implicated in the development of long-term diabetic complications and is compounded by smoking, alcohol and chronic inflammatory diseases.

Antioxidants work synergistically to modulate free radicals and chemicals generated by cell metabolism. Vitamins C, E, and A and some plant chemicals are naturally occurring antioxidants.

5.3 Obesity

Obesity is common in Type 2 diabetes. It occurs as a result of an imbalance between energy intake and output. It is not necessarily a result of excessive food intake and is a disease in its own right (Marks 2000). The demonstration of an obesity gene expressed in adipose tissue and the discovery of Leptin, a molecule thought to modulate appetite and the metabolic rate a few years ago, has changed the way obesity is viewed. The majority of obese people are deficient in Leptin and 40–60% of obesity is inherited.

People with central, or truncal obesity have the greatest risk of obesity-related diseases such as diabetes. Central obesity is associated with Type 2 diabetes, dyslipidaemia, and fatty liver and therefore carries a significant risk of cardiovascular disease.

The Body Mass Index is a simple method of assessing obesity and can be used by nurses. It is calculated using the following formula:

Weight in kilograms divided by height in metres squared.

Calculating the waist:hip ratio and measuring total body fat by Dual Energy X-ray Absorptiometry (DEXA) are other methods of determining obesity.

Obesity is a chronic condition and long-term solutions to its management are needed. Medication may be required. Expert dietary advice from a dietitian is essential. In the first instance, energy-dense food intake should be reduced and exercise increased. Very low calorie diets such as Modifast can be used in special circumstances. Surgery is an uncommon treatment.

The person's age and physical condition must be considered and because of the associated cardiovascular risks, exercise should be commenced gradually. Behaviour modification techniques can be beneficial.

If complications are present, drugs such as lipase inhibitors (Xenical) or serotonin reuptake inhibitors such as Sibutamide can be used, especially if the person is depressed.

The changing role of the nurse and the focus on the preventative aspects of healthcare mean that nurses have a responsibility to develop a knowledge of nutrition and its role in preventing disability and disease. It is integral to the adequate care of people with diabetes with respect to balancing energy intake, managing blood glucose and lipid levels and maintaining good nutrition.

Diseases such as diabetes, which are often associated with over-nutrition, may be prevented or ameliorated by avoiding excess weight. The recommended dietary guidelines, used in conjunction with the five food group plan for a nutritious diet, form the basis for dietary modification for diabetes. Diet is the mainstay and first line of treatment in the management of Type 2 diabetes.

An appropriate diet helps reduce the risk of developing diabetic complications, especially cardiovascular disease. The general dietary principles apply to all people with diabetes. Precise advice will vary according to individual lifestyle, eating habits, ethnic race and nutritional requirements. It is important that realistic targets be negotiated with the patient, particularly if weight control is necessary.

The effect of medications, fasting for procedures, and gastrointestinal disturbances such as diarrhoea and vomiting, on food absorption and consequently blood glucose levels is an important consideration. A basic screening tool to identify dietary and nutritional characteristics should therefore be part of the nursing assessment and patient care plan, and allows appropriate referral to the dietitian.

Optimal nutritional care is best achieved by interaction between nursing staff and the dietitian, their joint role effecting the most appropriate management regime. Nursing staff have the greatest continuous contact with the patient and so have an invaluable role in their nutritional management by:

(1) Identifying patients at high risk of nutritional deficiencies.
(2) Screening patients' nutritional characteristics to identify potential problems, e.g.:
    - inappropriate/erratic eaters
    - restricted eaters/overeaters
    - those with domestic/financial/employment problems.
(3) Providing ongoing monitoring of patients on a meal-to-meal basis.

This information provides the basis from which nursing staff can quickly and effectively refer patients to the dietitian, who can then support nursing staff by:

- Setting goals of diet management consistent with lifestyle and total healthcare goals.
- Identifying possible nutritional problems.
- Identifying causes of possible problems and suggesting strategies to overcome them.
- Counselling and educating the patient to best reduce the risks associated with these problems.
- Supporting nursing and medical staff on an ongoing basis to ensure most effective nutritional management has been achieved (Dunning & Hoy 1994).

Practice point

Dietary requirements change with increasing age, activity level, the degree of wellness, pregnancy, and lactation and for specific disease processes, e.g. renal and cardiac disease.

5.4 Method of screening for dietary characteristics and problems

5.4.1 Nutritional status

(1) Identify whether the person is overweight or underweight and whether the person's health is affected by their weight status.
(2) Calculate BMI and/or waist:hip ratio.
(3) Review any current haematological/biochemical measurements which reflect the

person's nutritional status (such as haemoglobin and serum levels of albumin, folate and cholesterol).

Recent research indicates malnourished patients have a longer length-of-stay, are older and have increased mortality rates compared with well-nourished patients. Most malnourished patients are not identified as being at risk (Middleton *et al.* 2001). Therefore, nurses have an important role in assisting the dietitian to manage the nutritional requirements of people with diabetes. Clues to nutritional deficiency are:

- Weight loss.
- Low lymphocyte count.
- An illness lasting longer than three weeks.
- Serum albumin < 3.5 g/dl.

If a patient is identified as being malnourished their nutritional status should be monitored by being weighed regularly, using the same scales and with the person wearing similar clothing, and by monitoring nitrogen balance. Nutritional supplements may be needed.

5.4.2 Dietary characteristics

Determine:

- The regularity/irregularity of meals and/or snacks.
- Whether the person consumes foods and fluids containing refined sugar.
- Whether the person omits any of the major food groups.

If one or more problems are identified by the nurse, they can then refer the person to the dietitian for confirmation and further dietary analysis and advice.

5.5 Principles of dietary management for people with diabetes

In general, the diet for people with diabetes should:

- Be high in complex carbohydrate (50–60% of total intake).
- Be low in fat (<10% of total energy value), especially saturated fat.
- Contain adequate protein (15% of total intake).
- Be low in simple sugar, less than 25 grams/day.
- Ensure a variety of food is eaten daily from each of the five food groups.
- Ensure that carbohydrate is consumed at each meal, especially for patients on insulin or diabetes medication.

The goals of dietary management are to:

- Improve the overall health of the patient by good nutrition.
- Attain optimal body weight.
- Attain acceptable lipid and blood glucose levels.
- Offer long-term support and education.
- Ensure normal growth and development in children.

- Decrease the risk of developing complications of diabetes.
- Identify nutrition-related disorders that can affect diabetes, e.g. anaemia.

5.5.1 Nursing responsibilities

(1) To assess dietary and nutritional characteristics and problems and refer to a dietitian as required, e.g. at a change from tablets to insulin, if there are frequent high or low blood glucose levels, or a diagnosis of a complication such as renal disease, if the patient displays inadequate knowledge, or when the person requests a referral.
(2) To observe and, if necessary, record food intake, with particular reference to carbohydrate intake of patients on diabetic medication.
(3) To promote general dietary principles to patients in accordance with accepted policies and procedures.
(4) To ensure the meals and carbohydrate content are evenly spaced across the day.
(5) To ensure adequate carbohydrate intake for fasting patients, and those with diminished intake, to avoid hypoglycaemia.
(6) Administer drugs at an appropriate time in relation to food.
(7) To know that the absorption of some drugs can be modified by food, especially antibiotics, and their effectiveness may be diminished or increased. These drugs are detailed in Table 5.1. The pharmacological response to drugs is influenced by the individual's nutritional status. In turn, drugs can affect the nutritional status. The sense of smell and taste play a significant role in adequate dietary intake. Both these senses diminish with age and can be changed by disease processes and drugs. Gastrointestinal (GIT) disorders can lead to malabsorption, pH changes, alter the bioavailability of nutrients and drugs, inhibit drug binding and chelation and impair the metabolism and excretion of drugs (NHMRC 1999).
(8) To observe for signs and symptoms of hyper- and hypoglycaemia, and correct same by appropriate nutritional management as part of the treatment strategy.

Inadequate nutrition and low protein stores can delay the healing process.

5.6 'Sugar-free' foods

'Sugar-free' usually refers to the sucrose content of foods. Other sugars are often used to sweeten foods labelled sugar-free (e.g. dextrose, fructose, maltose, lactose, galactose).

Table 5.1 Drugs whose absorption can be modified by food.

Reduced absorption	*Delayed absorption*	*Increased absorption*
Aspirin	Aspirin	Diazepam
Cephalexin	Cefaclor	Dicoumarol
Erythromycin	Cephalexin	Erythromycin
Penicillin V and G	Cimetidine	Hydrochlorothiazide
Phenacetin	Digoxin	Metoprolol
Tetracycline	Indoprofen	Nitrofurantoin
Theophylline	Metronidazole	Propranolol

They may not be appropriate for people with diabetes. Low calorie and artificially sweetened foods are generally recommended.

5.7 Non-nutritive sweeteners

Non-nutritive sweeteners are an acceptable alternative to sugar. For example:

- Saccharin
- Cyclamate
- Aspartame (Equal)
- Isomalt.

However, the excessive use of these sugar substitutes is not recommended.

Sorbitol is another sweetener often used in diabetic products. It is not generally recommended because of its potential to cause diarrhoea in some patients. In addition, it has the same caloric value as glucose, and in significant amounts can increase the blood glucose. Sorbitol is often used to sweeten biscuits and chocolates manufactured for people with diabetes and sold by pharmacies and health food shops. They are expensive and not recommended for people with diabetes.

Recently, Stevia (*Stevia rebaudiana*), a herb that is very sweet, is being promoted as a suitable sugar alternative for people with diabetes in Australia. Only very small quantities are required. It does not appear to affect blood glucose levels or have any side effects but it has not been extensively evaluated in clinical practice.

5.8 Carbohydrate modified foods

Foods labelled 'carbohydrate modified' often have a high fat content and are not generally recommended for people with diabetes.

5.9 Dietetic foods

Foods labelled 'dietetic' may not be suitable for people with diabetes. It is important to encourage people to read food labels.

5.10 Alcohol

It is recommended that alcohol consumption be limited because of its potential to affect blood glucose and contribute to, or mask, hypoglycaemia (see Chapter 8). Sweet alcoholic drinks can lead to *hyper*glycaemia, while the alcohol itself leads to *hypo*glycaemia. Alcohol should *never* be consumed on an empty stomach.

Alcohol supplies considerable calories and provides little or no nutritional value. In addition, alcohol clouds judgement and can lead to inappropriate decision making. Drunkenness can resemble hypoglycaemia and treatment of hypoglycaemia may be delayed. Appropriate education about hypoglycaemia risk with alcohol consumption is essential.

5.11 'Exchanges' and 'portions'

Exchanges and portions are ways of measuring the carbohydrate content of the diet. They help to ensure an even distribution of carbohydrate when planning meals for individual patients. The difference between the two terms relates to the amount of carbohydrate measured. An exchange is equal to 15 g and a portion 10 g. Exchanges are often used in the UK while Australia is increasingly using the glycaemic index.

5.12 Glycaemic index

The glycaemic index is a method of ranking foods based on their immediate effect on blood glucose levels. Foods that break down quickly are known as high glycaemic index foods (high GI), e.g. sugars, and foods that break down more slowly are known as low glycaemic index foods (low GI), e.g. cereals. The GI is the area under the glucose response curve measured after ingestion of a test food and multiplied by 100. Foods with a GI < 55 are classified as low, GI 56–69 as moderate and GI >70 are high GI foods. In general, the lower the GI, the smaller the impact on the blood glucose level.

However, many factors affect the rate at which carbohydrate is absorbed, including the types of sugar and starch in food, the degree of processing, cooking methods and the presence of other nutrients, e.g. fat and fibre and the particular combination of foods. Low GI foods are the preferred basis of a well-balanced diet. They slow food absorption from the gut so that the postprandial glucose load is reduced, cause satiety and help with weight control, reduce HBA1c, improve insulin sensitivity and help control lipids (Brand-Miller 1994).

People with diabetes are recommended to include low GI foods in at least one meal each day. Simple sugars do not have to be excluded using the GI food plan. Foods high in fat have a low GI because the fat delays their digestion and they are absorbed slowly. High fat foods are not recommended.

The move to GI-based diets is by no means universal and GI can be difficult for some people to understand. Generally if people are accustomed to working in portions or exchanges and have reasonable metabolic control they should not be expected to change, particularly if they are elderly.

5.13 Exercise/activity

Exercise has an important role in controlling the blood glucose and increasing overall fitness. It should be combined with a suitable diet. People commencing an exercise programme should first have a medical assessment. Before exercising they should check their blood glucose levels. It is important to make a gradual start to the exercise. Strenuous activity can cause hypoglycaemia; extra carbohydrate may be needed. The role of exercise in the management of diabetes is outlined in section 1.8.3.

5.14 Example questions to ask when taking a diet history

(1) Do you have a good breakfast?

- Poor morning appetite can indicate nocturnal hypoglycaemia and catecholamine production to maintain the falling blood glucose.

- People who do not eat breakfast often snack later in the day on energy-dense foods and can be protein deficient.
- Missing breakfast interferes with work performance.

(2) Do you eat takeaway foods?

- Takeaway foods tend to be high in fat, salt and sugar and low in fibre, protein and essential vitamins and minerals.

(3) Do you eat cream biscuits, chocolates or lollies?

- This question is a way of checking the individual's intake of sugar and fat.
- Questions should be asked sensitively as part of a nutritional assessment.

References

Australian Dietary Guidelines (1991) Australian Government Publications, Canberra.

Brand-Miller, J. (1994) Importance of glycaemic index in diabetes. *American Journal of Clinical Nutrition*, **59**, Suppl, 7475–7525.

British Diabetic Association Report (1992) Dietary recommendations for people with diabetes, *Diabetic Medicine*, **9**, 189–202.

Dunning, T. & Hoy, S. (1994) *What to Do till the Dietitian Gets There*. Servier Australia, Melbourne.

Marks, S. (2000) Obesity management. *Current Therapeutics*, **41**, 6.

Middleton, M., Nazarenko, G., Nivison-Smith, I. & Smerdely, P. (2001) Prevalence of malnutrition and 12-month incidence of mortality in two Sydney teaching hospitals. *Medical Journal of Australia*, **31**, 455–461.

NHMRC (National Health and Medical Research Council) (1999) *Diet for Older Australians*. Commonwealth of Australia, Canberra.

Sydney-Smith, M. (2000) Nutritional assessment in general practice. *Current Therapeutics*, **41**(9), 13–24.

Chapter 6
Oral Hypoglycaemic and Lipid Lowering Agents

6.1 Key points

- Review lifestyle, blood glucose monitoring technique and self-care potential before commencing.
- Administer 20 to 30 minutes before meals.
- Be aware of possible drug interactions.
- Presentation of hypoglycaemia may be atypical in people on oral hypoglycaemic agents.
- They are not insulin in oral form.

Rationale

Medications should be managed within the principles of the Quality Use of Medicines. Understanding the pharmacology of the different types of oral hypoglycaemic agents allows appropriate timing of meals and medication rounds and an understanding of how to monitor their effectiveness when assessing individual needs and metabolic response.

6.2 Introduction

Sulphonylureas were the first oral hypoglycaemic agents (OHA) to become available in the 1940s. The Biguanides followed them in 1950. The value of these drugs has been established and they have been consistently improved over that time and new generations of the original sulphonylureas introduced. In addition, three new classes of OHA have been released in the last five years. The newer OHAs might extend the life of the beta cells and delay the need for insulin (Dornhorst 2001).

OHAs do not contain insulin themselves. They should be used to supplement dietary measures. Excessive dosages are not recommended, nor are OHAs a substitute for proper dietary compliance. They are not suitable for Type 1 diabetes or during pregnancy.

OHAs target the different metabolic effects of Type 2 diabetes:

- Biguanides reduce insulin resistance and fasting glucose.
- Sulphonylureas and Glitinides are secretagogues that stimulate insulin production.

- Thiazolidinediones (TZI) decrease insulin resistance, reduce daytime preprandial hyperglycaemia and have some effect on the fasting blood glucose.
- Alpha-glucosidase inhibitors slow carbohydrate digestion and reduce postprandial glucose (Phillips 2000; Braddon 2001).

These drugs are effective alone, and can be used in combination. Multiple OHAs are often required because Type 2 diabetes is a slow progressive multifactorial disease. OHAs can also be effectively combined with insulin.

Blood glucose monitoring is essential to assess when, and which, agent should be commenced. When OHAs are started it is necessary to monitor the patient's response and tailor the dose. Key testing times are:

(1) Before breakfast (fasting) to assess the response of the liver to the prevailing insulin level.
(2) Postprandial, usually two hours after food, to assess glucose disposal.

Sometimes testing at both of these times will be required.

6.3 Sulphonylureas

They are usually well tolerated but there is a tendency for people to gain weight. Hypoglycaemia is a risk, especially in elderly people on long-acting agents such as Chlorpropromide (withdrawn in the UK and Australia), and Glibenclamide, and people with renal impairment. They are usually used in a daily or BD regime.

Sulphonylureas act by:

- Stimulating insulin secretion from the pancreatic beta cells.
- Increasing the effects of insulin at its receptor sites.
- Sensitising hepatic glucose production to inhibition by insulin.

6.3.1 Possible side effects

(1) Hypoglycaemia may result due to oversecretion of insulin if the dose of the OHA is increased, food is delayed, meals are missed or activity is increased.
(2) Liver dysfunction.
(3) Nausea, vomiting.
(4) Various skin rashes.
(5) Increased appetite.
(6) *Rarely*, agranulocytosis and red cell aplasia may also occur.

Note: (2) to (6) are very uncommon. Sulphonylureas are contraindicated in pregnancy. They are mostly metabolised in the liver and severe liver disease is a contraindication to their use. Caution should be taken in people who are allergic to the sulphur drugs because the sulphonylureas have a similar chemical makeup.

6.4 Biguanides

Biguanides are a useful first line treatment for overweight Type 2 diabetics. They act by:

- Impairing the absorption of glucose from the gut.
- Inhibiting gluconeogenesis (glucose production by the liver).
- Increasing glucose uptake into muscles and fat.
- Increasing the effects of insulin at receptor sites.
- Suppressing the appetite – mild effect.

There is some evidence that Biguanides cause malabsorption of vitamin B12 but they are old studies and the clinical relevance is not established. It could be an important consideration in people who are prone to malnourishment, e.g. the elderly and those with eating disorders.

Biguanides should be ceased for two days before IVP, a CAT scan and investigations that require IV-iodinated contrast media to be used (Calabrese *et al.* 2002).

Practice points

(1) Biguanides do not stimulate the production or release of insulin and therefore, are unlikely to cause hypoglycaemia.
(2) OHAs and drugs that interact with OHAs.
They have favourable effects on the lipid profile and slow glucose absorption from the intestine.
(3) They do not generally stimulate the appetite and are less likely to contribute to weight gain.

6.4.1 Possible side effects

(1) Nausea and/or diarrhoea may occur in 10–15% of patients. Most patients tolerate Biguanides if they are started at a low dose, the tablets are taken with or immediately after food and the dosage is increased gradually.
(2) Lactic acidosis may result if alcohol is consumed while taking Biguanides. This is rare with the Biguanides available in Australia but 57 cases have occurred since it was introduced, 16 were fatal and there were known risk factors present in 41 of the 57 cases (Jerrall 2002). The risk factors for lactic acidosis are shown in Chapter 10.
The risk of lactic acidosis is increased in people with liver, renal and cardiac disease. Early signs include:
    - anorexia
    - nausea and vomiting
    - abdominal pain
    - cramps
    - weight loss
    - lethargy
    - respiratory distress.
(3) Biguanides should not be prescribed:
    - during pregnancy
    - for patients with chronic renal failure because they are excreted unchanged in the urine; lactic acidosis may occur in these patients
    - Type 1 diabetes
    - impaired hepatic or cardiovascular function.

The commonly available OHAs are listed in Table 6.1.

6.5 Glitinides

These drugs increase insulin secretion at meal times and they should only be taken with meals, usually 2–3 times per day. They are short-acting drugs and have a low hypoglycaemic risk.

They target early phase insulin secretion, which is essential for postprandial glucose metabolism and deal with the meal-related glucose load (Dornhorst 2001). In this way they initiate an insulin response pattern close to normal. They can be used in combination with Biguanides and possibly TZIs.

6.6 Thiazolidinediones

The TZIs are given as a daily dose. They modify intracellular enzymes. It takes several days for their effects to show. They have a long duration of action with the main site of action in adipose tissue.

TZIs reduce muscle and liver insulin resistance, improve the blood glucose and lipid profiles, enhance insulin sensitivity and may restore the beta cell mass.

An early form of the drug was responsible for causing liver failure and was withdrawn from the market. This effect is unlikely with currently available preparations but it is recommended that liver function be monitored and caution be exercised in people with liver damage or whose albumin excretion rate is elevated.

Hypoglycaemia is possible because they reduce insulin resistance and enhance the effectiveness of endogenous insulin.

6.6.1 Side effects

- Localised oedema.
- Congestive cardiac failure and heart failure.
- Reduced red and white cell counts.
- Weight gain, especially deposition of subcutaneous fat, while visceral obesity is reduced.
- Hypercholesterolemia.
- Liver damage.
- Women with polycystic disease of the ovary should be counselled about contraception because TZIs improve fertility in these women.
- They are contraindicated in pregnancy and during breast feeding.
- Care should be taken in lactose intolerant people because TZIs contain a small amount of lactose.

TZIs are not authorised for use with insulin but they can be combined with other OHAs. However, the research indicates that they could be added to the insulin regime and improve glycaemic control (Raskin *et al.* 2001).

6.7 Alpha-glucosidase inhibitors

These drugs are usually taken in a TDS regime.

They act by reducing carbohydrate uptake from the gut and give normal glucose disposal mechanisms more time to deal with the postprandial glucose load, thereby reducing the postprandial glucose rise.

Table 6.1 Oral hypoglycaemic agents, dose range and frequency, possible side effects, the duration of action and main site of metabolism.

Drug	*Dose*	*Frequency*	*Possible side effects*	*Duration of action (DA)*	*Site of metabolism*
(1) *Sulphonylureas* Chlorpropamide Diabinese 250 mg	125–500 mg	Single dose taken with, or immediately after food	Hypersensitivity Hypoglycaemia (Rarely used in the elderly because of long duration of action and hypoglycaemia risk.) Transient: nausea anorexia vomiting GIT discomfort *May produce a disulfiram reaction with alcohol*	DA: 20–60 h Peak: 5–7 h	Liver
Glibenclamide Daonil 5 mg Euglocon 5 mg Glimel 5 mg	2.5–20 mg	Up to 10 mg as a single dose >10 mg in divided doses Taken with, or immediately before food	Side effects rarely encountered include: nausea anorexia skin rashes Severe hypoglycaemia especially in elderly and those with renal dysfunction	DA: 6–12 h Peak: 6–8 h	Liver
Glipizide Minidiab 5 mg	2.6–40 mg	Up to 15 mg as a single dose >15 mg in a twice daily dosage Taken immediately before meals	GIT disturbances Skin reactions Hypoglycaemia (rare)	DA: Up to 24 h Peak: 1–3 h	Liver

Tolbutamide					
Rastinon 0.5 g/1.0 g	0.5–3.0 g	1–3 times/day Taken immediately before food	Mild GIT disturbances Hypoglycaemia (rare)	DA: 8–12 h Peak: 5–7 h	Liver
Diamicron MR (a sustained release preparation	30–120 mgs Dose increments should be two weeks apart	Daily	Hypoglycaemia	Released over 24 hours	Liver
Glimepiride (Amaryl)	1–4 mgs	2–3/day	Hypoglycaemia	DA: 5–8 h	Liver
(2) *Biguanides* Metformin					
Diaformin 500 mg Diabex 500 mg Glucophage 500 mg	0.5–1.5 g May be increased to 3.0 g	1–3 times/day Taken with or immediately after food	GIT disturbances Lactic acidosis Hypoglycaemia with other OHAs Decrease B12 absorption	DA: 5–6 h	*Unchanged in urine*
(3) *Glitinides* (Repaglinide, Nataglitinide)	0.5–16 mgs	2–3/day	Hypoglycaemia with other OHAs Weight gain GIT disturbance		Liver
(4) *Thiazolidinediones* (Rosiglitazone, Pioglitazone)	4–8 mgs	Daily	Oedema Weight gain CCF, heart failure Raised liver enzymes Pregnancy risk in women with polycystic ovarian disease (Rosiglitazone)	DA: 24 h	Liver
(5) *Alpha-glucosidase inhibitors* (Acarbose)	50–100 mgs	TDS with food	GIT problems, e.g. flatulence, diarrhoea Hypoglycaemia		Faeces and urine

Their major side effects reflect the inhibition of carbohydrate absorption and the arrival of undigested carbohydrate in the lower bowel – bloating, flatulence and diarrhoea. These symptoms can be distressing and embarrassing and people often stop their medications because of these side effects.

Taking the drugs with meals, starting with a low dose and increasing slowly to tolerance levels and careful explanation to the patient can reduce these problems.

Hypoglycaemia is possible if they are combined with other OHAs.

Practice point

Oral glucose may not be an effective treatment for hypoglycaemia occurring in people on alpha-glucosidase inhibitors because absorption from the gut will be delayed. IM Glucagon is an alternative.

6.8 Drug interactions

Possible interactions between OHAs and commonly prescribed drugs are shown in Table 6.2.

Drug and OHA interactions are possible and can lead to hypo- or hyperglycaemia. A number of mechanisms for the interactions are known and they include:

- Displacement from binding sites;
- Inhibition or decreasing hepatic metabolism;
- Delayed excretion;
- Reducing insulin release;
- Antagonising insulin action.

Consideration should also be given to potential drug and herb or herb/herb interactions see Chapter 26.

Practice points

(1) The clinical relevance of some postulated drug interactions is uncertain.
(2) Other miscellaneous interactions that should also be considered are:
  - beta blockers can mask tachycardia and other signs of hypoglycaemia resulting in delayed recognition and treatment increasing the risk of hypoglycaemic coma;
  - chronic alcohol consumption can stimulate the metabolism of sulphonylureas and delay their effectiveness.

Potential interactions have not yet emerged for TZIs and the Meglitinides. Drugs that alter hepatic enzymes have the potential to cause interactions with these OHAs because they are metabolised in the liver.

Drugs that interfere with access to the gut by alpha-glucosidase inhibitors can inhibit their action, e.g. charcoal, digestive enzymes, cholestyramine and neomycin. GIT problems may be a contraindication to using these drugs.

Table 6.2 Potential drug interactions between oral hypoglycaemic agents and other drugs (based on Shenfield 2001).

Drug	*Possible mechanism*
Drugs that increase blood glucose	
Clonidine	Adrenergic response
Clozapine	Impaired insulin secretion
Corticosteroids	Oppose insulin action
Diuretics, especially Thiazides	Oppose insulin action
Nicotinic acid	Unknown
Nifedipine	Delays insulin action
Oral contraceptives	Unknown
Phenytoin	Impairs insulin secretion
Sugar-containing medicines, e.g. cough syrup	Increase blood glucose
Drugs that lower blood glucose	
ACE inhibitors	Enhance insulin action
Alcohol	Reduce hepatic glucose production
Fibrates	Unknown
MOA inhibitors	Unknown
Salicylates	Unknown

6.9 Combining OHAs

There is no real benefit in using a combination of two sulphonylureas since they both act by the same mechanism. Sulphonylureas can be prescribed with Biguanides for patients who have either primary or secondary failure with the sulphonylureas alone, especially if the patient is overweight.

Practice points

Medication rounds should be planned so that OHAs are given with, or before, meals to decrease the risk of hypoglycaemia.

6.10 Combining OHAs and insulin

In some patients a combination of insulin and sulphonylureas or Biguanides may help control the blood glucose. Since the results of the UKPDS in 1998, the combination of insulin and Biguanides is increasingly common. The time to commence insulin depends on the blood glucose profile. It is often commenced at bedtime to reduce fasting glucose levels. Combination therapy allows people to become accustomed to the need for insulin and helps preserve beta cell function. In many cases a small dose of intermediate/long-acting insulin is given at bedtime to help control the blood glucose overnight, and thus reduce fasting hyperglycaemia in the morning. It is often easier to control the blood glucose during the day if the pre-breakfast test is <10 mmol/L.

6.11 Lipid lowering agents

An essential part of the diabetes management plan is to reduce cardiovascular risk. People with diabetes, especially Type 2, are at significant risk of cardiovascular disease unless the blood glucose and lipids can be kept within normal limits. Lipid targets aim to reduce cholesterol, especially LDL and triglycerides, and increase HDL. HDL aids in the removal of LDL cholesterol. High LDL significantly increases the risk of myocardial infarction, but other risk factors are important and are often exacerbated by low levels of HDL (Colquhoun 2002).

Controlling blood glucose is integral to controlling lipids (Lipid Study Group 1998). Current lipid targets aim for total cholesterol < 5 and triglyceride and LDL < 3 in patients with existing heart disease (National Heart Foundation 2001).

6.11.1 Lipid management

Management strategies are based on the absolute risk rather than the lipid level alone. Individual risk assessment should include:

- Cardiovascular status, age, sex, presence of hypertension, smoking and family history of hypercholesteremia and cardiac disease.
- Dietary modification including reducing salt, alcohol and fat in the diet.
- Low dose aspirin to reduce platelet stickiness.
- ACE inhibitors to control blood pressure.
- Stop smoking.
- Lipid lowering agents. Most people will be commenced on a statin. Statins reduce recurrent coronary events and reduce the need for revascularisation, and the incidence of thromboembolic stroke (La Rosa *et al.* 1999).
- Coaching (see Chapter 11).

Table 6.3 depicts the major classes of lipid lowering agents (Colquhoun 2001).

6.11.2 Side effects

The main side effects:

- Occur in skeletal muscle and include myositis.
- GIT disturbances (Clofibrate).

Many people discontinue taking their lipid lowering agents because they are unconvinced about the need, perceive that they have poor efficacy or dislike the adverse events.

Nurses can play a key role in encouraging people to adhere to their medications by explaining the reason they need them and suggesting ways to limit minor side effects.

Practice points

(1) It is important to explain to the patient that Type 2 diabetes is a progressive disease and it is not their fault that insulin is required.
(2) People with Type 2 diabetes on insulin report a lower quality of life than those not on insulin, see Chapter 22.

Table 6.3 Lipid lowering agents.

Lipid lowering drug and main action	*Management considerations*
HMG-CoA reductase inhibitors: reduce LDL-c	Test liver function on commencing and in 6 months Use caution if liver disease is present Decrease the dose if the patient commences cyclosporine
Fibrates: Reduce cholesterol and triglycerides and increase HDL-c	Can be combined with HMG-CoA after a trial on monotherapy Monitor creatinine kinase and liver function at 6 weeks and then in 6 months
Resins (Cholestyramine, Colestipol): Enhance LDL-c lowering effects of HMG-CoA agents	Allows lower doses of the resins to be used Slows absorption of oral hypoglycaemic agents Increases hypoglycaemia risk when used with these agents
Low dose nicotinic acid	Can be given with HMG-CoA agents Enhance reduction of triglyceride and HDL-C
Statins: reduce LDL-c, have a moderate effect on tryglicerides, and increase HDL Increase bone mineral density	They can be used with a resin Monitor liver function

Source: Nicholson 2002.

References

Braddon, J. (2001) Oral hypoglycaemics: a guide to selection. *Current Therapeutics*, Suppl 13, 42–47.

Calabrese, A., Coley, K., Da Pos, S., Swanson, D. & Rao, H. (2002) Evaluation of prescribing practice: risk of lactic acidosis with Metformin. *Archives of Internal Medicine*, **162**, 434–437.

Colquhoun, D. (2000) Unstable angina – a definitive role for statins in secondary prevention. *International Journal of Clinical Practice*, **54**, 383–389.

Colquhoun, D. (2002) Lipid lowering agents. *Australian Family Physician*, **31** (1), 25–30.

Dornhorst, T. (2001) Insulinotropic meglitinide analogues. *Lancet*, **17** (358), 1709–1716.

Jerrall, M. (2002) Warning over Metformin use. *Archives of Internal Medicine*, **162**, 434–437.

La Rosa, J., He, J. & Vupputuri, S. (1999) Effect of statins on risk of coronary disease: a meta-analysis of randomised controlled trials. *Journal of the American Medical Association*, **282**, 2340–2346.

Lipid Study Group (1998) The long term intervention with pravastatin in ischaemic disease. Prevention of cardiovascular events and death with pravastatin in patients with coronary heart disease and a broad range of initial cholesterol levels. *New England Journal of Medicine*, **339**, 1349–1357.

National Heart Foundation (2001) *Lipid Management Guidelines*. National Heart Foundation, Melbourne.

Nicholson, G. (2002) Statins decrease fractures and increase bone mineral density. *Archives of Internal Medicine*, **163**, 537–540.

Phillips, P. (2000) Tablet tips for Type 2 diabetes. *Current Therapeutics*, **41** (9), 71–77.

Raskin, P., Rendell, M. & Riddle, M. (2001) A randomised trial of Rosiglitazone therapy in patients with inadequately controlled insulin treated Type 2 diabetes. *Diabetes Care*, **24** (7), 1226–1232.
Shenfield, G. (2001) Drug interactions with oral hypoglycaemic agents. *Australian Prescriber*, **24** (4) 83–84.

Chapter 7
Insulin Therapy

7.1 Key points

- Check dose and time of administration.
- Consider onset and duration of action when planning meal times and drug rounds.
- Monitor blood glucose profile.
- Only clear (short-acting) insulin is given IV.

Rationale

In Australia insulin should be managed according to the principles of the Quality Use of Medicines. This is also relevant to the UK since it refers to appropriate prescription, administration and monitoring of the person's response to medications. Understanding insulin action and the types of insulin preparations available allows appropriate timing of meals and administration of insulin. Blood glucose monitoring should be carried out to determine the effectiveness of the dose and regime.

7.2 Basic insulin action

Insulin is a hormone secreted by the beta cells of the pancreas. Normal requirements are between 0.5 and 1.0 units/kg/day. Insulin synthesis and secretion are stimulated by an increase in the blood glucose level after meals. Insulin attaches to insulin receptors on cell membranes to facilitate the passage of glucose into the cell for utilisation as fuel or for storage and decreases hepatic glucose production. Insulin also stimulates the storage of fatty acids and amino acids, and facilitates glycogen formation, and storage, in the liver and skeletal muscle and limits lipolysis and proteolysis. Therefore, an insulin deficiency results in altered protein, fat and carbohydrate metabolism.

Insulin is a very effective drug. It is vital for Type 1 diabetes and eventually required by ≥50% of people with Type 2 diabetes. Many people with Type 2 are reluctant to start insulin for a number of reasons including weight gain, needle fears and phobias, fear of hypoglycaemia and the mythology about disease severity, e.g. 'insulin is the end of the line'. Health professionals often contribute to the myth that diet and OHA controlled diabetes is milder than insulin-treated diabetes (Dunning & Martin 1999).

The possibility of insulin therapy should be raised early in the diabetes education process so the person understands that progression to insulin is an expected step in the diabetes management process. Unfortunately, people with Type 2 diabetes are often given the impression that insulin is a last resort to be used when all else fails and that they are to blame for that failure.

7.3 Objectives of insulin therapy

(1) To achieve blood glucose levels within an acceptable individual range by replacing absent insulin secretion in Type 1 and supplementing insulin production in Type 2 diabetes.
(2) To approximate physiological insulin secretion.
(3) To avoid the consequences of too much insulin (hypoglycaemia) or too little insulin (hyperglycaemia).
(4) Improve quality of life and reduce the risk of complications.

7.4 Types of insulin available

Insulin cannot be given orally at this stage. It is a polypeptide. Polypeptides are digested by gastric enzymes and do not reach the circulation. Research is currently under way to coat insulin in a substance that can withstand gastric juices and pass unchanged into the intestine before breaking down. Inhaled insulins are also the subject of research, see 7.17.

There are a number of different brands of insulins available, e.g. Novo Nordisk, Eli Lilly.

Animal insulins are rarely used nowadays but are still available in the UK. Insulin is manufactured by recombinant DNA technology (so-called 'human' insulin (HM)). The amino acid sequence of HM insulin is the same as that of insulin secreted by the beta cells of the human pancreas. HM is now the only widely available insulin, regardless of the brand used.

In the past few years insulin analogues have been developed that give a more physiologic response after injection and improve the blood glucose profile, e.g. Humalog, and more recently, insulin Aspart. The advantages of these insulins are reduced post-prandial hyperglycaemia and reduced risk of hypoglycaemia. Insulin Glargine will be introduced in Australia and in the UK in the near future. It gives a smooth peakless glucose profile for 24 hours (Buse 2001). Glargine is not widely available in some countries yet. These insulins allow for greater management flexibility and for the creation of insulin combinations to meet individual needs.

Practice point

Human insulin does not come from humans.

Insulin preparations vary in their duration of action.

7.4.1 Rapid acting insulin

Rapid acting insulin should be clear and colourless. Examples are:

- Lispro (Humalog)
- Novorapid.

They have a rapid onset of action, within 10 minutes, peak at 60 minutes and act for 2–4 hours.

They need to be given *immediately* before meals and are used in basal bolus regimes, in combination with intermediate acting insulin or used in combination with OHAs or in insulin pumps.

Combining them with alpha-glucosidase inhibitors, which reduce glucose absorption from the gut, can increase the risk of hypoglycaemia.

The first hour after injection and 2–3 hours after exercise are other peak times for hypoglycaemia.

7.4.2 Short-acting insulin

This should be clear and colourless. Examples are:

- Actrapid
- Humulin R, or Humulin S
- Hypurin neutral (beef).

They begin to take effect in 20 to 30 minutes, and act for about 4 hours. They can be used:

- Alone two to four times daily.
- In combination with intermediate or long-acting insulins.
- As IV insulin infusions.

7.4.3 Intermediate-acting insulin

This must be mixed gently before use and should be milky after mixing. Examples are:

- Protophane
- Humulin I/Humulin L
- Insulatard
- Hypurin (isophane).

They begin to act in 2 to 3 hours. The duration of action is 12 to 18 hours. Monotard preparations, however, last for up to 22 hours. They can be used:

- In combination with short-acting insulin – this is the usual method.
- Alone for patients who are sensitive to short-acting insulin, or in combination with oral hypoglycaemic agents.

7.4.4 Long-acting insulin

This must be mixed before use and should be milky after mixing. Examples are:

- Monotard
- Ultratard
- Humulin UL.

They begin to act in 4 to 6 hours. The duration of action is 30 to 36 hours. Uses:

- As for intermediate-acting insulins.

7.4.5 Biphasic insulins

Biphasic insulins are often prescribed for people with Type 2 diabetes. They allow people who find it difficult to mix insulins in syringes to continue to manage their own insulin therapy and remain independent.

These contain both short- and intermediate-acting insulins in various combinations. They must be mixed before using. They do not allow for independent adjustment of the short and intermediate components. Examples are:

- Mixtard 30/70
- Mixtard 50/50
- Mixtard 15/85
- Insulin Aspart (NovoMix 30)
- Humulin 20/80
- Humulin 50/50
- Humalog Mix 25

A range of devices is available to administer insulin. Frequently used devices are shown in Table 7.1. The range of Lilly insulins is shown in Figure 7.1 and the Novordisk range in Figure 7.2.

7.5 Storage of insulin

The temperature at which insulin is stored is important to maintaining its efficacy. Insulin should be stored according to the manufacturer's directions. Unopened vials should be stored in the refrigerator at 2–8°C. Insulin vials in use can be stored out of the refrigerator, e.g. in the patient's medication drawer, provided they are not stored near a source of heat (Campbell *et al*. 1993).

People with diabetes need to be educated about correct storage and handling of insulin as part of their education about insulin therapy.

Clinical observation

Hyperglycaemia associated with using incorrectly stored insulin and insulin that has passed the expiry date does occur.

Practice point

Do not freeze. Check expiry date. Discard if outdated.

7.6 Injection site and administration

Administer at the appropriate time before the meal. The abdomen is the preferred site; but upper arms, thighs and buttocks can also be used. Injection sites must be rotated to avoid lipoatrophy and lypodystrophy.

7.6.1 How to inject

The insulin injection technique can influence insulin absorption and, therefore, its action. Insulin should be administered subcutaneously. IM injections lead to unstable blood glucose levels (Vaag *et al*. 1990).

Table 7.1 Readily available insulin devices and some of the issues to be aware of with each device.

Device	*Issues to be aware of*
A) ***Syringes*** 30, 50 and 100 unit sizes	• There is still a place for syringes • Patients need to be able to recognise different dose increments on different sized syringes • Select size appropriate for dose • Needles are usually longer than other devices • Can be used with all available insulins
B) ***Insulin 'pens'*** There are 2 main manufacturers of insulin devices: Novo and Owen Mumford	• Insulin 'pens' are not suitable for people who need to mix insulins
1) *Novo Devices*	
NovoPen 3	• Dose range 2–70 units • Accurate dosing • Uses 3 ml insulin cartridges • Small, fine needles • Replacing the insulin cartridge can be difficult • Has a function to check the accuracy of the device • Pen is reusable
NovoPen Demi	• Similar to NovoPen 3, but $\frac{1}{2}$ unit dose increments are possible • Useful for children and insulin-sensitive patients who require very small doses
Novolet	• Preloaded disposable devices • Contain 3 ml of insulin • Range of insulins available • Small, fine needles • Dose range up to 78 units • Can be confusing to use and dose errors often occur especially with large doses • May be of benefit to people while travelling
INNOVO	• Dose range 1–70 units • Accurate dosing • Uses 3 ml insulin cartridges • Range of insulin available • Battery-operated, batteries last about 4 yr then the device needs to be replaced • Small, fine needles • A display indicates that insulin is being delivered, the number of units delivered, the dose given and time elapsed since the previous dose was administered • Can be difficult to use, especially if large doses are needed • May help people who forget whether they have taken their insulin • Reusable device

Cont'd

Table 7.1 *Cont'd*

Device	*Issues to be aware of*
INNOLET	• Dose range 1–50 units • Accurate dosing • Small, fine needles • Device is preloaded and disposable • Only Protaphane and Mixtard 30/70 insulin available in Australia, at this stage. Protaphane is not available in the UK • Contains 3 ml of insulin • Clear, easy to see numbers on the dose dial, which is an advantage for vision impaired people • Larger than other devices – takes up storage space in fridge
PenMate 3	• Automatic needle insertion device • Used with NovoPen 3 • Hides needle and injects insulin quickly and automatically • May benefit people with needle phobia and children
NovoMix 30 FlexPen	• Contains 3 ml of insulin • Disposable, preloaded device • Small, fine needles
Insulin Pumps	• Provide continuous basal insulin with a facility for giving bolus doses with meals • Uses only short-acting insulin • Uses small, fine needles • Expensive • Requires considerable expertise and time to be used effectively
Jet Injectors	• No needle required • Not widely used • Force insulin through skin under pressure • Bruising common • Sterilisation issues

- Pinch up a fold of skin (dermis and subcutaneous tissue) between the thumb and index finger.
- Inject at 90-degree angle. If the needle is long, pinch up may not be needed and a 45-degree angle can be used.
- Release the skin, remove the needle, and apply pressure to the site.
- Document dose and time of the injection.
- Injection sites should be regularly checked for swelling, lumps, pain or leakage of insulin.

Practice points

(1) A range of needle sizes is available. Needle size is important to people with diabetes.
(2) They usually prefer small, fine gauge needles.
(3) Injection with fine gauge needles is relatively painless.
(4) Giving the first injection is often very difficult for people with diabetes. Support and encouragement and allowing them to take their time and inject at their own pace is important.
(5) If insulin tends to leak after the injection, release the skin fold before injecting. Pressure from holding the skin fold sometimes forces the insulin back out of the needle track. Withdraw the syringe quickly to allow the skin to seal. Do not cover so that any insulin leakage can be observed.
(6) The loss of even small amounts of insulin can result in unpredictable increases in the blood glucose and inappropriate dose adjustment. Careful observation and estimation of the amount of insulin lost is necessary to make appropriate adjustments to the individual's injection technique – this applies to both patients and nurses.
(7) The larger the volume of insulin to be injected the greater the likelihood of some insulin leaking back along the needle track. Likewise, leakage can occur if the injection is too shallow, or given intradermally.
(8) To minimise the risk of insulin loss during injection, inject slowly and leave the needle in place for 3–6 seconds after the insulin is delivered.
(9) Long-acting and pre-mixed insulins for insulin pens must be mixed gently before administration.

Instructions for teaching people how to draw up and administer insulin appear in Chapter 23. Refer also to the manufacturer's instructions.

7.7 Mixing short- and long-acting insulins

7.7.1 General points

Mixing short- and long-acting insulins before injection may have the effect of diminishing the short-acting peak, which is more marked when there is substantially more long-acting insulin in the mixture (as is usually the case), especially if the insulin is left to stand for a long time before use.

The clinical significance of these changes is unknown. It is more likely to apply to in home situations where home-based nurses or relatives draw up doses for several days for patients to self-administer, see Chapter 25. This practice may not be ideal but it does allow people to retain a measure of independence where syringes are still the device of choice.

7.8 Common insulin regimes

7.8.1 Daily injection

A combination of short- and long-acting insulin usually given before breakfast. Insulin is often given at bedtime when it is combined with OHAs. Biphasic insulins such as Mixtard 30/70 and Humulin 20/80 can be used. Daily regimes are commonly used for:

- Elderly people.
- Those not willing to have more than one injection.
- Some situations where people are dependent on home nursing care.

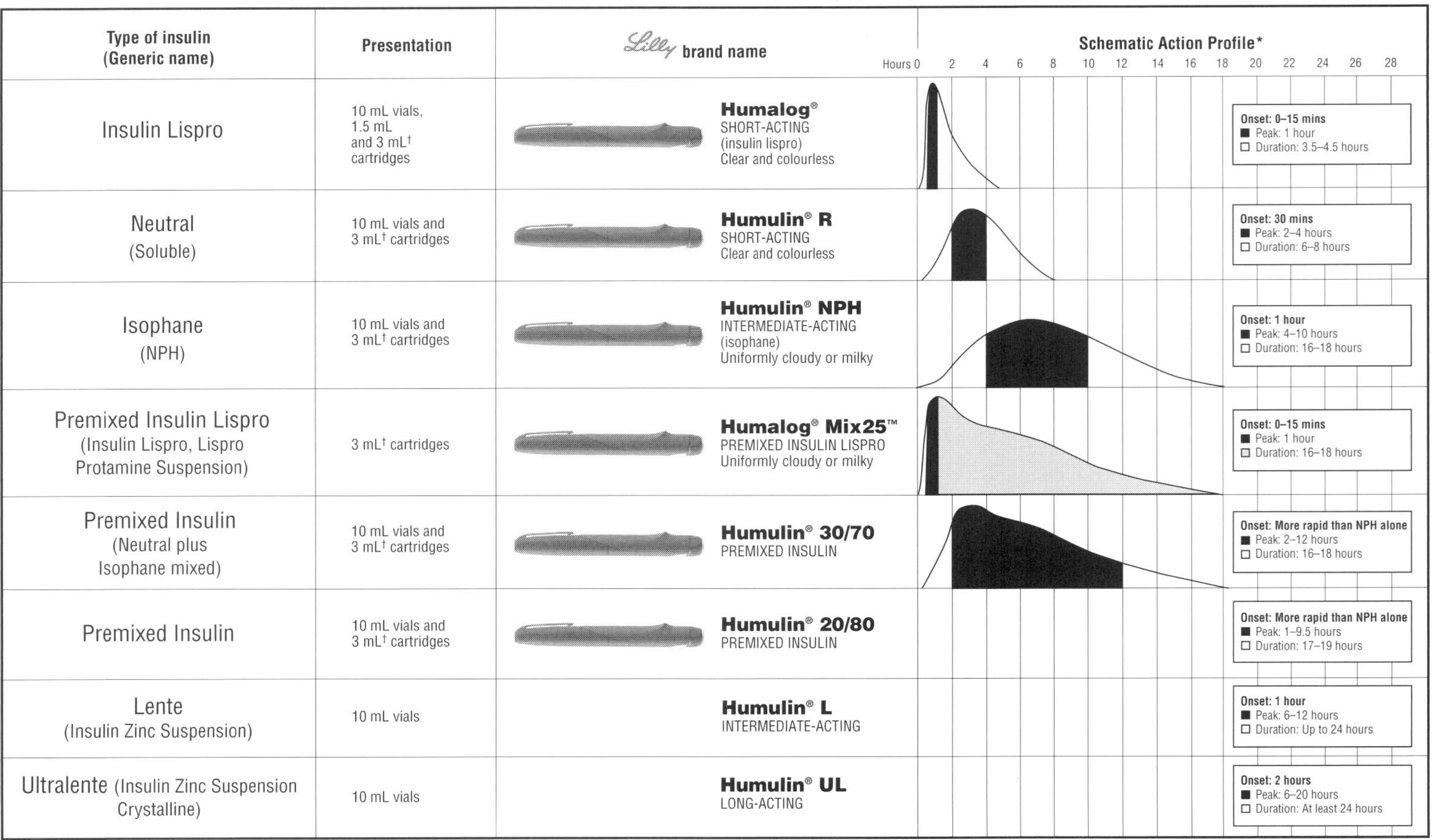

Figure 7.1 Range of Lilly insulins, their presentation and schematic action profiles. (Australia)

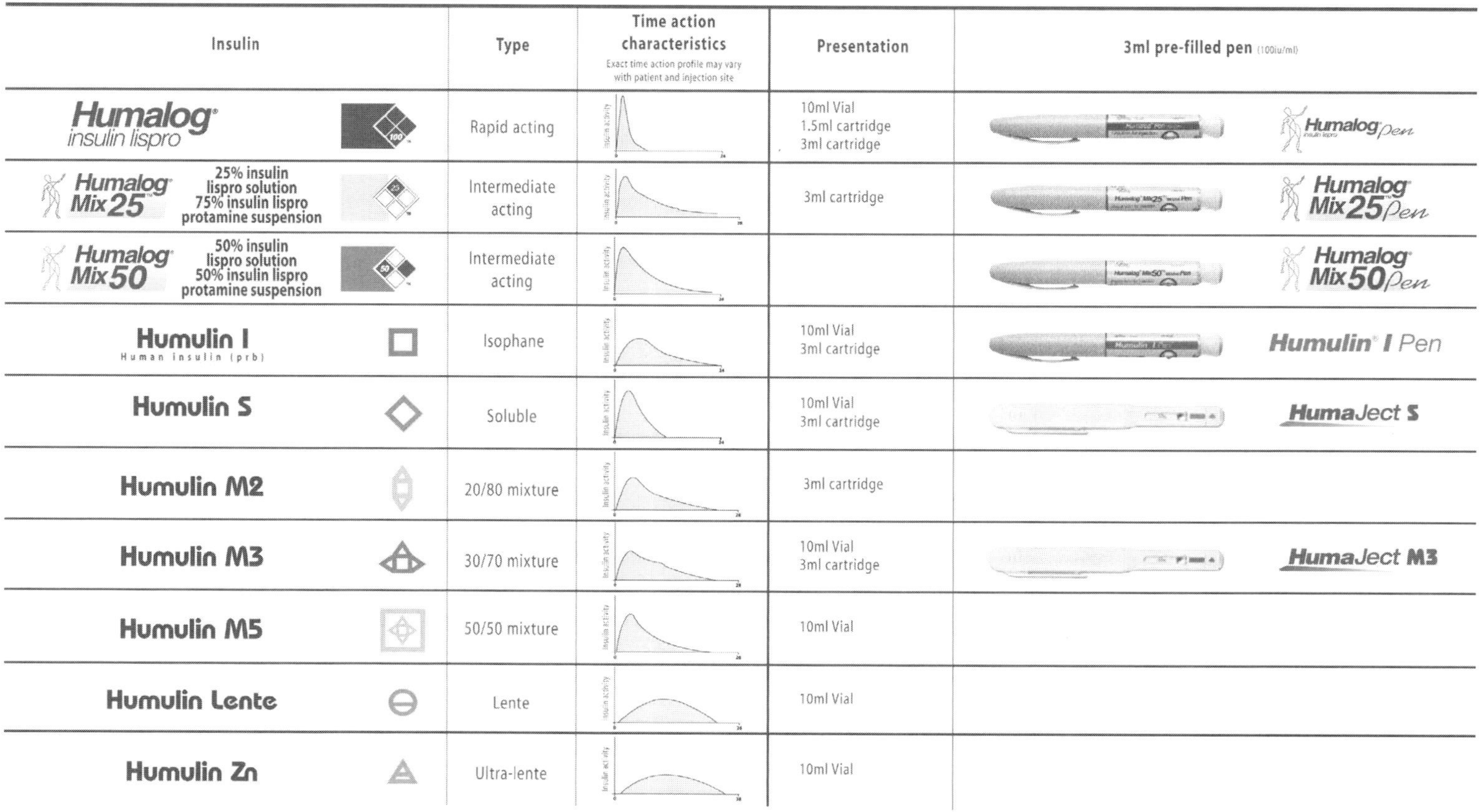

Insulin	Type	Time action characteristics Exact time action profile may vary with patient and injection site	Presentation	3ml pre-filled pen (100iu/ml)
Humalog® insulin lispro	Rapid acting		10ml Vial 1.5ml cartridge 3ml cartridge	Humalog Pen
Humalog® Mix25™ 25% insulin lispro solution 75% insulin lispro protamine suspension	Intermediate acting		3ml cartridge	Humalog® Mix25™ Pen
Humalog® Mix50™ 50% insulin lispro solution 50% insulin lispro protamine suspension	Intermediate acting			Humalog® Mix50™ Pen
Humulin I Human insulin (prb)	Isophane		10ml Vial 3ml cartridge	Humulin® I Pen
Humulin S	Soluble		10ml Vial 3ml cartridge	HumaJect S
Humulin M2	20/80 mixture		3ml cartridge	
Humulin M3	30/70 mixture		10ml Vial 3ml cartridge	HumaJect M3
Humulin M5	50/50 mixture		10ml Vial	
Humulin Lente	Lente		10ml Vial	
Humulin Zn	Ultra-lente		10ml Vial	

Figure 7.1 *cont'd* (UK)

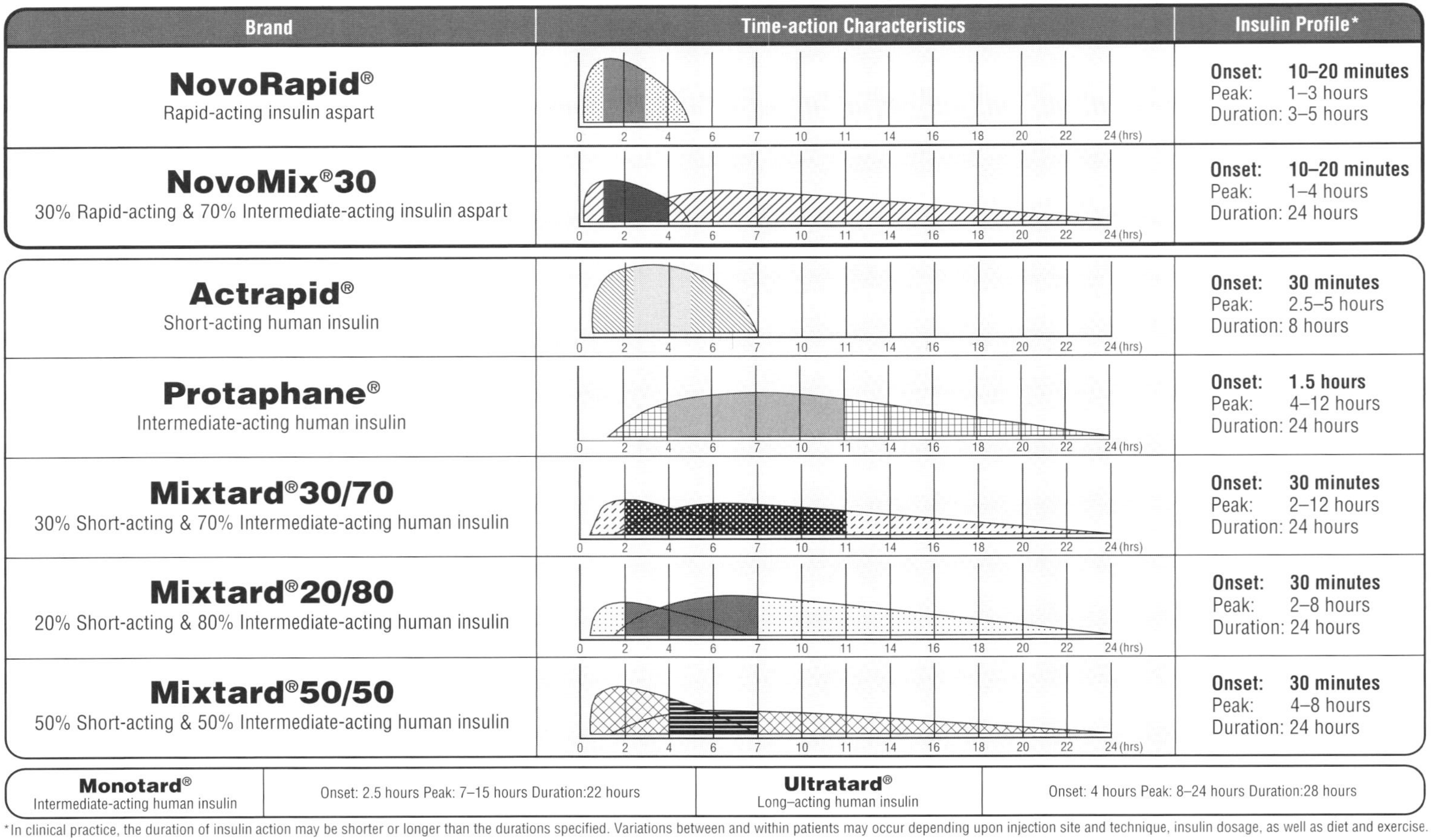

Brand	Time-action Characteristics	Insulin Profile*
NovoRapid® Rapid-acting insulin aspart	0 2 4 6 7 10 11 14 16 18 20 22 24 (hrs)	**Onset: 10–20 minutes** Peak: 1–3 hours Duration: 3–5 hours
NovoMix®30 30% Rapid-acting & 70% Intermediate-acting insulin aspart	0 2 4 6 7 10 11 14 16 18 20 22 24 (hrs)	**Onset: 10–20 minutes** Peak: 1–4 hours Duration: 24 hours
Actrapid® Short-acting human insulin	0 2 4 6 7 10 11 14 16 18 20 22 24 (hrs)	**Onset: 30 minutes** Peak: 2.5–5 hours Duration: 8 hours
Protaphane® Intermediate-acting human insulin	0 2 4 6 7 10 11 14 16 18 20 22 24 (hrs)	**Onset: 1.5 hours** Peak: 4–12 hours Duration: 24 hours
Mixtard®30/70 30% Short-acting & 70% Intermediate-acting human insulin	0 2 4 6 7 10 11 14 16 18 20 22 24 (hrs)	**Onset: 30 minutes** Peak: 2–12 hours Duration: 24 hours
Mixtard®20/80 20% Short-acting & 80% Intermediate-acting human insulin	0 2 4 6 7 10 11 14 16 18 20 22 24 (hrs)	**Onset: 30 minutes** Peak: 2–8 hours Duration: 24 hours
Mixtard®50/50 50% Short-acting & 50% Intermediate-acting human insulin	0 2 4 6 7 10 11 14 16 18 20 22 24 (hrs)	**Onset: 30 minutes** Peak: 4–8 hours Duration: 24 hours

Monotard® Intermediate-acting human insulin	Onset: 2.5 hours Peak: 7–15 hours Duration:22 hours	**Ultratard®** Long–acting human insulin	Onset: 4 hours Peak: 8–24 hours Duration:28 hours

*In clinical practice, the duration of insulin action may be shorter or longer than the durations specified. Variations between and within patients may occur depending upon injection site and technique, insulin dosage, as well as diet and exercise.

Figure 7.2 (a) Range of Novo Nordisk insulins with their time action characteristics and insulin profiles and (b) the delivery systems available with each insulin (Australia).

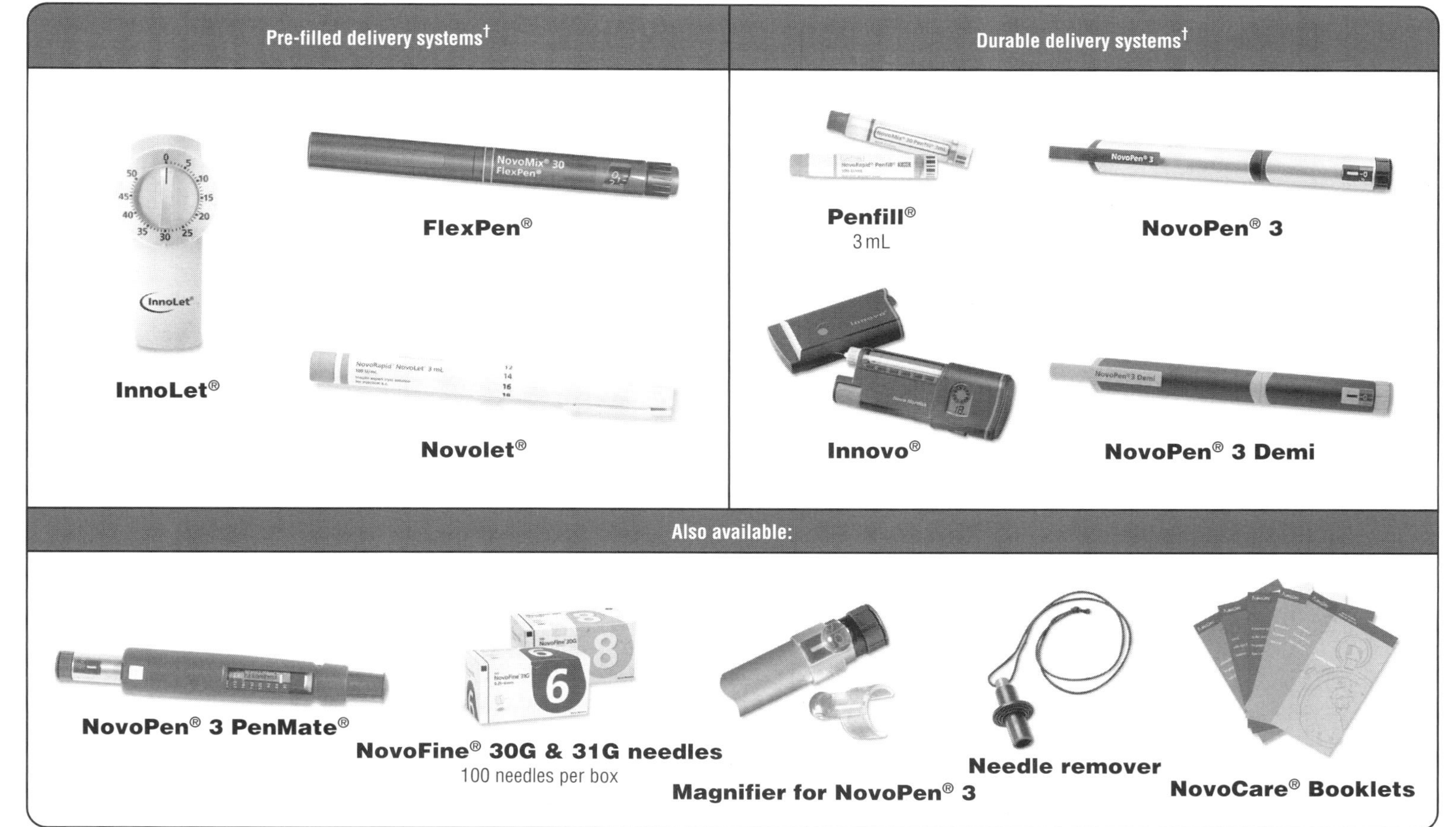

Figure 7.2 (b) *cont'd* (Australia)

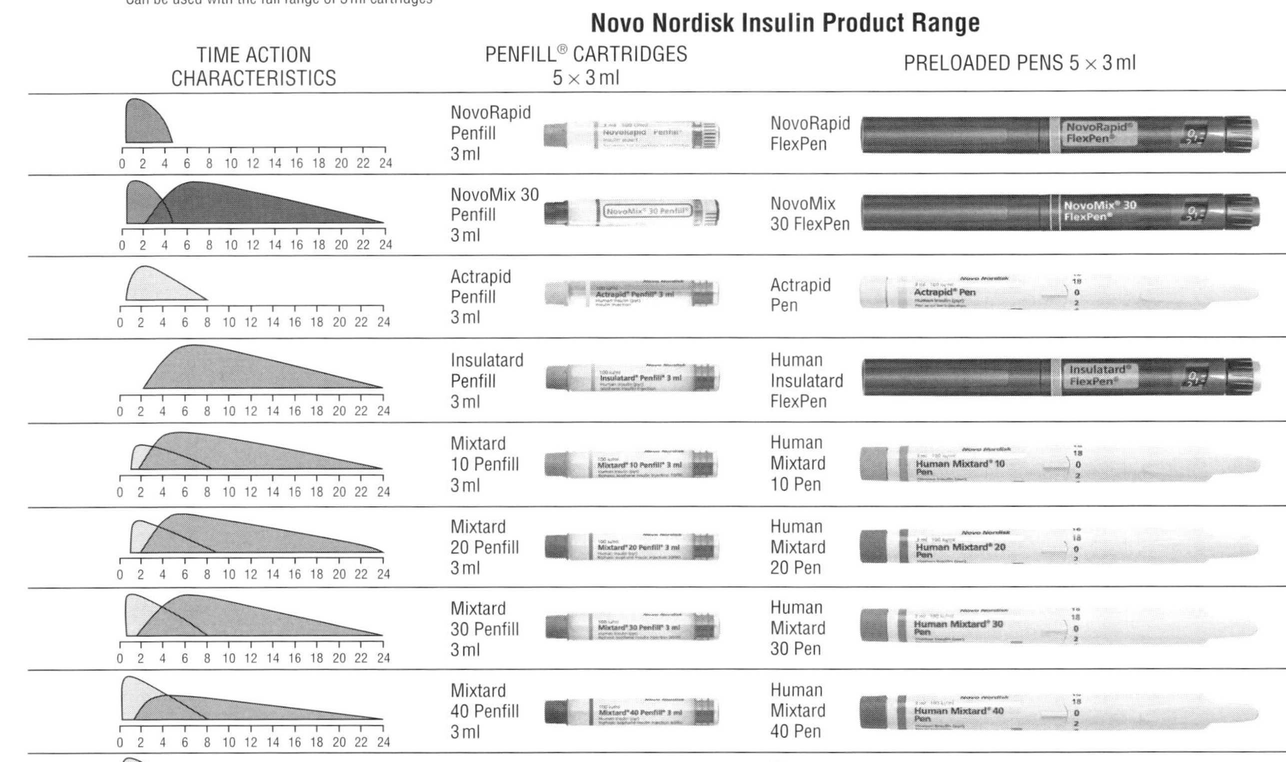

NovoRapid, Human Actrapid, Human Insulatard ge, Human Mixtard 30 ge, Human Mixtard 50, Human Velosulin®, Human Monotard®, Human Ultratard®, Pork Actrapid, Pork Insulatard and Pork Mixtard 30 are available in **10 ml vials.** Human Actrapid Penfill, Human Insulatard Penfill, Human Mixtard 10 Penfill, Human Mixtard 20 Penfill, Human Mixtard 30 Penfill, Human Mixtard 40 Penfill, Human Mixtard 50 Penfill are available in **1.5 ml cartridges.**

Figure 7.2 (a) *cont'd* (UK)

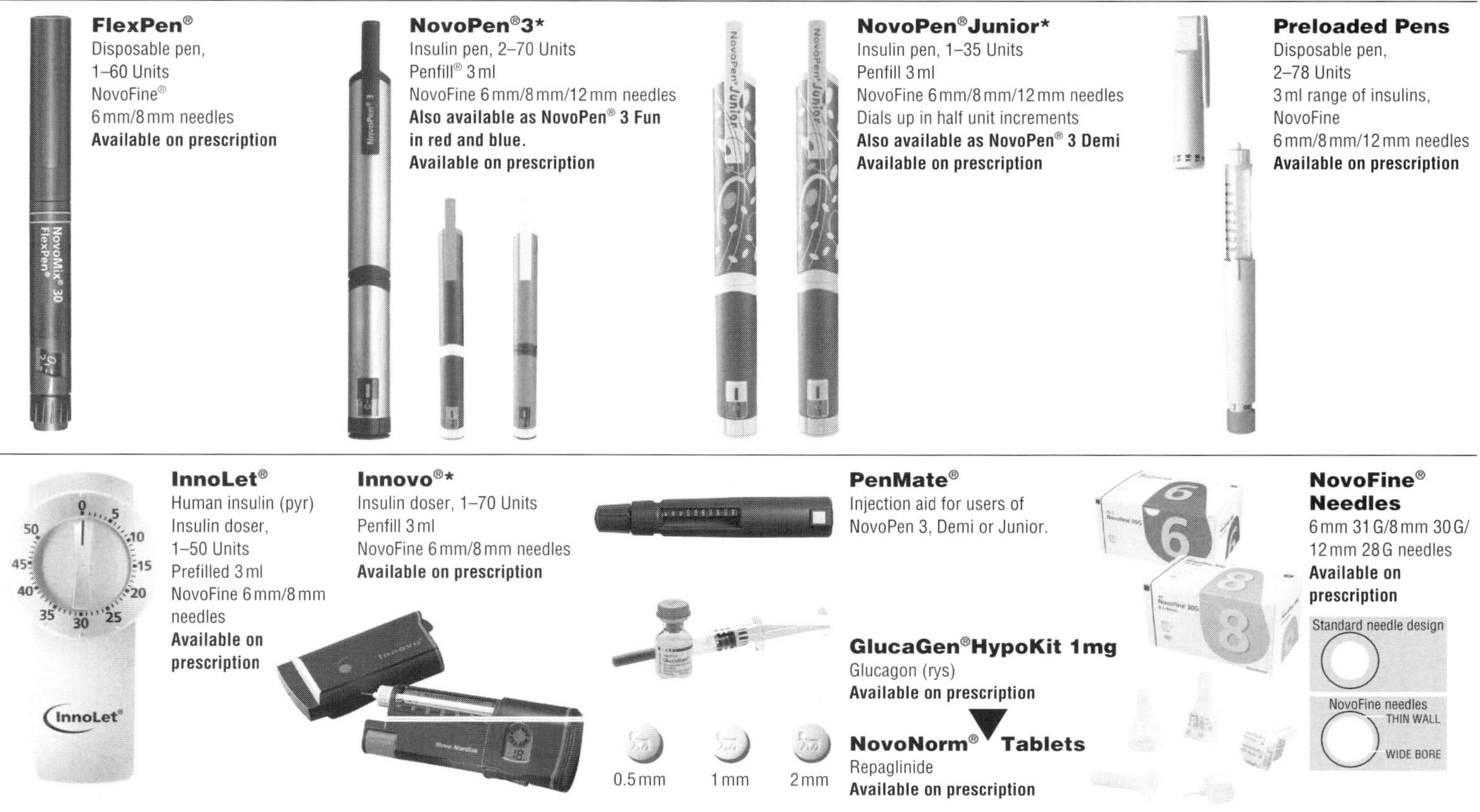

Figure 7.2 (b) *cont'd* (UK)

They are *not* recommended for young people with Type 1 diabetes. It can be difficult to attain good control using biphasic insulin because the amount of individual insulin in the mix cannot be altered. They can increase the risk of hypoglycaemia if eating is erratic, the carbohydrate intake is low or after vigorous exercise.

7.8.2 Twice daily regime

A combination of short- and longer-acting insulin is usually given before breakfast and before the evening meal. Biphasic insulins are commonly used. This does not allow a great deal of flexibility in adjusting doses but is more likely to control overnight hyperglycaemia. There is a risk of nocturnal hypoglycaemia, see Chapter 8. Usually two-thirds of the total dose is given in the morning and one-third in the evening.

Figure 7.3 depicts the insulin profiles of the various insulins and allows hypoglycaemia risk times to be identified. It gives an indication of which insulin to adjust when considered in conjunction with the blood glucose profile. Consideration should always be given to other factors that affect blood glucose levels, see Chapter 4.

Practice point

Rapid-acting insulins act very quickly. They should be given immediately before a meal, or within 15 minutes after the meal, to avoid hypoglycaemia.

7.8.3 Basal bolus regime

Basal bolus regimes simulate the normal pattern of insulin secretion, i.e. a small amount of circulating insulin is present in the blood and restrains gluconeogenesis and glycogenolysis, this is the basal insulin. A bolus amount of insulin is stimulated by the blood glucose rise after a glucose load. Bolus injections of short-acting insulin are given before each meal. The longer-acting insulin is given before bed to supply the basal insulin requirement. This regime offers more flexibility in insulin dose adjustment and meal times, and therefore lifestyle is less restricted. The amount of insulin given at each dose is usually small, therefore the likelihood of hypoglycaemia is reduced. It is commonly used for young people with Type 1 diabetes.

Insulin devices which are discreet and portable are often used for basal bolus regimes. Patients should continue to use their devices in hospital.

7.9 Continuous subcutaneous insulin infusion (CSII)

Insulin pumps continuously deliver subcutaneous insulin at a basal rate and can be programmed to give set bolus doses before meals. They allow a more physiological insulin profile to be attained and greater flexibility in meeting individual insulin requirements. They use short-acting insulin only, and therefore if they malfunction or are removed, e.g. for surgery, the patient must be given insulin via another method to avoid hyperglycaemia. This can be subcutaneously or via an IV depending on the circumstances.

Modern insulin pumps are generally reliable and have an inbuilt alarm system that identifies a number of faults such as kinks/blockages in the tubing, tubing disconnections from the pump and low batteries, so that malfunctions can be identified early and appropriate steps taken to avoid hyperglycaemia. Some do not alarm if the tubing

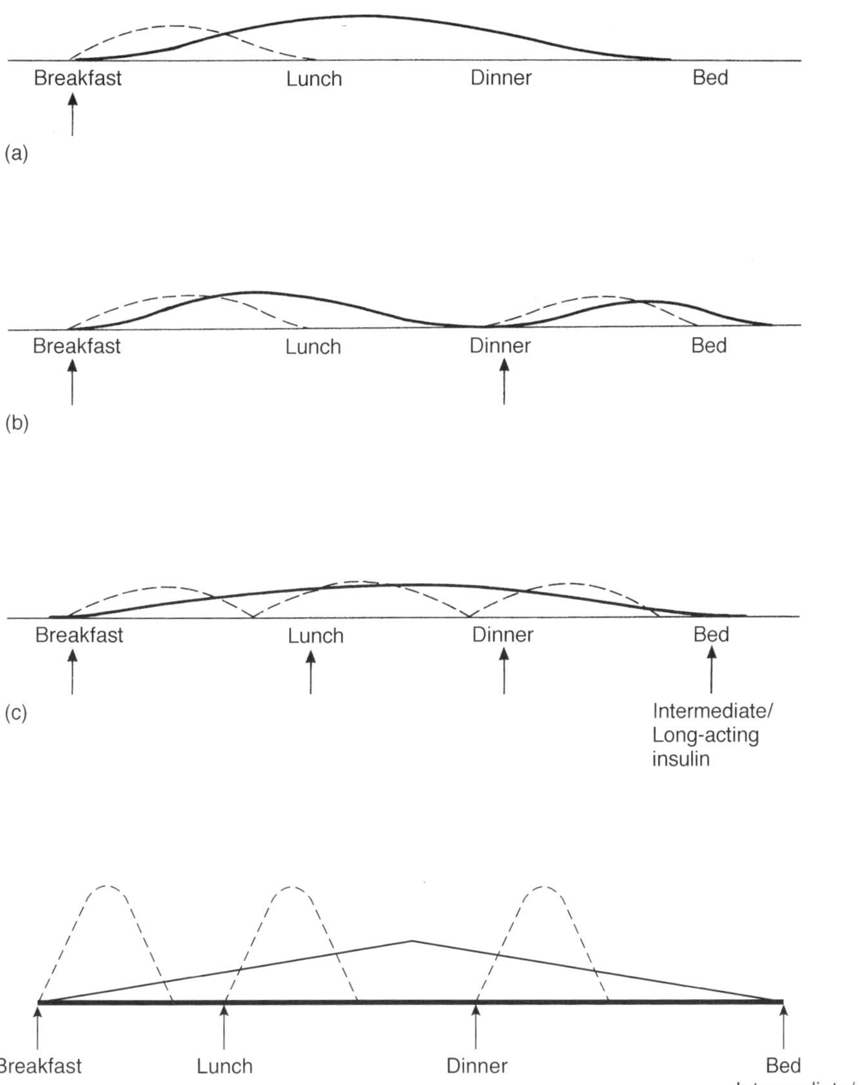

Figure 7.3 Diagrammatic representation of insulin action showing different regimes: (a) daily, (b) twice daily, (c) basal bolus using short-acting insulins and (d) basal bolus using rapid-acting insulins.

Note: The broken line depicts short-acting insulin, the unbroken line intermediate/long-acting insulin. The arrows indicate the time of injection.

disconnects from the insertion site. If this occurs insulin is not delivered and can go unnoticed until the blood glucose is tested. In people with Type 1 diabetes hyperglycaemia can occur quickly.

Pumps are expensive and require a great deal of commitment on the part of the person with diabetes to use them safely and effectively. Health professional support and the ready availability of advice are vital. People need time to adjust to the pump regime and become accustomed to not having intermediate-acting insulin. Pumps offer a great deal of flexibility and can have significant psychological benefits.

Practice points

(1) Insulin pumps are not a cure for poor metabolic control but they can help some people achieve better control.
(2) They allow the insulin regime to be matched to individual requirements.
(3) Blood glucose monitoring at least 4-hourly is necessary.
(4) Training and readily available support and advice from skilled pump experts are essential.
(5) People with existing psychological problems do worse on pumps than on other insulin regimes (DCCT 1993).
(6) Pumps are expensive to purchase and the ongoing cost of consumables is high. The cost is under review in both Australia and the UK with the hope that consumables will be subsidised by pharmaceutical benefits or similar schemes.

The choice of regime and insulin delivery system depends on personal preference, the degree of blood glucose control aimed for and the willingness and ability of the patient to monitor their blood glucose. Many factors can influence insulin absorption and consequently blood glucose; some of these factors are shown in Table 7.2.

Table 7.2 Some commonly encountered factors that affect insulin aborption.

Accelerated	*Delayed*
Exercise	Low body temperature
High body temperature	Poor circulation
Massage round injection site	Smoking
Depth of injection	Long-acting insulins

7.10 Sliding scale and top-up regimes

A sliding scale refers to insulin doses administered based on retrospective hyperglycaemia as opposed to anticipated insulin requirements (Hirsch *et al.* 1995). Insulin infusions do require a sliding scale, to be used effectively, and are considered separately, see 7.12.

Using subcutaneous sliding scales in day-to-day management can lead to disassociation between the insulin scale and other parameters that affect blood glucose such as the timing of meals, calorie-based activity, effects of illness, medications, e.g. steroids, and the onset of insulin action and is not generally recommended. Sliding scales can help maintain acceptable blood glucose levels if used appropriately in acute situations.

Using sliding scales to stabilise blood glucose for newly diagnosed, unstable or brittle diabetes is *not* generally recommended (Katz 1991).

An example of a sliding scale is given in section 7.12. Sliding scales are appropriately used in conjunction with intravenous insulin infusions, or when managing patients pre- and postoperatively.

It is preferable to monitor the blood glucose over 24–48 hours and adjust the insulin according to the emerging pattern and the daily, b.d. or basal bolus insulin regime chosen.

7.10.1 Top-up or stat doses

Top-up/stat doses of insulin refer to temporary supplementary doses of insulin, usually short-acting, to correct existing hyperglycaemia found on routine blood glucose monitoring. When needed, the extra insulin is best added to the next due dose of insulin rather than being given in isolation. The management regime and nursing/medical actions occurring at the time should be reviewed and may need adjusting if the situation occurs over several days.

One of the problems encountered in practice is that top-up doses often continue for days before the blood glucose profile is considered and insulin doses adjusted proactively rather than reacting to an abnormal reading.

Sliding and top-up scales are generally only used in hospital or managing unwell patients at home in special circumstances.

Practice point

The vision can deteriorate when insulin is commenced. Sight is not usually threatened but it is very distressing for the person with diabetes and they need a careful explanation and reassurance to help them understand. Activities of daily living such as reading and driving can be affected.

It occurs because the lens absorbs excess glucose in much the same way as sponge soaks up water. Changes in the amount of glucose in the lens can lead to blurred vision and can occur with high and low blood glucose levels.

This phenomenon is quite different from diabetic retinopathy, which can threaten the sight.

7.11 Intravenous insulin infusions

The IV route is preferred for very ill patients because the absorption of insulin is rapid and more reliable than from poorly perfused muscle and fat tissue. Absorption may be erratic in these patients, especially if they are hypotensive. The aims of the insulin infusion are to:

- Prevent the liver convering glycogen and fatty acids to glucose and therefore avoid hyperglycaemia.
- Prevent utilisation of fatty acids and therefore limit ketone formation.
- Decrease protein catabolism and therefore limit production of glucose substrate.
- Decrease peripheral resistance to insulin.

- Gradually decrease the blood glucose concentration to 10–12 mmol/L without subjecting the patient to hypoglycaemia.

The medication order for the infusion must be clearly and legibly written on the treatment sheet. Insulin doses for IV insulin infusions are usually 0.1 unit/kg/h. Sometimes an initial bolus of 5–10 units is given. In general, a low dose infusion such as this has been shown to reduce the blood glucose, ketosis and acidosis as effectively as high dose regimes, without the added risk of hypoglycaemia. The rate at which the insulin is to be administered should be written in ml/h and units to be delivered. Several protocols exist; the following is one example.

The infusion rate is adjusted according to the patient's blood glucose results (tested 2-hourly). This is a sliding scale of insulin. For example:

Blood glucose (mmol/L)	Insulin (units/h)
0–5.9	0
6–11.1	1
12–15.1	2
16–19	3
>19.1	4
>24	Notify doctor

The insulin order and blood glucose results should be reviewed regularly.

7.11.1 Preparing the insulin solution to be infused

Two people should check and make up the solution according to the medication order and hospital protocols.

Practice points

(1) Only clear short-acting insulin is used for insulin infusions. Solutions must be gently mixed and if not in haemaccel discard the first 50 ml through the giving set to allow insulin to bind to the plastic.
(2) All solutions must be discarded after 24 hours.

It has been well documented that insulin binds to plastic IV containers and tubing. Several methods have been used to minimise the binding. They include:

- Mixing insulin in haemaccel is expensive and the practice has been discontinued in many places.
- Flushing the infusion set with the insulin solution to saturate the binding sites before connecting it to the patient.

7.12 Uses of insulin infusions

7.12.1 General use (during surgical procedures)

Insulin is added to 4% dextrose in $\frac{1}{5}$ normal saline or 5% dextrose. The infusion is often given via *burette* or more commonly an IMED pump at 120 ml/h (i.e. 8-hourly rate; see previous example scale). Monitor blood glucose 2- to 3-hourly and review with medical staff *regularly*.

7.12.2 Special needs

- Myocardial infarction. In many areas an IV insulin infusion is commenced when the patient presents to the emergency department and continues for 24 hours, after which time subcutaneous insulin is commenced (Malmberg 1997), see Chapter 11.
- Open heart surgery.
- Ketoacidosis.
- Hyperosmolar coma.
- Intensive care unit (ICU) situations.

These situations always require the use of a controlled-rate infusion pump (IMED pump or syringe pump) to ensure accurate administration of the insulin. It is often necessary to limit the amount of fluid administered to avoid cerebral oedema in these situations especially in young children and the elderly. Standard regimes include:

(1) Haemaccel 100 ml + 100 Units Actrapid = 1 Units/1 ml, used in ICU and administered via IMED.
(2) Haemaccel 500 ml + 100 Units Actrapid = 1 Units/5 ml via IMED.

People who are insulin-resistant, such as those who:

- have liver disease
- are on steroid therapy
- are obese
- have a serious infection.

may require more insulin, i.e. a high-dose infusion (more units per hour).

Practice points

(1) Subcutaneous insulin must be given before removing the infusion and the patient must be eating and drinking normally to avoid hyperglycaemia because of the short half-life of insulin given IV.
(2) Ceasing the infusion before a meal allows a smooth transition to subcutaneous insulin.

7.13 Risks associated with insulin infusions

- Hypoglycaemia
- Cardiac arrhythmias
- Sepsis at IV site
- Fluid overload.

7.14 Factors affecting insulin delivery via infusion

- Accuracy of system, including blood glucose testing.
- Stability of solution.
- Circulatory insufficiency.

7.15 Mistakes associated with insulin infusions

(1) Where a burette is used and if insulin is added to the burette rather than the bag of IV fluid, refilling the burette from the bag results in no insulin being administered and hyperglycaemia results.
(2) An incorrect amount of insulin added to the bag/burette can be a result of inadequate checking, not using an insulin syringe to draw up the insulin or failing to check illegible medical orders, especially where insulin doses are written as U/s instead of 'units' and the dose is misinterpreted.
(3) Problems can arise if the insulin infusion is run at the same time as other intravenous fluids, e.g. 4% dextrose in $\frac{1}{5}$ normal saline. The most common method is to infuse the different fluids through the one IV cannula using a three-way adaptor (octopus), see Figure 7.4.

Clinical observation

Indicating insulin doses by writing U/s is common practice and can be very unclear when written by hand. Incorrect, usually excess, insulin has been administered where this is common practice and serious hypoglycaemia resulted. In one case, in Australia, in a care home for the elderly, a patient died and a court case ensued. Both the nurse who administered the insulin and the doctor who wrote the prescription were found to have contributed to the death. There were other issues involved with the particular patient but the case highlights the importance of accurate documentation and the nurse's responsibility to check.

Insulin doses should always be indicated by writing 'units' after the amount to be given.

Usually the dextrose or saline is running at a faster rate than the insulin infusion. Problems can arise if there is a complete or partial blockage of the cannula. The force of gravity pushing the fluid towards the vein can actually cause the dextrose/saline to flow back up the slower-flowing insulin line resulting in high blood glucose levels. Figure 7.4 depicts the result of a blockage in the IV cannula and three-way adaptor during the concurrent administration of insulin and dextrose/saline.

If hyperglycaemia occurs during an insulin infusion check:

- That the tubing and adaptors are patent;
- That insulin has been added to the burette/bag;
- That the amount of insulin added is correct;
- Possible sources of infection, e.g. UTI, the feet.

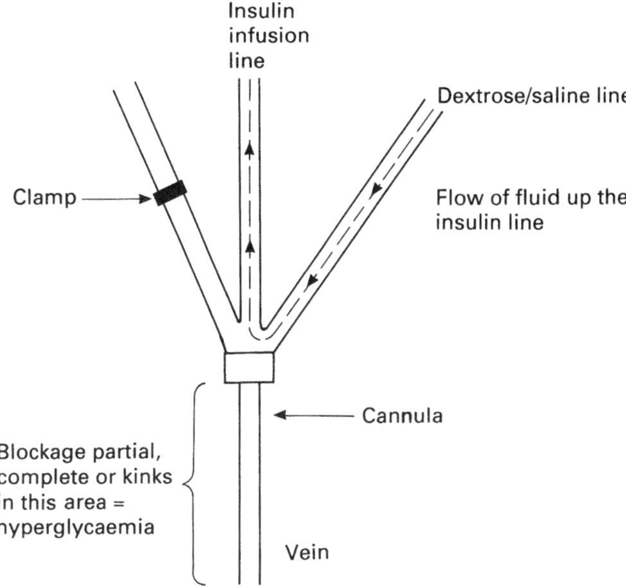

Figure 7.4 Possible results of a blockage in the IV cannula and three-way adaptor during the concurrent administration of insulin and dextrose/saline.

7.16 Inhaled insulin

Significant amounts of insulin can be absorbed through the skin and nose if enhancers are used. The alveoli are permeable to large polypeptides such as insulin. Clinical research involving inhaled insulin has been under way for a number of years but it is not yet widely available. The technology is now available to create a dry powder insulin aerosol that can deliver insulin directly into the lungs.

Inhaled insulin appears to be well tolerated without causing short-term lung problems. Long-term effects are not known at this stage. Reasonable glycaemic control has been achieved in Type 1 and Type 2 diabetes.

The insulin is administered using a spacer device and approximately 10% of the dose is absorbed systemically. The peak action and duration of effect are closer to the rapid-acting analogues, being shorter than subcutaneous insulin administration.

At present, inhaled insulin can only partially replace subcutaneous insulin and long-acting insulin is still required because long-acting nasal insulin preparations are not available. Inhaled insulin could be of most benefit to people with needle phobias, although usually subcutaneous long-acting insulin is still required (Cefalu *et al.* 2001; Skyler *et al.* 2001).

The inhaler device is very large and may be unattractive to some people accustomed to small devices. However, the benefits of fewer injections might balance this concern and devices are likely to become smaller with time.

7.17 Insulin allergy

Insulin allergies are rare with modern, highly purified insulins but they do sometimes occur.

Two types of reaction have been reported:

(1) Localised weal and flare with itching due to antihistamine reactions;
(2) Generalised anaphylaxis, which is rare.

Allergic reactions are most likely to occur where people have been on insulin previously, e.g. during GDM, surgery or acute illness in people with Type 2 diabetes where insulin is used intermittently, e.g. during surgery and with steroid medications, and when injection sites are not rotated.

To diagnose insulin allergy a careful case history is required. The person should be given insulin and observed where resuscitation equipment is available. Any reaction should be carefully documented. Blood test for IgG and other immune response factors can be helpful.

If insulin allergy is present a desensitisation programme may be required. Local reactions can be managed by using a different insulin and antihistamine creams (Williams 1993; Dunning *et al.* 1998).

7.18 Pancreas transplants

Pancreas transplants of either the whole pancreas or islet cells or the pancreas and kidneys is available to some people with diabetes and end stage renal failure. It requires major surgery and is usually reserved for Type 1 people. Immunosuppresive therapy is required and if rejection does not occur the response is good. The transplanted pancreas secretes insulin and HBA1c normalises in three months.

Obtaining pancreases for transplantation is difficult and other options are under study. For example, islet cells are injected into the portal vein but the success rate is low. Beta cell engineering and stem cell cloning are other areas of study. Islet cell transplants have been undertaken successfully in Canada, and in the UK an islet cell consortium has been established to try to reproduce positive results.

References

Buse, J. (2001) Insulin analogues. *Current Opinion in Endocrinology*, **8** (2), 95–100.

Campbell, M., Anderson, D., Holcombe, J. & Massey, E. (1993) Storage of insulin: a manufacturer's view. *Practical Diabetes*, **10** (6), 218–220.

Cefalu, W., Skyler, J., Kourides, I., Landschulz, W., Balagatas, C. & Cheng, S. (2001) Inhaled insulin treatment in patients with Type 2 diabetes. *Annals of Internal Medicine*, **134**, 242–244.

DCCT (Diabetes Control and Complications Trial Research Group) (1993) Effects of intensive insulin therapy on the development and progression of long-term complications in IDDM. *New England Journal of Medicine*, **329**, 977–986.

Dunning, T. & Martin, M. (1997) Using a focus group to explore perceptions of diabetes severity. *Practical Diabetes International*, **14** (7), 185–188.

Dunning, T. & Martin, M. (1999) Health professional's perceptions of the seriousness of diabetes. *Practical Diabetes International*, **16** (3), 73–77.

Dunning, T., Rosen, S. Alford, F. (1998) Insulin allergy: a diagnostic dilemma. *Journal of Diabetes Nursing*, **26**.

Hirsch, I., Paaun, D. & Brunzell, J. (1995) Inpatient management of adults with diabetes. *Diabetes Care*, **18** (6), 870–877.

Katz, C. (1991) How efficient is sliding scale insulin therapy? Problem with a 'cookbook' approach in hospital patients. *Postgraduate Medicine*, **5** (5), 46–48.

Malmberg, K. (1997) Prospective randomised study of intensive insulin treatment on long-term survival after acute myocardial infarction. *British Medical Journal*, **314**, 1512–1515.

Skyler, J., Cefalu, W., Kourides, I., Landschulz, W., Balagatas, C. & Cheng, S. (2001) Efficacy of inhaled human insulin in Type 1 diabetes mellitus. *Lancet*, **357**, 331–335.

Vaag, A., Handberg, A., Lauritzen, M., Henriksen, J., Pedersen, K. & Beck-Neilsen, H. (1990) Variation in insulin absorption of NPH insulin due to intramuscular injection. *Diabetes Care*, **13** (1), 74–76.

Williams, P. (1993) Adverse effects of exogenous insulin: clinical features, management and prevention. *Drug Safety*, **8**, 427–444.

Chapter 8
Hypoglycaemia

8.1 Key points

- Recognise early.
- Treat promptly.
- Treat adequately.
- Monitor recovery.
- Seek cause.
- Document episode.
- Educate patient.
- Recognise the psychological impact on the person's quality of life.

Rationale

Hypoglycaemia can be prevented by an appropriate nursing care plan, early recognition of impending hypoglycaemia and appropriate management.

8.2 Introduction

Some nursing staff find it difficult to distinguish between hypoglycaemia and hyperglycaemia. Many journal articles and reference texts discuss these topics together under headings such as 'The diabetic comas', which often adds to the confusion. A state of hypoglycaemia or hyperglycaemia (including ketosis) can occur without the patient being comatose or unconscious. The only conclusive method of distinguishing between the two is to perform a blood glucose test. Results of <3 mmol/L in people taking insulin or oral hypoglycaemic agents indicate hypoglycaemia.

My preference has been to consider these two very different entities requiring different management in separate chapters.

8.3 Definition of hypoglycaemia

Hypoglycaemia occurs when the blood glucose falls low enough to cause signs and symptoms. It is usually defined as a blood glucose level of <3.0 mmol/L in people with diabetes treated with insulin or oral hypoglycaemic agents.

Practice point

Diabetic patients who are managed by diet alone do not usually require treatment of low blood glucose levels.

Age, sex and associated medical conditions such as liver disease, cerebrovascular disease and autonomic neuropathy and the rate at which the glucose falls may influence the development and recognition of symptoms. In general, a rapid decrease in blood glucose results in the development of the classic symptoms of hypoglycaemia described in Table 8.1. The classic presentation is more likely to occur in insulin-treated patients.

The focus on achieving tight blood glucose control or normoglycaemia since the DCCT by intensifying management and transferring people with Type 2 diabetes onto insulin sooner has increased the possibility of hypoglycaemia. Education and strategies to prevent/manage hypoglycaemia should accompany medication management changes and include family and significant others.

8.4 Recognising hypoglycaemia

Some, or all, of the signs and symptoms listed in Table 8.1 can be present. Symptoms may be less obvious in people treated with OHAs, where hypoglycaemia tends to develop much more slowly and the classic oral hypoglycaemic associated signs may not be present or not recognised. The patient may complain of lethargy, tiredness or dizziness. Severe cases may present as a cerebrovascular accident resulting in misdiagnosis and delayed treatment. This happens less frequently now because all unconscious patients presenting to the emergency department have a capillary blood glucose test performed. Hypoglycaemia may be prolonged and can recur or become chronic.

Table 8.1 Signs and symptoms of hypoglycaemia.

*Sympathetic adrenergic**	*Neuroglycopaenic†*
Weakness	Headache
Sweating	Hypothermia
Tachycardia	Visual disturbances
Palpitations	Mental dullness
Tremor	Confusion
Nervousness	Amnesia
Irritability	Seizures
Tingling of mouth and fingers	Coma
Hunger	

*Caused by increased activity of the autonomic nervous system triggered by a rapid fall in blood glucose.
†Caused by decreased activity of the central nervous system because of very low blood glucose.

Nausea and vomiting may occur but are unusual.

Table 8.2 The counter-regulatory hormonal response to hypoglycaemia.

Hormone	*Action*
Glucagon	Increased glucose output from liver and muscle (glycogenolysis)
Adrenaline and noradrenaline	Enhanced glycogenolysis in liver and muscle Enhanced gluconeogenesis Decreased insulin secretion Causes many of the signs and symptoms of hypoglycaemia (sympathetic response; see Table 8.1)
Cortisol	Mobilises the substrates for gluconeogenesis
Growth hormone	Acts with cortisol and adrenaline to inhibit peripheral glucose utilisation

8.5 Counter-regulatory hormonal response to hypoglycaemia

The brain requires 120–140 g glucose per day to function normally and has a very limited capacity to manufacture its own glucose. Therefore it is dependent on adequate levels of circulating blood glucose. When the blood glucose falls below normal the body releases hormones to counteract the effects of hypoglycaemia. This is known as the counter-regulatory response. Glycogen stores are liberated and new glucose is formed in the liver from precursors e.g. fatty acids and protein. The hormones released are shown in Table 8.2, along with their resultant action, the nett result being an increase in blood glucose.

8.6 Objectives of care

To be alert to the possibility of hypoglycaemia in all patients on insulin or OHAs, and should it occur to:

(1) Supply quick-acting carbohydrate to immediately raise blood glucose levels.
(2) Maintain blood glucose levels within the acceptable range of 4–10 mmol/L.
(3) Ascertain the cause of the hypoglycaemic episode.
(4) Limit further episodes of hypoglycaemia.
(5) Allay fear and anxiety including that of relatives.
(6) Prevent trauma occurring as a result of hypoglycaemia.
(7) Assess knowledge and educate if necessary.

8.7 Treatment

Rapid treatment is important.

8.7.1 Conscious patient

Test and record the blood glucose level.

First: give quick-acting sugar or other high glycaemic index food to raise the blood glucose immediately, e.g.:

3 level teaspoons sugar in $\frac{1}{2}$ cup water, tea or coffee
or 1 cup orange juice
or $\frac{1}{2}$ regular sugary/soft drink (*not low calorie* (joule))
or proprietary glucose preparation such as glucose gels/tablets or person's usual remedy.

Second: follow with long-acting carbohydrate to maintain blood glucose until the next meal time, e.g.:

$\frac{1}{2}$ sandwich
or 2 to 4 dry biscuits (unsweetened)
or 1 piece of fruit
or 2 plain sweet biscuits.

Check blood glucose in one hour then as necessary. The next dose of insulin or OHA is not usually withheld following a mild hypoglycaemic episode. However, if hypoglycaemia occurs frequently, the diabetic regime might need to be adjusted, e.g. extra carbohydrate in the diet, reduction in medication dose.

8.7.2 Impaired conscious state

Note: Do not give anything by mouth.

(1) Place patient on side.
(2) Clear airway.
(3) One nurse notify doctor.
(4) Second nurse test blood glucose level and confirm with chemical pathology (i.e. urgent glucose).
(5) Assemble glucagon and IV tray containing 50% dextrose. Instructions for glucagon administration appear in section 8.14.
(6) Give complex carbohydrate low glycaemic index food to maintain the blood glucose level when consciousness returns. The patient may still be confused and may need to be reminded to chew and swallow.
(7) Repeat fingerprick in one hour then as necessary, but not less than 4-hourly.

Patient should be monitored for at least 36 hours. Ascertain the time and dose for the next insulin injection/OHA dose.

8.7.3 In both cases

Recovery should be rapid. If recovery does not occur in 10–15 minutes, exclude other causes of unconsciousness.

(1) Record episode and blood glucose level on diabetic chart and in patient unit record.
(2) Monitor progress/recovery from episode.
(3) Look for cause of hypoglycaemia, e.g. meal delayed or missed, inadequate intake of carbohydrate, unaccustomed activity, excessive medication, drug/drug, drug/herb or herb/herb interactions.
(4) Reassure the patient and relatives.

(5) Ensure patient has an understanding of causes and management of hypoglycaemia (refer to diabetes nurse specialist/diabetes educator).
(6) See Chapter 18 for information about managing hypoglycaemia in the elderly.

8.8 Nocturnal hypoglycaemia

The blood glucose may drop during the night, often around 2 to 3 AM and hypoglycaemia can go unnoticed by the patient.

People with diabetes and their relatives are very fearful of hypoglycaemia at any time, but particularly at night, and careful explanations about the possible causes and suggestions to prevent nocturnal hypoglycaemia are essential. Families/significant others need to know how to manage the hypoglycaemia by maintaining the person's airway and calling an ambulance. If they have Glucagon at home they should give it.

8.8.1 Indicators of nocturnal hypoglycaemia

- Night sweats.
- Nightmares.
- Unaccustomed snoring.
- Morning lethargy.
- Headaches.
- Depression.
- High blood glucose before breakfast (Somogyi effect).
- Morning ketonuria.

The Somogyi effect refers to prebreakfast hyperglycaemia following an overnight hypoglycaemic episode.

If any of the above symptoms occur, the blood glucose should be measured at 2 to 3 AM over several nights to establish if nocturnal hypoglycaemia is occurring. The insulin is then adjusted accordingly by decreasing the morning long-acting dose for those on a daily insulin, the afternoon long-acting dose for those on b.d. insulin or the pre evening meal or bedtime dose for basal bolus regimes.

Clinical observation

(1) Sometimes the evening short-acting insulin, rather than the intermediate-acting insulin, causes the hypoglycaemia episode.
(2) Stress is usually associated with hyperglycaemia; however, stress can induce hypoglycaemia in Type 1 diabetes. The mechanism is not known.

Practice point

The Somogyi effect should be distinguished from another condition that results in morning hyperglycaemia, the 'dawn phenomenon'. The dawn phenomenon refers to a situation where insulin requirements and blood glucose concentration increase between 5 AM and 8 AM. It occurs in up to 75% of diabetic patients. Treatment consists of *increasing* the insulin dose.

Many other hormones have a normal physiological rise in the early morning, e.g. testosterone, which causes early morning erections.

8.9 Chronic hypoglycaemia

In elderly people, especially those on OHAs, hypoglycaemia can become chronic and present as failing mental function, personality changes or disordered behaviour. Accurate monitoring of the blood glucose levels is important to detect chronic hypoglycaemia. Management consists of revising the care plan and checking:

- That carbohydrate intake is adequate and evenly distributed;
- The ability of the individual to accurately prepare and administer their insulin;
- Commencement of any new medications or complementary therapies;
- Teeth/dentures to ensure there is no infection or mouth ulcers and that false teeth fit and are worn;
- Presence of diabetic complications or comorbidities that can affect self-care ability.

8.10 Relative hypoglycaemia

People who are accustomed to high blood glucose levels for long periods of time may experience the symptoms of hypoglycaemia when blood glucose control improves and blood glucose levels normalise. In general it is not necessary to treat the symptoms once the blood glucose is recorded, but reassurance, support and education are necessary until the patient adapts to the new blood glucose range.

8.11 Drug interactions

Some commonly prescribed drugs can interact with the sulphonylurea prescribed to control the blood glucose and increase the possibility of hypoglycaemia (see Table 8.3).

Table 8.3 **Commonly prescribed drugs which can increase the hypoglycaemic effect of sulphonylurea agents.**

Drugs	*Means of potentiation*
Sulphonamides Salicylates Warfarin Clofibrate Phenylbutazone	Displaces sulphonylureas from protein binding sites
Coumarin derivatives Chloramphenicol Phenylbutazone	Inhibits/decreases hepatic metabolism of the sulphonylurea
Probenecid Salicylates Tuberculostatics Tetracyclines	Delays urinary excretion of the sulphonylurea
MAO inhibitors	Increases action by an unknown mechanism

Practice point

Consider complementary therapy use, e.g. herbs, supplements, relaxation therapies. These therapies can exert hypoglycaemic effects themselves, interact with conventional treatments or cause liver or renal damage that alters drug metabolism and predisposes the person to hypoglycaemia (see Chapter 26).

8.12 Patients most at risk of hypoglycaemia

(1) Those taking insulin or OHAs.
(2) Those with renal or hepatic disease.
(3) Those with long-standing diabetes who no longer recognise sympathetic warning signs usually as a result of existing autonomic neuropathy or changed symptomatology.
(4) People fasting for a procedure/surgery or religious reasons, e.g. Ramadan.
(5) People with diarrhoea and vomiting.
(6) Those with an impaired conscious state.
(7) Those sedated or on narcotic infusions.
(8) Those on long-acting diabetic medications (e.g. chlorpropamide, Ultratard).
(9) The elderly.
(10) Those beginning an exercise/diet regime or excessive exercise.
(11) Alcohol may also cause hypoglycaemia, particularly if food is not eaten at the same time. The hypoglycaemia can occur hours after consuming alcohol.
(12) People taking a lot of medications and complementary therapies.

Practice points

(1) The signs of alcohol intoxication can make hypoglycaemia difficult to recognise. Alcohol impairs cognitive function and reduces the ability to recognise hypoglycaemia. Self-care and diet are often inadequate. In addition, chronic alcohol abuse leads to malnutrition and limited glucose stores to mount an effective counter-regulatory response.
(2) People with chronic alcohol addiction are very difficult to manage because OHAs are often contraindicated and insulin puts them at high risk of hypoglycaemia.

8.13 Psychological effects of hypoglycaemia

Hypoglycaemia is feared and hated by many people with diabetes and the effects are often underrated by health professionals. The importance of recognising and accepting these concerns cannot be overemphasised. Hypoglycaemia has profound effects on people's quality of life, social activities, e.g. driving and work, and they fear brain damage and death from hypoglycaemia. It is not unusual for people to deliberately run their blood glucose levels high to avoid hypoglycaemia (Dunning 1994) (see Chapter 22). They can then be termed 'non-compliant' and placed in a conflict situation. Commonly expressed concerns are:

- Loss of control of the situation;
- Reminder that they have diabetes;

- Losing face and making a fool of themselves;
- Swinging too high after treatment;
- Sustaining brain damage;
- Recovery can take days following serious hypoglycaemia;
- Dying.

Hypoglycaemia can lead to decreased confidence in the ability to cope. Support and understanding, and exploring all of the issues, physical, mental and social that are an important part of management, are vital.

Clinical observation

There have been several media reports in the last few months about pet dogs recognising their owner's hypoglycaemia and alerting them in time to be able to treat it early or rouse another family member.

8.14 Guidelines for the administration of glucagon

Glucagon is a hormone produced by the alpha cells of the pancreas. It acts on the liver to release glucose stores. Glucagon is available in a single dose pack containing one vial of glucagon hydrochloride powder (1 mg) and a glass syringe prefilled with sterile water (water for injection).

8.14.1 Indication

Glucagon is used to treat severe hypoglycaemia in people with diabetes treated with insulin or OHAs, primarily those unable to take glucose orally who are unconscious or uncooperative.

8.14.2 Instructions for use

(1) Individual patients must be assessed to determine the appropriate dose and route of administration. Glucagon is given according to body weight and muscle bulk (intramuscular or subcutaneously). The buttock is the ideal injection site.
(2) The intravenous route may be the preferred route in profound hypoglycaemia to ensure rapid absorption but is usually only administered by doctors.
(3) Check the expiry date. Glucagon should be used soon after reconstitution. Do not use if reconstituted solution is not clear and colourless.
(4) Follow the instructions in the package to prepare the injection and the medical order for the dose.
(5) Record the time and route of administration, the dose, and the patient's response.

8.14.3 Dosage

- Adults and children of weight >25 kg full dose (1/1).
- Children of weight <25 kg half dose (1/2).

Practice points

(1) Glucagon can be repeated; however, repeated injections can cause nausea, making subsequent food intake difficult.
(2) If recovery does not occur within 10–15 minutes IV glucose might be required. It could indicate limited glucose stores but other causes of unconsciousness should be considered. A second dose is not usually recommended because it can cause nausea making oral intake difficult on recovery.
(3) Glucagon may be contraindicated where glycogen stores are low, e.g. in fasting states, chronic hypoglycaemia, chronic adrenal insufficiency and malnutrition where the individual is unable to mount an effective counter-regulatory response.

8.15 Adverse reactions

These are rare. Occasionally transient nausea occurs that can make it difficult to take in sufficient oral carbohydrate, which is necessary to avoid the blood glucose dropping again. Vomiting occurs occasionally, usually only after a second dose.

Glucagon is a peptide so theoretically hypersensitivity is possible and is more likely in atopic patients.

Clinical observation

Hypothermia can prolong recovery from hypoglycaemia especially in the elderly in winter. Management of the hypothermia as well as the hypoglycaemia is usually required.

References

Dunning, P. (1994) Having diabetes: young adult perspectives. *The Diabetes Educator*, **21** (1), 58–65.

National Health and Medical Research Council (1991) *Hypoglycaemia and Diabetes*. Australian Government Printers, Canberra.

Chapter 9
Stabilisation of Diabetes

9.1 Key points

- Outpatient stabilisation is preferred.
- Encourage independence.
- Allow patient to perform own self-care tasks.
- Provide support and encouragement.
- Explore psychological and quality of life issues.

Rationale

Optimal blood glucose control can prevent or delay the onset of long-term complications. Insulin is frequently required by people with Type 2 diabetes to achieve optimal control.

Stabilisation of diabetes refers to the process of achieving an optimal blood glucose range, appropriate diabetes knowledge and managing diabetic complications, either acute or chronic, and usually specifically refers to commencing insulin (NHMRC 1991a). Stabilisation may occur at initial diagnosis of diabetes, when a change of treatment is indicated, e.g. transfer from oral agents to insulin therapy, and for antenatal care.

In most cases, stabilisation of diabetes can be achieved without admitting the person to hospital. Managing diabetes in primary care settings as far as possible is a core component of both the Australian and UK diabetes management strategies (MacKinnon 1998; NDS 1998). This process is known as outpatient stabilisation. Outpatient stabilisation requires specialised staff, specific protocols and ample time if it is to be successful. It can result in considerable cost benefits, and reduces the stress and costs associated with a hospital admission.

There are considerable psychological and quality of life benefits for the person with diabetes. Home/outpatient stabilisation allows insulin to be adjusted according to the individual's usual lifestyle and reduces the risk of the person having to assume 'sick role' behaviours.

However, some patients will continue to be admitted to hospital for stabilisation of their diabetes, for example, complex issues that cannot be identified in outpatient settings, where clinical observation is necessary, for patient convenience or where the person is admitted with a concurrent illness or is diagnosed during an admission and commences insulin while in hospital.

9.2 Stabilisation of diabetes in hospital

People admitted to improve their metabolic control (stabilisation) are not generally ill and should be encouraged to:

- Keep active;
- Wear clothes instead of pyjamas;
- Perform diabetes self-care tasks such as blood glucose monitoring and insulin administration.

They will require support, encouragement and consistent advice. The time spent in hospital should be kept to a minimum.

9.2.1 Nursing responsibilities

(1) Inform the appropriate staff about the person's admission especially the diabetes nurse specialist/diabetes educator, specialist team, and dietitian soon after they are admitted.
(2) Assess the patient carefully (refer to Chapter 2).
(3) Monitor blood and urine glucose according to usual protocols; for example, 7 AM, 11 AM, 4 PM and 9 PM. In some cases postprandial levels are also performed (see Chapter 4).
(4) Supervise and assess the patient's ability to test their own blood glucose and/or administer insulin, or teach these skills if the person is newly diagnosed.
(5) Ensure diabetes knowledge is assessed and updated, and select an appropriate diet: new learning may include insulin techniques, sharps disposal, hypoglycaemia and home management during illness.
(6) TPR daily, or every second day.
(7) BP, lying and standing, daily.
(8) Ensure all blood samples, urine collections and special tests are performed accurately. The opportunity is often taken to perform a comprehensive complication screen while the person is in hospital, especially if they often miss appointments or it has not been performed for some time. Inspection of injection sites and assessment of the person's psychological status should be included. These tests include ECG, eye referral, 12- or 24-hour urine collection for creatinine and microalbumin.
(9) Ensure the patient has supplies, e.g. test strips, lancets, insulin device, before discharge and that the appropriate follow-up appointments have been made.
(10) Ensure they have a contact telephone number in case they need advice.

9.3 Outpatient stabilisation

The types of outpatient service provided for people with diabetes include:

- Diabetes education;
- Commencement on diabetes medication (oral agents, insulin);
- Complication screening and assessment;
- Blood glucose testing;
- Consultations with dietitian, diabetes nurse specialist/diabetes educator or diabetes specialist;
- Clinical assessment;
- Education is a key factor in a person's understanding and acceptance of diabetes.

Diabetes educators often know the person well from the outpatient service and can assist ward nurses to plan appropriate nursing care and understand the person's needs.

Practice point

The specific protocol and policy of the employing institution should be followed and all contacts including telephone advice documented. The following is an example protocol for insulin stabilisation on an outpatient basis.

9.3.1 Objectives of outpatient stabilisation onto insulin

Short-term objectives

(1) To reassure the individual and their family and allay the fear that everything about diabetes must be learned at once.
(2) Lifestyle should be modified as little as possible.
(3) To establish trust between the patient and the diabetes team.
(4) To gradually normalise blood glucose.
(5) To teach the 'survival skills' necessary for the person to be safe at home:
   - how to draw up and administer insulin;
   - blood glucose monitoring;
   - recognising and treating hypoglycaemia;
   - how to obtain advice – contact telephone number.

Long-term objectives
The aim in the long term is for the patient to:

(1) Accept diabetes as part of their life and recognise their part in the successful management of the diabetes.
(2) Be able to make appropriate changes in insulin doses, carbohydrate intake and activity to maintain acceptable blood glucose levels.
(3) Be able to maintain an acceptable range of blood glucose, HbA1c and lipids.
(4) Be able to maintain a healthy weight range.
(5) Modify risk factors to prevent or delay the onset of the long-term complications of diabetes and therefore the need for hospital admissions.
(6) Attend regular medical/education appointments.
(7) Receive ongoing support and encouragement from the diabetes team.
(8) Maintain psychological wellbeing and quality of life.

Clinical observations

People are often overwhelmed, unsure what to do and confused by conflicting or inaccurate advice given by health professionals, family and friends and the media or obtained on the Internet.

These issues frequently need to be addressed and clarified before commencing the insulin stabilisation process.

The therapeutic relationship and trust between health professional and the person with diabetes is a vital aspect of their adjustment to having diabetes and changes in their diabetic management or status. Therapeutic relationships should be cultivated and treasured.

9.3.2 Rationale for choosing outpatient stabilisation

Outpatient stabilisation onto insulin is preferred for the following reasons:

(1) To avoid the 'sick role' which is often associated with a hospital admission.
(2) It is cost effective, i.e. does not require a hospital bed.
(3) It involves less time away from work and usual activity for the patient, who can therefore be stabilised according to their usual routine, rather than hospital routines and food.
(4) To encourage self-reliance and confidence.

Practice point

Outpatient stabilisation is labour-intensive; however, unhurried time is necessary if the process is to be successful.

9.3.3 Criteria for patient selection for outpatient stabilisation

The patient must be:

- Able to attend daily for the required period, which depends on the individual. In some cases twice daily visits may be necessary. Telephone contact should be maintained as long as necessary;
- Physically and mentally capable of performing blood glucose monitoring and insulin administration, or have assistance to do so.

In addition, some social/family support is helpful.

9.3.4 The process of stabilisation

(1) It should involve members of the diabetes team as appropriate.
(2) Communication, especially between the doctor, diabetes nurse specialist/diabetes educator, dietitian and patient, is essential.
(3) Patients should be assessed on an individual basis, so that appropriate education goals and blood glucose range can be determined. The insulin regime and insulin delivery system will depend on individual requirements; follow-up advice and early assessment must be available.
(4) Formal teaching days should not include weekends or public holidays unless staff are available.
(5) Adequate charting and documentation of progress should be recorded after each session: blood glucose results, ability to manage insulin technique, goals of management.

A sample protocol for outpatient stabilisation is shown at the end of this chapter. This is a comprehensive protocol and will usually be the responsibility of the diabetes nurse specialist/diabetes educator and dietitian. It is included here to give nurses an overview of the kind of information required and the complex issues people with diabetes have to deal with, often when they feel vulnerable.

Practice points

(1) People of all ages forget how to manage emergencies. Health professionals and well-meaning family and friends often give inaccurate advice that either confuses the person with diabetes or causes them to ignore all advice.
(2) People with Type 1 diabetes are at risk of ketoacidosis but often do not have ketone testing equipment at home or if they do it is out of date (Sumner *et al.* 2000; Tay *et al.* 2001). Constant, diplomatic reminders are important. An episode in hospital is one such opportunity.

Traditionally, initiation of insulin occurred on an individual basis. Recent reports suggest that group education programmes for commencing insulin can be effective and achieve reductions in HbA1c and competent insulin self-care by individuals (Almond *et al.* 2001). Such programmes could be a cost effective way to manage the increasing numbers of people being commenced on insulin as a result of the DCCT and UKPDS trials, provided competent facilitation is available.

References

Almond, J., Cox, D., Nugent, M., Day, J., Rayman, G. & Graham, A. (2001) Experience of group sessions for converting to insulin. *Journal of Diabetes Nursing*, **5** (4), 102–105.

MacKinnon, M. (1998) *Diabetes Care in General Practice*. Class Publishing, London.

NDS (1998) *National Diabetes Strategy and Implementation Plan*. Diabetes Australia, Canberra.

NHMRC (National Health and Medical Research Council) (1991a) *Stabilisation of Diabetes*. National Health and Medical Research Council, Canberra.

NHMRC (National Health and Medical Research Council) (1991b) *The Role of Ambulatory Services in the Management of Diabetes*. Document No. 1. Australia.

Sumner, J., Baber, C. & Williams, V. (2000) What do people with Type 1 diabetes know about hypoglycaemia? *Practical Diabetes International*, **17** (6), 187–190.

Tay, M., Messersmith, R. & Lange, D. (2001) What do people on insulin therapy remember about safety advice? *Journal of Diabetes Nursing*, **5** (6), 188–191.

Example protocol for outpatient stabilisation onto insulin

SUGGESTED PROTOCOL

These are guidelines only and should be
modified to suit individual needs

Day One

Aim to commence at 7.30–8 AM. The length of stay will depend on the individual and the insulin regime decided upon. If a full day stay is envisaged a 2–3 hour break in the middle is usually necessary.

(1) Introduce the diabetes team and area facilities.
(2) Test blood glucose.
(3) Insulin dose/frequency is determined in consultation with the doctor.
(4) Educator prepares and gives the insulin and explains the procedure to the patient.
(5) Breakfast.
(6) It is important to encourage the patient to discuss their feelings about diabetes and to assess current diabetes knowledge, learning capacity, style, psychological status and social situation.

Education Goals

(1) To give a basic explanation of what diabetes is and what an acceptable blood glucose range is.
(2) To explain the reason for instituting insulin therapy.
(3) To explain the effects of insulin on blood glucose levels, i.e. insulin action and the role of long- and short-acting insulin in control of blood glucose levels.
(4) To explain insulin technique:
- preparing the dose depending on the insulin delivery system chosen
- sites for injection
- expiry dates of insulin bottles/cartridges
- care and storage
- appropriate sharps disposal.

(5) To explain why insulin must be given by injection and allow patient to handle insulin device and bottles and practise preparing the insulin dose.
(6) To explain hypoglycaemia:
- recognising symptoms of low blood glucose levels
- causes and prevention
- effective management
- patient should carry carbohydrate for 'emergencies'.

(7) Blood glucose monitoring should be encouraged, to provide feedback to the patient and enable them to telephone in the afternoon with a result if necessary. The role of monitoring should be explained as well as the timing of testing and how to record results.
(8) Basic introduction to a food plan: role of carbohydrate in blood glucose control and the need to reduce fat and the need for regular meals.
(9) If on twice-daily insulin, the injection and dinner may be given before the patient leaves, or the insulin can be drawn up for the patient to give at home.
(10) Explain and enrol the patient in the National Diabetes Supply Scheme*

**Point (10) above:* the National Diabetes Supply Scheme only applies in Australia.

Example protocol for outpatient stabilisation *cont'd*

(11) Ensure patient has the equipment to administer insulin and monitor blood glucose and knows how and where to obtain future supplies and knows who to contact for advice.

Day Two (if required)

(1) Patient comes at 8 AM and stays 2–3 hours. If on twice-daily insulin the patient may return in the afternoon or give own dose after telephoning staff with blood glucose result; depending on accuracy of insulin technique and personal confidence/preference.
(2) Test blood glucose and document.
(3) Insulin dose is determined (consultation with doctor may be necessary). Patient to prepare and give own injection under supervision. Document in patient record.

Education Goals

(1) Revision of day one and answer any questions the patient may have.
(2) Detailed revision of blood glucose monitoring and insulin technique.
(3) Explanation of testing for ketones in Type 1 diabetes.
(4) Detailed food plan and revision of role of carbohydrate and sweeteners: with dietitian if possible.

Days Three, Four and Five (if required)

As for day two. Revision of previous day's information and questions answered. Patient should be testing own blood glucose and giving own insulin injection under supervision if necessary.

Education Goals

(1) Discuss how to manage illness at home, in relation to:
- who to contact
- effects of illness on blood glucose
- emergency diet
- monitoring and recording of blood glucose and urine or blood ketones
- adjusting/continuing insulin
- need to rest.

(2) Discuss precautions to be taken relating to driving, work, etc.
(3) Discuss the role of exercise/activity in controlling blood glucose levels.
(4) Prescriptions for insulin, test strips, pen syringes, etc. should be finalised.
(5) Complete food plan.
(6) Encourage patient to wear some form of identification.
(7) Ensure that patient has a contact telephone number and knows who to contact for advice.
(8) Provide appropriate follow-up appointments for doctor, nurse specialist/educator according to patient needs.
(9) Provide ongoing individual teaching as required.
(10) Ensure patient knows about other services available for people with diabetes, e.g. Diabetes Associations and relevant support groups.
(11) Arrange for consultation with family if necessary.

Chapter 10
Hyperglycaemia, Diabetic Ketoacidosis (DKA), Hyperosmolar Coma and Lactic Acidosis

10.1 Key points

- Ketoacidosis and hyperosmolar coma are serious short-term complications of diabetes, even if they are managed competently.
- Meticulous attention to detail reduces morbidity and mortality.
- Monitor rehydration closely.
- Gradually decrease blood glucose.
- Monitor ketone clearance in urine and/or blood.
- Educate patient.
- Consider psychological issues.

Rationale

Hyperglycaemia, DKA and HONK are preventable short-term complications of diabetes. When hyperglycaemia does occur, effective nursing care can reduce the progression to DKA and HONK and limit the attendant metabolic derangements should these conditions occur.

10.2 Hyperglycaemia

Hyperglycaemia refers to an elevated blood glucose level (>10 mmol/L) due to a relative or absolute insulin deficiency. The symptoms of hyperglycaemia usually occur when the blood glucose is persistently above 15 mmol/L; see section 1.3. In people with an established diagnosis of diabetes the cause of the hyperglycaemia should be sought, and corrected to avoid the development of diabetic ketoacidosis (DKA) or hyperosmolar coma. Hyperglycaemia, DKA and hyperosmolar coma are often referred to as short-term complications of diabetes. DKA develops over a short time. HONK evolves over several days to weeks.

10.3 Diabetic ketoacidosis (DKA)

Diabetic ketoacidosis is a life-threatening complication of diabetes. The basic pathophysiology consists of a reduction in the effective action of circulating insulin and the increase in counter-regulatory hormones. Glucose is unable to enter the cells and accumulates in the blood. Insulin deficiency leads to catecholamine release, lipolysis and the mobilisation of free fatty acids and subsequently ketone bodies, B-hydroxybutyrate, and acetoacetate resulting in metabolic acidosis (ADA Position Statement 2002). Protein catabolism also occurs and forms the substrate for gluconeogenesis, further increasing the blood glucose, at the same time glucose utilisation in tissues is impaired. DKA usually only occurs in Type 1 patients, but may occur in Type 2 people with severe infections or metabolic stress. The mortality rate in expert centres is <5% but is higher at the extremes of age and if coma and/or hypotension are present (Malone *et al.* 1992).

Diabetic ketoacidosis is characterised by hyperglycaemia, osmotic diuresis, metabolic acidosis, glycosuria, ketonuria and dehydration. The definition by laboratory results is blood glucose >17 mmol/L; ketonaemia, (ketone bodies) >3 mmol/L; acidosis, pH <7.30 and bicarbonate <15 mEq/L.

The signs, symptoms and precipitating factors for DKA are shown in Table 10.1, while Figure 10.1 outlines the physiology, the signs and symptoms which occur as a result of decreased utilisation of glucose and the biochemical manifestations found on blood testing.

Table 10.1 Signs, symptoms and precipitating factors in diabetic ketoacidosis (DKA).

Symptoms and signs	*Precipitating factors*
Thirst	(1) Newly diagnosed IDDM (20–30%)
Polyuria	(2) Omission of insulin therapy
Fatigue	(3) Inappropriate dose reduction
Weight loss	(4) Relative insulin deficiency
Nausea and vomiting	(a) Acute illness:
Abdominal pain	Infection (50% of cases)
Muscle cramps	Myocardial infarction
Tachycardia	Trauma, acute stress
Kussmaul's respirations	Cerebrovascular accident
(early sign)	(b) Endocrine disorders (rare):
	Hyperthyroidism
	Pheochromocytoma
	Acromegaly
	Cushing's disease
	(c) Drugs:
	Cortisone
	Thiazide diuretics
	Sympathomimetic agents
	Alcohol[a]

10.3.1 Late signs, i.e. severe DKA

The initial signs and symptoms of DKA (polyuria, polydipsia, lethargy and Kussmaul's respirations) are an attempt by the body to compensate for the acidosis. If treatment is delayed the body eventually decompensates. Signs of decompensation (late signs) include:

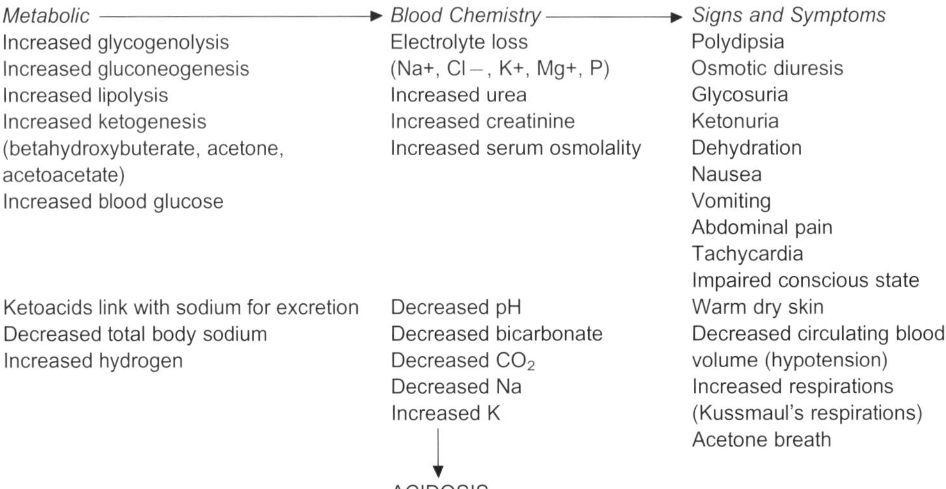

Figure 10.1 An outline of the physiology, signs and symptoms and biochemical changes occurring in the development of diabetic ketoacidosis (DKA).

- Warm, dry skin.
- Hypothermia.
- Hypoxia and decreased conscious state.
- Decreased renal output (oliguria).
- Decreased respirations – absence of Kussmaul's respirations.
- Bradycardia.

10.3.2 Differential diagnosis

- Starvation ketosis, which can be determined by taking a careful clinical history of the presentation.
- Alcoholic ketosis where the blood glucose is usually only mildly elevated to low.

The implications of the metabolic and physiological changes associated with DKA are shown in Table 10.2.

10.3.3 Assessment

The following factors should be established:

- Whether the person has known diabetes;
- Usual insulin dose, regime and type of insulin;

Table 10.2 The metabolic consequences of diabetic ketoacidosis and associated risks.

Metabolic consequences of ketoacidosis	*Associated risk*
Increased blood fats	Embolism
Dehydration, haemoconcentration and coagulation changes	Myocardial infarction, stroke, thrombosis
Gastric stasis	Inhalation of vomitus, aspiration pneumonia
Changes in intra- and extracellular potassium	Cardiac arrhythmias
Hyperglycaemia	Infection, thrombosis, low mood, visual changes
Abdominal pain	Unnecessary surgery, inappropriate pain relief causing further respiratory distress
	Death

- The time the last dose was taken and amount administered;
- Whether the person is taking OHAs. DKA is rare in Type 2 diabetes but it can occur;
- Presence of fever, which can be a sign of myocardial infarction as well as infection;
- Duration of the deteriorating control/illness;
- Remedial action taken by the patient;
- Whether the person has taken any other medications, complementary therapies, alcohol or illegal drugs;
- Conscious state.

A thorough physical assessment should be undertaken and blood taken to establish the metabolic and infection status of the patient. An ECG may be done and a chest X-ray when the condition is stable.

10.3.4 Aims of treatment of DKA

Treatment aims to:

(1) Correct:
   - dehydration
   - electrolyte imbalance
   - ketoacidosis
   - hyperglycaemia (to slowly decrease blood glucose to 7–10 mmol/L). Hyperglycaemia, relative insulin deficiency, or both, predispose people with and without diabetes to complications such as severe infection, polyneuropathy, multiorgan failure and death (Van den Bergh *et al*. 2001).

(2) Reverse shock.
(3) Ascertain the cause of DKA and treat appropriately.
(4) Prevent complications of treatment (see Section 10.3.6).
(5) Educate/re-educate the patient and their family/carers.

10.3.5 Objectives of nursing care

To support the medical team to:

(1) Restore normal hydration, euglycaemia and metabolism.
(2) Prevent complications of DKA including complications occurring as a result of management.
(3) Pay meticulous attention to detail.
(4) Document progress of recovery.
(5) Re-educate/educate the patient and their family/carers about the management of illness at home or general diabetes education if a new diagnosis. Patient education about managing diabetes during illness can be found in Chapter 23.
(6) Ensure follow-up care after discharge, in particular: review of diabetes knowledge, nutritional assessment and physical and psychological assessment.

10.3.6 Preparation of the unit to receive the patient

Assemble:

(1) Oxygen and suction (tested to ensure they are in working order).
(2) Intravenous trolley (IV) containing:
    - dressing tray and antiseptic solution
    - local anaesthetic
    - selection of intravenous cannulae
    - IV fluids – normal saline, SPPS
    - giving sets, burette
    - IMED pump or syringe pump
    - clear short-acting insulin, preferably in an IV infusion
    - blood gas syringe
    - blood culture bottles.
(3) Cot sides and IV pole.
(4) Blood glucose testing equipment (cleaned, calibrated).
(5) Ketone testing equipment: urine and/or blood strips.
(6) Appropriate charts:
    - fluid balance
    - diabetic record
    - conscious state.
(7) Urinary catheterisation equipment.
(8) Nasogastric tubes are not usually required.
(9) Initial care in the intensive care unit is preferable.

If the patient is admitted to the intensive care unit, central venous pressures, continuous blood gas and electrocardiogram monitoring is usually performed.

Practice point

Short-acting insulin has a rapid onset of action and quickly promotes transport of glucose into the cells. Intravenous administration is preferred because absorption is more predictable than by the subcutaneous route.

10.3.7 Nursing care/observations

The nursing management of DKA involves traditional nursing actions as well as monitoring of the responses to medical therapy.

Initial patient care

Initial patient care is often given in the intensive care unit. The procedure is:

- Maintain the airway.
- Nurse the patient on their side, even if the patient is conscious, because gastric stasis and inhalation of vomitus is a possible and preventable complication of DKA.
- Ensure strict aseptic technique.

Nursing observations (1–2 hourly)

(1) Observe 'nil orally'. Provide pressure care especially in the elderly patient.
(2) Provide mouth care to protect oral mucous membranes and relieve the discomfort of a dry mouth.
(3) Administer IV fluid according to the treatment sheet.
(4) Administer insulin according to the treatment sheet; it is usually given via an insulin infusion adjusted according to blood glucose tests, see Chapter 7. Intensive insulin therapy to maintain the blood glucose within a narrow range and thereby reduce the morbidity and mortality associated with critical illness (Van den Burghe *et al.* 2001). In some cases short-acting insulin is given intramuscularly, usually in remote areas where ICU units are not available.
(5) Replace serum potassium. If the initial biochemical result is >5.0 mmol/L potassium is not required initially. It should be added to the second or third litres of IV fluid or when levels fall to <4.5 mmol/L depending on expected potassium loss, e.g. from vomiting.
(6) There is general agreement that bicarbonate replacement is not required if the pH is >7.0. There is no consensus about pH <7.0. Some experts state that bicarbonate should be given to minimise respiratory decompensation. Others believe bicarbonate automatically corrects as the acidosis resolves with fluid and insulin (Hamblin 1995).
(7) Estimate blood glucose levels and confirm biochemically in the early stages.
(8) Observe strict fluid balance. Record second hourly subtotals of input/output *from admission*. Urine output should be >30 ml per hour measured hourly in a calibrated collecting device. Report a urine output of <30 ml per hour. Measure specific gravity (SG).
    - *Heavy* glycosuria invalidates SG readings.
    - Test for ketones.
    - Record fluid loss, e.g. vomitus.
(9) Monitor central venous pressure.
(10) Monitor conscious state.
(11) Record pulse, respiration and blood pressure. Fever associated with DKA indicates sepsis. But it should be noted that an elevated white cell count can be due to metabolic abnormalities and does not necessarily indicate the presence of infection.
(12) Administer oxygen via face mask or nasal catheter.
(13) Monitor and report all laboratory results (electrolytes and blood gases).

(14) Report any deterioration of condition immediately.
(15) Physiotherapy may be helpful to prevent pneumonia and emboli due to venous stasis, and to provide passive mobilisation.
(16) Administer other drugs as ordered (potassium, calciparine, antibiotics).
(17) Reposition and provide skin care to avoid pressure areas and/or venous stasis.

Subsequent care
As the patient's condition improves:

- Review the frequency of blood glucose testing, decreasing to 4-hourly including the night time.
- Allow a light diet and ensure the patient is eating before the IV is removed.
- Administer subcutaneous insulin before the IV is removed.
- Continue to monitor temperature, pulse and respiration every 4 hours.
- Provide support and comfort for the patient.
- Establish the duration of deteriorating control and identify any precipitating factor such as infection.

Plan for:

- Medical follow-up appointment after discharge.
- Nutrition review.
- Education/re-education about appropriate management (for days when the patient is unwell); see Chapter 23.
- Review of medication dosage, especially insulin.
- Consider sexual assault. Sexual assault is an uncommon but important cause of DKA and should be considered when repeated admissions occur. This is a difficult area to assess and should be undertaken by people with the appropriate skills and with consideration of the legal implications and the effect on the individual and their family.

Practice point

Psychiatric consultation should be considered if a patient repeatedly presents in DKA. Eating disorders complicate 20% of recurrent cases of DKA (Polonsky *et al.* 1994). People, especially young women, reduce their insulin doses to avoid weight gain and hypoglycaemia. Reducing or stopping insulin is also a form of risk taking and rebellion at having diabetes (Dunning *et al.* 1994).

10.3.8 Complications which can occur as a result of DKA

Most complications of DKA are due to complications of treatment and most are avoidable:

(1) Hypoglycaemia due to overzealous treatment.
(2) Inhalation of vomitus – aspiration pneumonia.
(3) Hypokalaemia which may lead to cardiac arrhythmias.
(4) Cerebral oedema is rare and often fatal. It occurs in 0.7–10% of children especially on the first presentation of diabetes and any morbidity that occurs is permanent (Rosenbloom 1990).

(5) Myocardial infarction.
(6) Deep venous thrombosis.
(7) Adult respiratory distress syndrome.

Be extra vigilant with:

(1) Elderly patients, especially those with established vascular and coronary disease. Risks include myocardial infarction and deep venous thrombosis.
(2) Children are at increased risk of cerebral oedema, which has a high mortality rate in this group of patients.

10.4 Hyperosmolar non-ketotic coma (HONK)

Hyperosmolar non-ketotic coma is a metabolic disturbance characterised by a marked increase in serum osmolality, the absence of ketones, hyperglycaemia (usually >40 mmol/L) and extreme dehydration caused by inadequate insulin levels to allow glucose utilisation but adequate enough to prevent lipolysis and ketoacidosis (Kitabchi *et al.* 1994). It occurs in people with Type 2 diabetes, but also in people with no previous diagnosis of diabetes. Dehydration is usually severe. The patient is often confused, and focal and general neurological signs are usually present.

Practice point

People with Type 2 diabetes usually still have sufficient endogenous insulin production to prevent the formation of ketones.

HONK predominantly occurs in older people and is often a new diagnosis of diabetes. The onset is associated with severe stress such as infection, extensive burns, myocardial infarction or decreased fluid intake. People in care facilities for the elderly are at risk because they are often unaware of thirst and are not always offered fluids in hot weather. Other precipitating factors include:

- Some medications: thiazide diuretics, steroids, immunosuppressants.
- Peritoneal dialysis.
- Parenteral nutrition.

There is a high mortality rate associated with HONK. It has decreased since the 1960s but is still ≥15% (ADA 2002).

The nursing care and objectives are similar to those for DKA, but extra vigilance is needed because of the age of these patients.

Monitor closely:

- Record strict fluid balance.
- IV fluid rate.
- Blood glucose may fall with rehydration alone over the first 1–3 hours.
- ECG.
- Urine output.
- Neurological observations.
- Skin integrity.

Observe for deep venous thrombosis or embolism. Subsequent care is as for DKA.

Education may be more difficult because of the age of these patients. It may be difficult to assess the mental state of the patient because of the dehydration. Ensuring that the family/caregivers understand how to care for the patient is important.

Figure 10.2 is an outline of the factors involved in the development of hyperosmolar coma. There are similarities with DKA, with some important differences. Ketone production is absent or minimal, because the patient is usually producing enough endogenous insulin to allow the ketone bodies to be metabolised and utilised. The degree of dehydration is often greater in HONK and the serum and urine osmolality is increased.

Practice point

Glass thermometers should not be placed in the mouth if the conscious state is impaired. They can be bitten and break, causing local trauma.

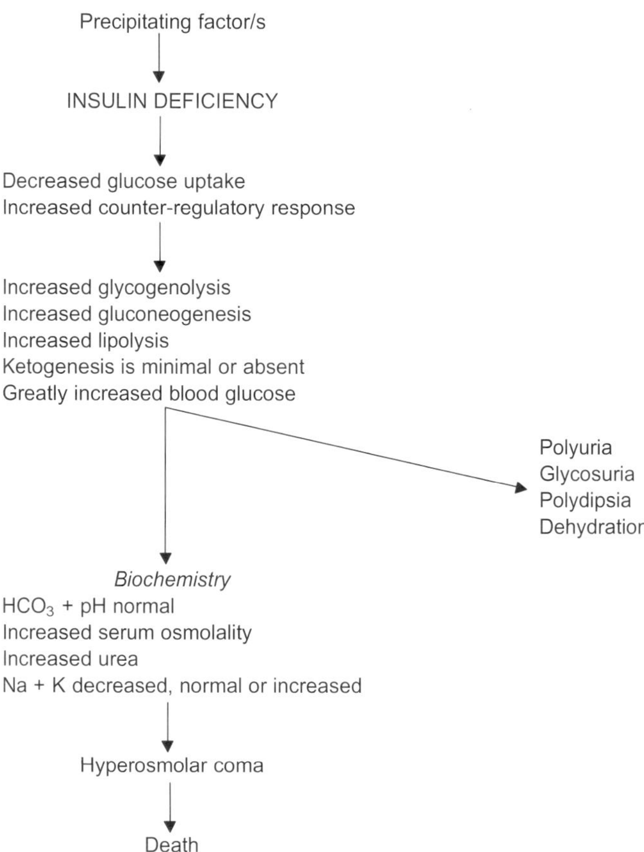

Figure 10.2 An outline of the development of hyperosmolar coma.

10.5 Prevention

Prevention of all three abnormalities is desirable and possible. It requires:

- Early recognition of new presentations of diabetes.
- Good access to competent medical and nursing care and ongoing education.
- Good knowledge on the part of people with diabetes and health professionals.
- Good communication/therapeutic relationship between the person with diabetes and their health professionals (see Munro *et al.* 1973: this is an old reference but it is still pertinent in the light of the frequent presentation to hospital of hyperglycaemia-associated conditions).
- Psychological screening to be incorporated into routine complication assessment programmes (Ciechanowski *et al.* 2000; Dunning 2001).

10.6 Euglycaemic DKA

Munro *et al.* originally documented euglycaemic DKA in 1993. Euglycaemic DKA refers to ketoacidosis in the setting of near normal blood glucose levels. This condition indicates that the blood glucose level and development of DKA do not necessarily correlate. De & Child (2001) postulated that heavy glycosuria triggered by counter-regulatory hormone activity or reduced hepatic glucose production could result in lower than expected blood glucose levels. Although euglycaemic DKA is a rare condition it highlights the importance of monitoring serum ketones and blood gases and using low dose IV insulin infusions in all people with diabetes during illness.

Ketosis without hyperglycaemia occasionally occurs postoperatively in the presence of repeated vomiting. Rehydration with dextrose/saline and control of vomiting are required to restore depleted hepatic glycogen stores.

10.7 Lactic acidosis

Lactic acidosis is another uncommon coma sometimes associated with diabetes. It should be considered in people with diabetes who are very ill, vasoconstricted, hypotensive and with underlying diseases such as:

- Cirrhosis
- Occult infection
- Renal or hepatic impairment.

Lactic acidosis should also be considered if Biguanides are used in cardiac disease, and in cases of renal and hepatic impairment. Biochemistry shows low pH, usually <7.1 but only moderate, if any, ketones and mildly elevated blood glucose, usually <20 mmol/L.

Lactic acidosis should be managed in ICU settings.

10.7.1 Management

Management consist of:

- IV fluid replacement to maintain the circulating volume and tissue perfusion.
- Oxygen therapy.

- Bicarbonate given early in large doses.
- IV insulin at a rate of 10–12 units/hour in dextrose.
- The mental status should be monitored as well as monitoring the physical status.

References

ADA (American Diabetes Association) (2002) *Hyperglycaemic Crisis in Patients with Diabetes Mellitus*. American Diabetes Association, USA.

Ciechanowski, P., Katon, W., Russo, J. (2000) Depression and diabetes. Impact of depressive symptoms on adherence, function and costs. *Archives of Internal Medicine*, **160**, 3278–3285.

De, P. & Child, D. (2001) Euglycaemic ketoacidosis – is it on the rise? *Practical Diabetes International*, **18** (7), 239–240.

Dunning, T. (2001) Depression and diabetes, summary and comment. *International Diabetes Monitor*, **13** (5), 9–11.

Dunning, P., Ward, G. & Rantzau, C. (1994) Effect of alcohol swabbing on capillary blood glucose measurements. *Practical Diabetes*, **11** (4), 251–254.

Hamblin, S. (1995) Diabetic ketoacidosis. *Australian Diabetes Educator's Association Journal*, Spring, 17.

Kitabchi, A., Fisher, J., Murphy, M. & Rumbak, M. (1994) Diabetic ketoacidosis and the hyperglycaemic hyperosmolar nonketotic state. In: *Joslin's Diabetes Mellitus* (eds C. Kahn & G. Weir), pp. 738–770. Lea & Febiger, Philadelphia.

Malone, M., Gennis, V. & Goodwin, J. (1992) Characteristics of diabetic ketoacidosis in older versus younger adults. *Journal of the American Geriatric Society*, **40**, 1100–1104.

Munro, J., Campbell, I., McCuish, A. & Duncan, L. (1973) Euglycaemic ketoacidosis. *British Medical Journal*, **2**, 578–580.

Polonsky, W., Anderson, B., Lohrer, P., Aponte, J., Jacobson, A. & Cole, C. (1994) Insulin omission in women with IDDM. *Diabetes Care*, **17**, 1178–1185.

Rosenbloom, A. (1990) Intracerebral crises during treatment of diabetic ketoacidosis. *Diabetes Care*, **13**, 22–33.

Van den Berghe, M., Wouters, P., Weekers, F. *et al.* (2001) Intensive insulin in critically ill patients. *New England Journal of Medicine*, **345**, 1359–1367.

Chapter 11
Cardiovascular Disease and Diabetes

11.1 Key points

- Cardiovascular disease is the leading cause of death in industrialised countries.
- Treat all people with diabetes as if they have heart disease.
- Chest pain may be atypical in people with diabetes.
- Watch for weakness, fatigue, increased blood glucose, congestive cardiac failure (CCF).
- Counsel about risk factors.
- Smoking increases micro- and macrovascular damage.
- Offer support.
- Transient ischaemic attacks (TIA) may indicate impending stroke.

Rationale

Cardiovascular disease is a major cause of hospital admissions and mortality in people with diabetes. It is often associated with diabetic renal disease. Complex metabolic abnormalities are present and the need for surgical intervention is high. Autonomic neuropathy can give rise to atypical presentations of cardiovascular disease and heart attack and lead to delayed treatment.

The major clinical manifestations of cardiovascular disease involve:

- The heart and coronary circulation
- The brain and cerebral circulation
- The lower limbs – peripheral vascular disease (see Chapter 19).

Cardiac disease is a common complication of diabetes, and carries a higher mortality rate than for people without diabetes. There is an association among increasing age, duration of diabetes, the presence of other complications and mortality. Cardiac disease is associated with diffuse atherosclerosis, coexisting cardiomyopathy, autonomic neuropathy, hyperglycaemia and hyperlipidaemia, the metabolic consequences being hypercoaguability, elevated catecholamines and insulin resistance. Atherosclerosis is more frequent and more severe in people with diabetes. It occurs at a lower age than in people without diabetes and is more prevalent in women.

Cardiac disease accounts for >50% of deaths in Type 2 diabetes (Standl & Schnell 2000; Huang *et al.* 2001) and half of these die before they reach hospital. The mortality rate has not been reduced despite new therapeutic measures and preventative health programmes.

A number of clinical trials demonstrate the importance of reducing lipids, blood pressure and blood glucose to reduce the risk of cardiovascular disease (Hansson *et al.* 1998; UKPDS 1998). Hypertension leads to thicker, less elastic blood vessel walls and increases the strain on the heart. There is a linear relationship between the diastolic blood pressure and the eventual outcome of Type 2 diabetes. Reducing the blood pressure below 90 mmHg significantly improves the outcome.

Subtle changes occur in the heart as a result of ischaemia-induced remodelling and the effects of hyperglycaemia on the endothelium of large blood vessels that predispose the heart to failure (Standl & Schnell 2000). Heart muscle metabolism is critically dependent on glucose during ischaemia, and heart muscle performance is improved in the presence of insulin, which stimulates glucose uptake supporting the use of IV insulin in acute myocardial infarction (Malmberg *et al.* 1995). However, impaired heart performance is multifactorial and blood pressure, lipids, and prothrombin imbalance all play a part. Table 11.1 outlines some of the diabetic-specific abnormalities linked to the development of cardiovascular disease.

Myocardial infarction is 'silent' in 32% of people with diabetes, which leads to delay in seeking medical attention and may be a factor in the increased mortality rate. 'Silent' infarct means that the classic pain across the chest, down the arm and into the jaw is absent. Only mild discomfort, often mistaken for heartburn, may be present. The atypical nature of the chest pain may make it difficult for people to accept that they have had a heart attack. Risk factor modification may not be seen as essential. The person may present with hypertension, heart failure, cardiogenic shock or, in the elderly, diabetic ketoacidosis or hyperosmolar coma.

Diabetes may be diagnosed at the time of an infarct or during cardiac surgery. Emotional stress, and the associated catecholamine response, leads to increased blood glucose levels in 5% of patients admitted to coronary care units (CCUs). The blood glucose

Table 11.1 Diabetes-specific cardiovascular abnormalities that predispose an individual to heart disease.

Abnormality	*Relevance to cardiovascular disease*
Microvascular disease	Nephropathy, frequently in association with retinopathy
Autonomic neuropathy	Postural hypotension Abnormal cardiovascular reflexes Loss of sinus arrhythmia Resting sinus tachycardia Painless myocardial ischaemia and infarction Increased anaesthetic risk Sudden death
Endothelial damage in membrane or outer lining of large blood vessels	Weak vessel walls Impaired blood flow Reduced tissue oxygenation and nourishment
Hypertension	Thickening of blood vessel walls Increased strain on the heart

may normalise during convalescence; however, counselling about diabetes and its management is important. Tact and sympathy are necessary when informing the patient about the diagnosis of diabetes in these situations.

Patients will usually be cared for in CCUs, but patients in other wards may develop cardiac problems. A longer stay in CCU may be indicated for people with diabetes, because 35% of patients die, often in the second week after the infarct (Karlson *et al.* 1993).

Short- and long-term morbidity and mortality can be improved by IV insulin/glucose infusion followed by multidose subcutaneous insulin injections (Malmberg *et al.* 1995). Acute myocardial infarction causes a rapid increase in catecholamines, cortisol and glucagon. Insulin levels fall in the ischaemic myocardium and tissue sensitivity to insulin falls and impairs glucose utilisation by cardiac muscle. Free fatty acids are mobilised as fuel substrates and potentiate ischaemic injury by direct toxicity or by increasing the demand for oxygen and inhibiting glucose oxidation. IV insulin during acute episodes and subcutaneous insulin for three months after the infarct may restore platelet function, correct lipoprotein imbalance, reduce plasminogen activator inhibitor-1 activity and improve metabolism in non-infarcted areas of the heart.

11.2 Objectives of care

Nursing care should be planned to avoid constant disturbance of the patient and allow adequate rest and sleep. The objectives of care are to:

- Treat the acute attack according to medical orders and standard protocols.
- Stabilise cardiac status and relieve symptoms.
- Prevent extension of the cardiac abnormality and limit further episodes.
- Retain independence as far as possible.
- Achieve and maintain euglycaemia.
- Provide psychological support.
- Prevent complications while in hospital.
- Counsel about risk factor modification.
- Educate/re-educate about diabetes.

11.3 Nursing responsibilities

(1) To be aware that myocardial infarction can present atypically in diabetes with CCF, syncope, vomiting, abdominal pain, and fatigue that improves with rest. An ECG should be performed urgently if any of these symptoms are present.

(2) To provide psychological, educational and physical care.

(3) To monitor blood glucose, 2–4 hourly depending on stability and route of insulin administration.

(4) To provide adequate pain relief, and to control vomiting, which can exacerbate high blood glucose levels.

(5) To perform treatment according to the medical orders for the specific cardiac abnormality.

(6) To administer insulin:

   - Many patients on OHAs are changed to insulin during the acute phase to improve blood glucose control.

- Insulin is usually administered via an infusion at least for the first 48 hours. Only clear insulin is used. Insulin infusions are discussed in Chapter 7. The patient should be eating and drinking normally before the infusion is removed, and a dose of subcutaneous insulin given to prevent hyperglycaemia developing.

Some endocrinologist/cardiologist teams have adopted Malmberg *et al.*'s recommendations, the so-called DIGAMI protocol, or some variation of it. This usually involves commencing an IV insulin infusion for people with diabetes presenting with myocardial infarction from the time of presentation in the emergency room. IV insulin is usually continued for 24 hours after which time subcutaneous insulin is commenced and maintained for three months.

The aim of the DIGAMI regime is to normalise glucose utilisation in the myocardium, achieve normoglycaemia and reduce morbidity and mortality.

(7) Medications: OHAs should be stopped while the patient is having insulin to reduce the risk of hypoglycaemia and lactic acidosis. Thiazide diuretics can:
- increase blood glucose levels.
- cause hypokalaemia.
- Beta blockers reduce mortality by >30%. Ace inhibitors improve blood pressure and cardiac remodelling and stabilise the rate of progression of renal disease. There is a close association between cardiac and renal diseases in diabetes (see Chapter 16).

Non-cardiac-specific beta-blocking agents may mask the signs of hypoglycaemia. Patients who are normally tablet controlled will require support and education about the use of insulin. It should be explained that insulin is being given to increase the glucose available to the myocardium and decrease free fatty acids in the blood. Units where the DIGAMI regime is used usually discharge the patient on subcutaneous insulin that is continued for three months then reassessed.

(8) Physical status:
- Monitor fluid balance and maintain accurate charts, to help assess kidney function.
- Monitor blood pressure, lying and standing. Some antihypertensive medications can cause orthostatic hypotension. Counsel the patient to change position gradually, especially on getting out of bed or out of a chair.
- Monitor ECG.
- Observe for weakness, fatigue, CCF or unexplained hyperglycaemia which may indicate a further infarct.
- Provide appropriate skin care to prevent dryness and pressure areas.

(9) Blood tests:
- Monitor serum electrolytes, cardiac enzymes, blood gases and potassium levels. Report abnormalities to the doctor promptly. Fluctuating potassium levels can cause or exacerbate cardiac arrhythmias.
- Prevent hypoglycaemia by careful monitoring of blood glucose and carbohydrate intake.

(10) Thrombolytics are beneficial to reduce plaque. Low dose aspirin reduces emboli and reduces the risk of cardiac disease and stroke.

Clinical observation

Introducing the DIGAMI protocol requires collaboration between the cardiology, emergency room and endocrinology teams. It does increase the workload of nurses especially diabetes nurse specialists/diabetes educators, but the benefits to the person with diabetes are significant.

In many cases previous metabolic control has been suboptimal and insulin therapy indicated for some time before the infarct occurred.

Some OHAs are contraindicated if cardiac, renal and/or liver disease is present (see Chapter 6).

Practice points

(1) The patient may not recognise the signs of hypoglycaemia if:
- Autonomic neuropathy is present.
- Non-selective beta-blocking agents are used.

(2) Neuroglycopenic signs of hypoglycaemia (confusion, slurred speech or behaviour change) may predominate.

11.4 Medical tests/procedures (see Chapter 13)

(1) The eyes should be assessed *before* thrombolytic medications are commenced. If proliferative retinopathy is present, bleeding into the back of the eye may occur, requiring urgent treatment.

(2) Diagnostic procedures which require the use of contrast dyes, e.g. angiograms, have been associated with renal complications.
Ensure adequate hydration before and after procedures and monitor urine output, especially in elderly people or those with renal disease.

(3) There is a high prevalence of cardiovascular disease in people with renal disease (Levin 2001).

11.5 Rehabilitation

(1) Encourage activity within tolerance limits. Refer for physiotherapy/occupational therapy.

(2) Encourage independence.

(3) Counsel about resumption of normal activity, including sexual intercourse, after discharge home.

(4) Ensure diabetic education/re-education is available. Refer to diabetes nurse specialist/diabetes educator, dietitian and physiotherapist. Education should include the need to protect kidney function and also address the risk factors involved in the development of cardiac disease (see section 11.6). Particular areas of concern are:
- recognition of hypoglycaemia.
- correct insulin technique.
- correct blood glucose monitoring technique.
- possible indicators of further cardiac problems.
- dietary assessment and advice.
- risk factor modification.

(5) Explain the need for multidrug therapy.

11.6 Modification of risk factors associated with the development of cardiac disease

Patients require both information and support to motivate them to:

- Stop smoking.
- Avoid high calorie foods and high fat intake to achieve sensible weight reduction.
- Increase regular exercise/activities.
- Achieve acceptable blood glucose levels.
- Reduce blood fats.
- Reduce blood pressure by an appropriate diet and exercise and stopping smoking. Tight blood pressure control is important and people are often prescribed three or more antihypertensive agents. The choice of medication is individualised and includes reducing blood glucose as part of a comprehensive cardiovascular risk management plan (Lowe 2002).

11.7 Coaching

Coaching patients with coronary heart disease and suboptimal lipids improves adherence to drug therapy and dietary advice. It contributes to an improved lipid profile and could be an important aspect of cardiac rehabilitation programmes (Vale *et al*. 2002).

11.8 Cerebrovascular disease

The brain is supplied with blood by four main arteries: two carotids and two vertebral arteries. The clinical consequences of cerebrovascular disease depend on the vessels or combination of vessels involved.

Transient ischaemic attacks (TIAs) arise when the blood supply to a part of the brain is temporarily interrupted without permanent damage. Recovery from a TIA usually occurs within 24 hours. If TIAs occur frequently they can indicate impending stroke. Small repeated strokes that cause progressive brain damage can lead to multi-infarct dementia, which is common in diabetes. Signs that this is occurring are:

- Gradual memory loss.
- Diminished intellectual capacity.
- Loss of motor function.
- Incontinence.

Strokes are classified as thrombotic or haemorrhagic and occur when a major vessel is blocked. They frequently cause permanent damage requiring prolonged rehabilitation and often significantly reduced self-care potential and quality of life. In these cases diabetes management should be discussed with the family or carers who will be responsible for assisting the person with diabetes.

11.8.1 Signs and symptoms

- A careful history will elicit failing mental function.

- Carotid bruits are usually present and can be evaluated using Doppler studies.
- Angiography is required in symptomatic cases.

11.8.2 Management

The preventative measures outlined for cardiovascular disease apply to cerebrovascular disease. Carotid endarterectomy is indicated if the carotid arteries are significantly narrowed. Low dose aspirin may be beneficial.

Nursing responsibilities include care during investigative procedures (see Chapter 13). Rehabilitation focuses on returning the person to optimal functioning and independence within their capabilities.

References

Huang, E., Meigs, J. & Singer, D. (2001) The effect of interventions to prevent cardiovascular disease in patients with Type 2 diabetes. *American Medical Journal*, **11** (8), 663–642.

Karlson, B., Herlitz, J. & Hjalmarson, A. (1993) Prognosis of acute myocardial infarction in diabetic and non-diabetic patients. *Diabetic Medicine*, **10**, 449–454.

Larkins, R. (1995) Aspirin: the effects are complex. *Diabetic Communication*, **10** (3), 5–6.

Lowe, J. (2002) Hypertension in diabetes. *Australian Prescriber*, **25** (1), 8–10.

Malmberg, K., Ryden, L., Efendic, S., Herlitz, J., Nicol, P. & Waldenstrom, A. (1995) Randomised trial of insulin–glucose infusion followed by subcutaneous insulin treatment in diabetic patients with acute myocardial infarction (DIGAMI study) effects on mortality at 1 year. *Journal of the American College of Cardiology*, **26**, 57–65.

Standl, E. & Schnell, O. (2000) A new look at the heart in diabetes: from ailing to failing. *Diabetalogia*, **43**, 1455–1469.

UKPDS Group (1998) Intensive blood glucose control with sulphonylureas or insulin compared with conventional treatment and risk of complications in patients with Type 2 diabetes (UKPDS 33). *Lancet*, **352**, 837–853.

Vale, M., Jelinek, M., Best, J. & Santamaria, J. (2002) Coaching patients with coronary heart disease to achieve cholesterol targets: a method to bridge the gap between evidence-based medicine and the 'real world' – randomized controlled trial. *Journal of Clinical Epidemiology*, **55**, 245–252.

Chapter 12
Management During Surgical Procedures

12.1 Key points

- Surgery is a stressful experience that can increase the blood glucose to 6–8 times normal.
- Morning procedure is desirable.
- Insulin should never be omitted in people with Type 1 diabetes.
- The blood glucose should be controlled and complications stabilised before surgery.
- Cease oral agents 24–36 hours preoperatively before the procedure and before discharge.
- Ascertain if the person is taking any complementary therapies especially herbal medicines.
- Instruct patient carefully before the procedure and before discharge.

Rationale

Anaesthesia and surgery are associated with a complex metabolic and neuroendocrine response that involves the release of counter-regulatory hormones and glucagon leading to insulin resistance, gluconeogenesis, reduced glucose use and hyperglycaemia. This response also occurs in people without diabetes but is more pronounced and difficult to manage in people with diabetes.

12.2 Introduction

People with diabetes undergo surgery for the same reasons as those without diabetes; however, because of the long-term complications of diabetes they are more likely to require:

- Cardiac procedures
- Angioplasty
- Bypass surgery
- Amputations (toes, feet)
- Eye surgery such as cataracts, retinal detachment or carpal tunnel decompression.

Surgery results in endocrine, metabolic and long-term effects that have implications for the management of people with diabetes undergoing surgery. Different types of surgery present specific risks as does the age of the person, with the very young and the elderly being particularly at risk. These effects are summarised in Table 12.1. These factors must be controlled in order to prevent ketoacidosis and hyperosmolar coma, to promote healing and reduce the risk of infection postoperatively. Hyperglycaemia affects white cell function and coagulability (Kirschner 1993).

Surgery is increasingly performed as day procedures often without appropriate consideration of the effects of surgical and the related psychological stress on metabolic control. A multidisciplinary approach to planning is important.

Table 12.1 Hormonal, metabolic and long-term effects of surgery.

Hormonal	*Metabolic*	*Long-term effects*
↑ secretion of epinephrine, norepinephrine, ACTH, cortisol and growth hormone ↓ secretion of insulin Insulin resistance	Hyperglycaemia ↓ glucose utilisation ↑ gluconeogenesis ↑ protein catabolism ↑ lipolysis with ↑ ↓ insulin release production of free fatty acids and ketone bodies ↑ risk of cerebrovascular accident, myocardial arrhythmias infarction Electrolyte disorders ↑ metabolic rate ↑ blood pressure and heart rate ↓ peristalsis	Loss of lean body mass – impaired wound healing, ↓ resistance to infection Loss of adipose tissue Deficiency of essential amino acids, vitamins, minerals, and essential fatty acids

The magnitude of the metabolic/hormonal response depends on the severity and duration of the surgical procedure and the presence of complications such as sepsis, acidosis, hypotension and hypovolaemia (Marks *et al.* 1998). Metabolic disturbances can be present in euglycaemic states (De & Child 2001).

12.3 Aims of management

(1) To achieve normal metabolism by supplying sufficient insulin to counterbalance the increase in stress hormones during fasting and surgery (blood glucose between 5 and 10 mmol/L) and avoid the need for prolonged fasting.
(2) To achieve this with regimes which minimise the possibility of errors.
(3) To supply adequate carbohydrate to prevent catabolism and ketosis.
(4) To ensure that the patient undergoes surgery in the best possible physical condition.
(5) To prevent:
- hypoglycaemia, children <5 years are prone to hypoglycaemia during anaesthetics and surgery (Kirschner 1993)
- hyperglycaemia predisposing the patient to ketoacidosis, especially Type 1
- complications of surgery
- electrolyte imbalance

- worsening of pre-existing diabetic complications
- infection.

(6) To avoid undue psychological stress.

12.4 Preoperative nursing care

Good preoperative nursing care is important for both major and minor procedures. Preadmission clinics have an important role in identifying and managing preventable surgical risks. Only rarely, these days people are admitted 2 to 3 days before the operation to stabilise glucose levels. Because many procedures require a day admission only, careful explanation about what is required and *written* instructions about medication adjustment/withdrawal are vital. The individual's blood glucose profile needs to be reviewed and their diabetes regime adjusted to achieve good control prior to surgery. Erratic control could indicate the presence of infection that should be treated prior to surgery. If possible, schedule for a morning procedure to avoid the need for prolonged fasting and counter-regulatory hormone release that leads to hyperglycaemia.

12.4.1 Nursing actions

(1) Confirm time of operation.
(2) Explain procedure and postoperative care to patient. Those patients controlled OHAs or diet may require insulin *during surgery and immediately postoperatively*. They should be aware of this possibility. Insulin during the operative period does not mean that diet- or tablet-controlled patients will remain on insulin when they recover from the procedure.
(3) Ensure all documentation is completed:
    - consent form
    - medication chart
    - monitoring guidelines
    - chest X-ray and other X-rays, scans, MRI (magnetic resonance imaging)
    - ECG.
(4) Sulphonylureas are usually ceased 24 hours preoperatively; metformin and chlorpropamide 36 hours preoperatively. Check medical orders. Metformin should be withdrawn 3 days before surgery because any deterioration in renal function predisposes the patient to lactic acidosis (Gill 1997), see Chapter 10. Insulin therapy must be initiated before the procedure in people with Type 1 diabetes.
(5) Encourage patients who smoke to stop.
(6) Assess:
    - metabolic status: blood glucose control, ketones in blood and urine, hydration status, nutritional status, presence of anaemia, diabetic symptoms
    - educational level and understanding of diabetes
    - family support
    - any known allergies or drug reactions, which should include asking about complementary therapies, particularly herbal therapy use, because some herbs predispose the person to haemorrhage and should be stopped at least 7 days prior to surgery (see Chapter 26)
    - presence of diabetic complications and other comorbidities, e.g. renal, hepatic, cardiac disease (ECG for people >50 years to detect the risk of silent infarction is performed in some units), presence of neuropathy. Patients with autonomic

neuropathy pose special problems while under the anaesthetic: gastroparesis delays gastric emptying and the stomach can be full despite fasting and increases the possibility of regurgitation and inhalation of vomitus; or the vasoconstrictive response to reduced cardiac output may be absent and they may not recognise hypoglycaemia
- current medications
- presence of infection; check feet.
- self-care potential and home support.

Note: Complications should be managed before the operation where possible.

12.5 Major procedures

12.5.1 Day of operation

Premedication and routine preparation for the scheduled operative procedure should be performed according to the treatment sheet and standard protocols.

Where insulin is required, e.g. Type 1 diabetes, major surgery and poor control, an IV infusion is the preferred method of delivering the insulin. The insulin should be balanced with adequate calories to prevent starvation ketosis, e.g. saline/dextrose delivered at a rate that matches the insulin dose (Gill 1997).

Morning procedure

(1) Ensure oral medications have been ceased.
(2) Fast from 12 midnight.
(3) Ascertain insulin regime: commence insulin infusion (see Chapter 7).
(4) Monitor blood glucose 2-hourly.

Afternoon procedure

(1) Fast after an early light breakfast.
(2) Ensure oral medications have been ceased.
(3) Ascertain insulin dose, usually $\frac{1}{2}$ to $\frac{1}{3}$ of usual dose (best given after an IV has been commenced).
(4) It is preferable for IV therapy to be commenced in the ward to:
    - prevent dehydration
    - decrease the risk of hypoglycaemia.

    This will depend on the surgical and anaesthetic team and usual hospital procedure.
(5) Monitor blood glucose.

The anaesthetist is usually responsible for the intraoperative blood glucose monitoring. The patient is dependent on this monitoring to detect hypo- or hyperglycaemia. The usual signs of hypoglycaemia will be masked by the anaesthetic. Precautions are needed to avoid regurgitation and aspiration, cardiac arrhythmias and postural hypotension in young children and patients with autonomic neuropathy. Hypoglycaemia increases the risk of seizures. In all cases careful explanation to the patient and their family/carers is essential.

12.6 Postoperative nursing responsibilities

12.6.1 Immediate care

(1) Monitor and record vital signs.
(2) Maintain an accurate fluid balance.
(3) Monitor blood and urinary glucose/ketones initially 2-hourly.
(4) Observe dressings for signs of haemorrhage or excess discharge.
(5) Ensure drain tubes are patent and draining.
(6) Document all information relating to input and output, especially:

Input	**Output**
IV fluid	Drainage from wound
Oral	Vomitus
EN and TPN	Diarrhoea
	Urine

(7) Maintain care of IV insulin infusion.
(8) Ensure vomiting and pain are controlled.
(9) Ensure psychological needs are addressed, e.g. body image change.
(10) Ensure referral to appropriate allied health professional, e.g. physiotherapist.
(11) Insulin therapy is continued for tablet-controlled patients until they are eating a normal diet and blood glucose levels are stabilised.

12.6.2 Ongoing care

(1) Document all data accurately on the appropriate charts.
(2) Prevent complications:
- infection – aseptic dressing technique including IV sites
- venous thrombosis – anti-embolic stockings, physiotherapy, early ambulation
- hypo/hyperglycaemia.

(3) Diabetes education, instruct patient and their family/carers in wound care and medication management.
(4) Rehabilitation.

Antibiotics and heparin should be administered according to individual patient requirements and medical orders.

Clinical observation

People often have a sore throat for 24 hours after a general anaesthetic. They need to be reassured that this is normal and resolves spontaneously but advised to seek medical advice if it persists.

12.7 Minor procedures

Minor surgery may be performed on an outpatient basis. The metabolic risks are still a consideration if the patient is expected to fast for the procedure. Ensure that the procedure is fully explained to the patient at the time of making the appointment. Give *written* instructions about insulin, oral agents and other medications. Preoperative care is the same as for major surgery on the day of operation as regards:

- Diabetes medications.
- Complications screening and management when present.
- Morning procedure is preferred.

Guidelines for patient instructions
Examples of patient instructions for people undergoing outpatient procedures can be found in Example Instruction Sheets 2 (a) and (b).

N.B. These are examples only and protocols in the nurse's place of employment should be followed. Adjusting medications for investigations and day procedures is becoming more complex as the types of insulin available increase, and multiple injections become common practice.

It is important to consider the individual's blood glucose pattern, the medication regime they are on and the type of procedure they are having when advising them about their diabetes medications.

Where people are on basal bolus regimes and scheduled for a morining procedure, the bedtime insulin dose may need to be reduced and the morning dose omitted. If the procedure is scheduled for the afternoon the morning dose may be given and the lunchtime dose omitted.

When people are on a combination of insulin and oral hypoglycaemic agents the oral agents are usually withheld on the night before the procedure and the morning dose of insulin will be withheld for morning procedures. A reduced dose of insulin will usually be given if the procedure is scheduled for the afternoon.

Practice point

Advice about medications should also include information about medications and complementary therapies the person may be taking besides insulin and oral hypoglycaemic agents.

Morning procedure

(1) Withhold insulin in the morning on the day of the procedure.
(2) Test blood glucose before coming to hospital.
(3) Fast from 12 midnight.
(4) Bring insulin to hospital.
(5) Advise patient to have someone available to drive them home after the procedure.

Afternoon procedure

(1) Light breakfast (e.g. tea and toast).
(2) Fast after this breakfast.
(3) Test blood glucose and ketones in Type 1 before coming to hospital.
(4) Give insulin dose according to blood glucose test as ordered by the doctor.
(5) Explain before discharge:
    - the risk of hypoglycaemia if not eating
    - what to take for pain relief
    - when to recommence OHAs/insulin

- what and when to eat
- any specific care, e.g. wound dressings or care of a biopsy site.

In both cases

(1) Test blood glucose at the end of the procedure and before discharge and administer OHA or insulin dose.
(2) Ensure the patient has appropriate doctor's appointments.
(3) Ensure the patient has someone to accompany them home.
(4) Allay concerns about the procedure.
(5) Provide appropriate care according to the medical orders.
(6) Inspect all wounds before discharge.
(7) It is not advisable to drive, operate machinery or drink alcohol until the following day.

Clinical observations

It is important to ensure the patient and their family/carers understand what is meant by 'fasting' and 'light breakfast'. People have stated that they will 'come as fast as I can but I can only move slowly because of my hips'.

12.8 Emergency procedures

The specific management will depend on the nature of the emergency. If possible the metabolic status should be stabilised before surgery is commenced. The minimum requirements are:

(1) Adequate hydration.
(2) Freedom from hyperglycaemia and especially ketoacidosis (DKA). If the patient presents with an abdominal emergency ensure that it is not due to DKA before operating.

Specific treatment depends on:

- The nature of the emergency
- The time of the last food intake and the presence of autonomic neuropathy/gastric stasis.
- The time and type of the last insulin dose
- Blood glucose levels
- Complications such as cardiac arrhythmias and renal disease.

References

De, P. & Child, D. (2001) Euglycaemic ketoacidosis – is it on the rise? *Practical Diabetes International*, **18** (7), 239–240.

Gill, G. (1997) Surgery and diabetes. In: *Textbook of Diabetes* (eds. G. Williams & J. Pickup), Blackwell Science, Oxford, pp. 820–825.

Kirschner, R. (1993) Diabetes in paediatric ambulatory surgical patients. *Journal of Post Anaesthesia Nursing*, **8** (5), 322–326.

Marks, J., Hirsch, J. & de Fronzo, R. (eds) (1998) *Current Management of Diabetes Mellitus*, C.V. Mosby, St Louis, pp. 247–254.

Example Instruction Sheet 2(a): Instructions for diabetic patients on oral hypoglycaemic agents having procedures as outpatients under sedation of general anaesthesia

INSTRUCTIONS FOR DIABETIC PATIENTS ON ORAL HYPOGLYCAEMIC AGENTS HAVING PROCEDURES AS OUTPATIENTS UNDER SEDATION OR GENERAL ANAESTHESIA

Patient's Name: . . . . UR: . . . .

Time & Date of Appointment: . . . .

IT IS IMPORTANT THAT YOU INFORM NURSING AND MEDICAL STAFF THAT YOU HAVE DIABETES

Morning

If your diabetes is controlled by diet and/or diabetic tablets and you are going to the operating theatre in the morning:

- take nothing by mouth from midnight
- test your blood glucose
- omit your morning diabetic tablets.

Afternoon

If your diabetes is controlled by diet and/or diabetic tablets and you are going to the operating theatre in the afternoon:

- have a light breakfast only (coffee/tea, 2 slices of toast with spread), and nothing by mouth after that
- test your blood glucose
- omit your morning diabetic tablets.

If you have any questions:

Contact: . . . . Telephone: . . . .

Note: The inappropriate paragraph can be deleted or, better still, separate forms can be produced for morning and afternoon procedures.

Example Instruction Sheet 2(b): Instructions for diabetic patients on insulin having procedures as outpatients under sedation or general anaesthesia

INSTRUCTIONS FOR DIABETIC PATIENTS ON INSULIN HAVING PROCEDURES AS OUTPATIENTS UNDER SEDATION OR GENERAL ANAESTHESIA

Patient's Name: . . . . UR: . . . .

Time & Date of Appointment: . . . .

IT IS IMPORTANT THAT YOU INFORM NURSING AND MEDICAL STAFF THAT YOU HAVE DIABETES

Morning

If your diabetes is controlled by insulin and you are going to the operating theatre in the morning:

- take nothing by mouth from midnight
- test your blood glucose
- omit your morning insulin.

Afternoon

If your diabetes is controlled by insulin and you are going to the operating theatre in the afternoon:

- have a light breakfast only (coffee/tea, 2 slices of toast with spread), and nothing by mouth after that
- test your blood glucose
- take . . . . units of insulin.

If you have any questions:

Contact: . . . . Telephone: . . . .

Note: The inappropriate paragraph can be deleted or, better still, separate forms can be produced for morning and afternoon procedures.

Chapter 13
Care During Investigative Procedures

13.1 Key points

- Careful preparation and explanation to the patient and their family/carers.
- Never omit insulin in Type 1 diabetes.
- Radio-opaque dyes may cause tubular necrosis in the elderly diabetic; monitor fluid balance.
- Complementary therapies especially herbs and topical aromatherapy may need to be stopped.

Rationale

Metabolic stress occurs to a lesser degree during investigative procedures than during surgical procedures but still occurs and needs to be managed appropriately to limit adverse outcomes.

Clear written instructions about managing medications and any specific preparation required can improve the individual's understanding and compliance with instructions.

Management protocols for patients undergoing medical tests/procedures such as X-rays, gastroscopy or laser therapy are not as intricate as those for ketoacidosis or major surgery. However, vigilant nursing care is equally important to prevent excursions in blood glucose levels and consequent metabolic effects, and psychological stress.

N.B. Morning procedures are preferred.

13.2 The objectives of care

(1) As for surgical procedures, see Chapter 12.
(2) To ensure correct preparation for the test.
(3) To ensure the procedure has been explained to the patient.
(4) To provide written instructions for the patient if the test is to be performed on an outpatient basis. These instructions should include what to do about their diabetes medications (insulin and oral agents) and any other medications they are taking and how to recognise and manage hypoglycaemia should it occur while the person is fasting.

Usually the doctor referring the person for a procedure should explain the procedure to the individual as part of the process for obtaining informed consent from them to undertake the procedure. It is the nurse's responsibility to ensure instructions have been given and were followed.

13.3 General nursing management

(1) Insulin/oral hypoglycaemic agents:
- insulin is *never omitted* in Type 1 diabetics
- if the patient needs to fast, insulin should be adjusted accordingly
- OHAs are usually withheld on the morning of the test
- ensure written medical instructions are available, including for after the procedure.

(2) Aim for a morning procedure if fasting is required and avoid prolonged fasting that results in a catabolic state and counter-regulatory hormone release (see Chapters 1 and 12).

(3) Monitor blood glucose before and after the test and during the night (3 AM) if fasting and in hospital.

(4) Observe for signs of dehydration. Maintain fluid balance chart if:
- fasting is prolonged
- bowel preparations are required (some may lead to a fluid deficit)
- an IV infusion is commenced
- dehydration in elderly people may predispose them to kidney damage if a radio-opaque contrast medium is used.

An IV infusion may dilute some radio-opaque dyes. The advice of the radiographer should be sought if IV therapy is necessary. Continue IV infusions and oral fluids after the procedure to wash out dyes and contrast medium.

(5) Control nausea and vomiting and pain which can increase the blood glucose level.

(6) Ensure the patient can eat and drink normally after the procedure to avoid hypoglycaemia.

(7) Assess puncture sites (e.g. angiography) before discharge.

(8) Recommence medications as per the medical order.

13.4 Colonoscopy

(1) Iron, aspirin and arthritis medications may need to be stopped one week before the procedure. Diabetes medications should be adjusted according to the procedures outlined for day procedures in Chapter 12.

(2) The day before the colonoscopy clear fluids only are permitted and some form of bowel preparation is usually required to clean out the bowel and allow a better view of the lining. Bowel preparations should be diluted in water because cordial can contribute to diarrhoea. The elderly are at risk of dehydration and should be carefully monitored. Modern preparations are not absorbed and do not usually lead to significant electrolyte disturbances.

(3) Fasting for at least 6 hours is usually necessary.

13.5 Eye procedures

People with diabetes are more prone to visual impairment and blindness than the general population. The eye manifestations of diabetes can affect all ocular structures. The time of appearance, rate of progression and severity of eye disease vary between individuals. However, most patients have some evidence of damage after 25 years of diabetes and vision is threatened in 10% of people with diabetes.

Retinopathy is symptomless and may remain undetected if the eyes are not examined regularly by an ophthalmologist. Fluorescein angiography and retinal photography may aid in determining the severity of the disease. Management aims at conserving vision, and laser therapy is often effective in this respect.

Risk factors for eye disease include hypertension, pregnancy, nephropathy, hyperlipidaemia and smoking.

13.5.1 Care of patient having fluorescein angiography

Fluorescein angiography is usually an outpatient procedure. The reasons for the test and the procedure should be carefully explained to the patient. They should be aware that:

- Transient nausea may occur.
- The skin and urine may become yellow for 12–24 hours.
- Drinking adequate amounts of fluid will help flush the dye out of the system.
- The dye is injected into a vein.

13.5.2 Care of the patient having laser therapy (photocoagulation)

'Laser' is an acronym for light amplification stimulated emission of radiation. There are many types of laser. The ones that are used to treat diabetic patients are the argon, krypton and diode lasers. The lasers absorb light, which is converted to heat, which coagulates the tissue. Laser therapy is frequently used to treat diabetic retinopathy and glaucoma.

Goals of photocoagulation
To maintain vision:

- By allowing fluid exchange to occur and reducing fluid accumulation in the retina.
- By photocoagulating the retina, which is ischaemic, and thereby causing new vessels that are prone to haemorrhage, to regress.

Laser therapy is usually performed on an outpatient basis. Fasting is not required and medication adjustment is unnecessary.

Practice point

Laser therapy may not increase vision, but can prevent further loss of vision.

Nursing responsibilities
Ensure the purpose of laser therapy has been explained to the patient.

(1) Before the procedure the patient should know that:
- the procedure is uncomfortable
- the pupil of the eye will be dilated
- anaesthetic drops may be used
- the laser beam causes bright flashes of light

- vision will be blurred for some time after the laser treatment
- they should test their blood glucose before and after laser treatment
- they should not drive home.

(2) After the procedure the patient should know that:
- sunglasses will protect the eye and help reduce discomfort
- spots can be seen for 24–48 hours
- there can be some discomfort for 2–3 weeks
- headache may develop after the procedure
- paracetamol may be taken to relieve pain

Practice point

Aspirin is best avoided because of its anticoagulant effect. If new vessels are present due to retinopathy they can bleed and threaten sight.

- activities which will increase intraocular pressure for 24–36 hours, e.g. lifting heavy objects, straining at stool, should be avoided
- night vision may be temporarily decreased
- vision to the side may be permanently diminished; this is known as 'tunnel vision'.

Practice point

Blurred vision does not necessarily indicate serious eye disease. It can occur during both hypo- and hyperglycaemia. Vision often also becomes worse when diabetic control is improved, e.g. after commencement of insulin therapy. Although this is distressing for the patient, vision usually improves in 6–8 weeks. Prescriptions for glasses obtained in these circumstances may be inappropriate. Glasses are best obtained when the eyes settle down.

The nursing care of people who are vision impaired is discussed in Chapter 14.

13.6 Care of the patient having radiocontrast media injected

Radiocontrast media are excreted through the kidneys. Fasting is often required. The patient can become dehydrated, especially if kept waiting for long periods, and kidney complications can occur. Patients most at risk:

- Are over 50 years old
- Have established kidney disease
- Have had diabetes for more than 10 years
- Are hypertensive
- Have proteinuria
- Have an elevated serum creatinine.

Kidney problems caused by radiocontrast media may not produce symptoms. A decreased urine output following procedures requiring radiocontrast media may indicate kidney damage and should be investigated.

13.6.1 Management

(1) Ensure appropriate preparation has been carried out.
(2) Ensure the patient is well hydrated before the procedure (intravenous therapy may be needed).
(3) Maintain an accurate fluid balance chart.
(4) Avoid delays in performing the procedure.
(5) Monitor urine output after the procedure.
(6) Assess serum creatinine after the procedure.
(7) Maintain good diabetic control.
(8) Encourage the patient to drink to help flush out the contrast media.

Chapter 14

Special Situations and Unusual Conditions Related to Diabetes

Introduction

This chapter outlines some specific conditions that are encountered in the care of people with diabetes. They are often managed in specialised services and some are very rare. A basic knowledge about these conditions can alert nurses to the possibility that they could be present, allow appropriate nursing care plans to be formulated and facilitate early referral.

The conditions covered in this chapter are:

14a: Enteral and parenteral nutrition
14b: Diabetes and cancer
14c: Autonomic neuropathy
14d: Corticosteroids
14e: Brittle diabetes
14f: Teeth and gums
14g: Haemochromotosis and iron overload
14h: Breast mastopathy

Practice point

The policies and procedures of the employing institution for the care of central lines, dialysis equipment and nasogastric tubes should be adhered to.

14a Enteral and parenteral nutrition

14.1 Key points

- Strict asepsis is important.
- Ensure patency of tubes.
- Weigh regularly.
- Maintain accurate fluid balance chart.
- Monitor blood glucose.
- Monitor serum electrolytes, albumin, urea and lipids to ascertain nutritional status (see Chapter 5).

Enteral and parenteral nutrition supply nutritional requirements in special circumstances such as malnourished patients admitted with a debilitating disease and where there is a risk of increasing the malnourishment, e.g. fasting states. Malnourishment leads to increased mortality and morbidity thus increasing length of stay (Middleton *et al.* 2001). Often the patient is extremely ill or has undergone major gastrointestinal, head or neck surgery or has gastroparesis diabeticorum, a rare complication specific to diabetes that leads to delayed gastric emptying and can result in hypoglycaemia due to delayed food absorption, bloating and abdominal pain and is very distressing for the patient (see Section c).

14.2 Aims of therapy

(1) Decrease anxiety associated with the procedure by thorough explanation.
(2) Prevent sepsis.
(3) Maintain an acceptable blood glucose range (4–10 mmol/L).
(4) Maintain normal urea, electrolytes, LFTs and blood gas levels.
(5) Supply adequate nutrition in terms of protein, fat and carbohydrate.
(6) Achieve positive nitrogen balance.
(7) Prevent complications of therapy.
(8) The long-term aim of enteral/parenteral feeding is the return of the patient to oral feeding. However, in some cases with reduced life expectancy or the elderly it may be permanent.

14.2.1 Complications of enteral nutrition

(1) Mechanical problems such as aspiration, poor gastric emptying and reflux can occur especially if the person has altered mental status and a suppressed gag reflex.
(2) Metabolic consequences include hyperglycaemia and hypernatraemia depending on the feed used, the supplements added to the feed and with high feeding rate. Feeding into the small bowel rather than the stomach can minimise these disturbances. People who cannot indicate that they are thirsty and who have altered mental status, particularly the elderly, are at risk of these metabolic consequences.

    Hypoglycaemia can occur if food is not absorbed, the calorie load is reduced and if there are blockages in the feeding tubes.
(3) Gastrointestinal problems, the most common is diarrhoea, which is usually osmotic in nature.

14.3 Routes of administration

14.3.1 Enteral feeds

This route supplies nutrients and fluids via an enteral tube when the oral route is inadequate or obstructed. Feeds are administered via a nasogastric, duodenal, jejunal or gastrostomy tube.

Enteral feeding is preferred over parenteral feeding when the gut is functioning normally and oral feeds do not meet the patient's nutritional requirements (McClave *et al.* 1999). Nasogastric tubes may be used in the short term. Nasogastric feeds have a significant risk of pulmonary aspiration. The tubes are easily removed by confused patients and cause irritation to the nasal mucosa and external nares that can be uncomfortable and is an infection risk in immunocompromised patients.

Duodenal and jejunal tubes do not carry the same risk of pulmonary aspiration but the feeds can contribute to gastric intolerance and bloating.

Gastroscopy tubes are used in the long term where the stomach is not involved in the primary disease. This may preclude their use in people with established autonomic neuropathy that involves the gastrointestinal tract. The tubes can be inserted through a surgical incision and the creation of a stoma. A second, increasingly common method uses percutaneous endoscopic techniques (PEG) (Thomas 2001). In these procedures an artificial tract is made between the stomach and the abdominal wall through which a tube is inserted. The tube can be a balloon tube or a button type that is more discrete and lies flat to the skin. An extension tube is inserted into the gastroscopy tube during feeding.

14.3.2 Gastrostomy (PEG) feeds

Feeds can usually be undertaken 12–24 hours after the insertion of the tube. They can be given as early as 4–6 hours in special circumstances. The initial feed may be water and or dextrose saline depending on the patient's condition.

Mode of administration

(1) Bolus instillation – may result in distension and delayed gastric emptying. Aspiration can occur. Diarrhoea may be a complication. *This method is not suitable for people with diabetes who have autonomic neuropathy, especially gastroparesis.*
(2) Continuous infusion – via gravity infusion or pump. This can lead to hyperinsulinaemia in Type 2 diabetes because glucose-mediated insulin production occurs. Administering insulin via the IV route allows the caloric input to be balanced with the insulin requirements but is not suitable for long-term use.

The strength of the feeds should be increased gradually to prevent a sudden overwhelming glucose load in the bloodstream. An IV insulin infusion is an ideal method to control blood glucose levels.

The feeds usually contain protein, fat and carbohydrate. The carbohydrate is in the form of dextrose, either 25% or 40%, and extra insulin may be needed to account for the glucose load. A balance must be achieved between caloric requirements and blood glucose levels. Patients who are controlled by OHAs will usually need insulin while on enteral feeding.

14.3.2 Parenteral feeds

This is administration of nutrients and fluids by routes other than the alimentary canal, i.e. intravenously via a peripheral or central line.

Mode of administration
Parenteral supplements are either partial or total.

(1) Peripheral – used after gastrointestinal surgery and in malabsorption states. Peripheral access is usually reserved for people in whom central access is difficult or sometimes as a supplement to oral/enteral feeds. It is not suitable if a high dextrose supplement is needed because dextrose irritates the veins, causing considerable discomfort.
(2) Central – supplies maximum nutrition in the form of protein, carbohydrate, fats, trace elements, vitamins and electrolytes. For example, in patients with cancer or burns, larger volumes can be given than via the peripheral route. Provides long-term access because silastic catheters can be left *in situ* indefinitely. If patients are at risk of sepsis, the site of the central line is rotated weekly using strict aseptic technique. Insulin can be added to the bag (*clear* insulin only). The use of a central line allows the patient to remain mobile, which aids digestion.

14.4 Choice of formula

The particular formula selected depends on the nutritional assessment and absorptive capacity of the patient. It is usual to begin with half strength formula and gradually increase to full strength as tolerated. The aim is to supply adequate:

- Fluid
- Protein
- Carbohydrate
- Vitamins and minerals
- Sodium spread evenly over the 24 hours.

Nutritional requirements can vary from week to week and careful monitoring of the patient and formula adjustment are essential.

Diabetes medication, insulin or oral agents, are adjusted according to the pattern that emerges in the blood glucose profile. The dose depends on the feeds used as well as the person's condition. Generally the medication dose is calculated according to the caloric intake.

14.5 Nursing responsibilities

14.5.1 Care of nasogastric tube

(1) Explain purpose of tube to patient.
(2) Check position of the tube regularly to ensure it is in the stomach and prevent pulmonary aspiration.
(3) Confirm position with X-ray.
(4) Change position in nose daily to avoid pressure areas.
(5) Flush regularly to ensure patency.

(6) Check residual gastric volumes regularly to avoid gastric distension and the possibility of aspiration, especially if gastroparesis is present.

14.5.2 Care of PEG tubes

The same care required for nasogastric tubes applies. Additional care:

(1) Monitor gastric aspirates at least daily.
(2) Elevated the head of the bed where there is a risk of pulmonary aspiration.
(3) Weigh the patient to ensure the desired weight outcome is achieved.
(4) Monitor nutritional status, see Chapter 5.
(5) Manage nausea and vomiting if they occur because they increase the risk of aspiration and are uncomfortable for the patient. Record the amount and type of any vomitus. Antinausea medication may be required. Warm herbal teas such as chamomile, peppermint or ginger may be non-drug alternatives for some people.
(6) If the PEG tube blocks it can sometimes be cleared with a fizzy soft drink but local protocol should be followed because fizzy drinks can lead to electrolyte imbalances if used frequently.
(7) Ensure there is adequate fluid in the feeds to avoid dehydration and the consequent risk of hyperosmolar coma, see Chapter 10 (Thomas 2001).

14.5.3 Care of IV and central lines

(1) Dress regularly.
(2) Check position of central line on chest X-ray.
(3) Maintain strict aseptic technique.
(4) Maintain patency, usually by intermittent installation of heparinised saline (weekly or when line is changed).
(5) Patients should be supine when the central catheter is disconnected and IV giving sets should be carefully primed to minimise the risk of air embolism.
(6) Check catheter for signs of occlusion (e.g. resistance to infusion or difficulty in withdrawing blood sample). Reposition patient: if occlusion still present consult doctor.
(7) Observe exit site for any tenderness, redness or swelling. If bleeding occurs around suture or exit apply pressure and notify doctor.
(8) Monitor the patient for signs of infection, e.g. fever.

14.5.4 General nursing care

(1) Ensure dietitian referral.
(2) Maintain an accurate fluid balance chart, including loss from stomas, drain tubes, vomitus and diarrhoea.
(3) Monitor serum albumin, urea and electrolytes to determine nutritional requirements, nitrogen balance and energy requirements.
(4) Weigh regularly (weekly) at the same time, using same scales and wearing similar clothing to ensure energy balance and sufficient calories are supplied. Excess calories leads to weight gain and hyperglycaemia. Insufficient calories leads to weight loss and the risk of hypoglycaemia.
(5) Monitor blood glucose regularly, at least 4-hourly, initially. If elevated, be aware of possibility of a hyperosmolar event (see Chapter 10). If stable, monitor less frequently.

(6) Record temperature, pulse and respiration and report if elevated (>38°C) or if any respiratory distress occurs.
(7) Check the date and appearance of all infusions before administration.
(8) Medications are given separately from the formula except insulin and anti-coagulants, which can be added to the formula. Follow pump instructions carefully.
(9) Skin fold thickness and mid-arm muscle circumference measurement can also be useful to ascertain weight loss/gain.
(10) Skin care around tube insertion sites and stoma care for gastrostomy tubes to avoid infection.

14.5.5 Care when recommencing oral feeds

(1) Monitor blood glucose very carefully. Long-acting insulin is usually commenced at this time so there is a risk of hypoglycaemia.
(2) Monitor any nausea or vomiting, describe vomitus.
(3) Maintain accurate fluid balance chart, usually 2-hourly subtotals.

References

McClave, S., Snider, H. & Spain, D. (1999) Use of residual volume as a marker for enteral feeding intolerance: prospective blinded comparison with physical examination and radiographic findings. *Journal of Parenteral and Enteral Nutrition*, **16**, 64s–70s.

Middleton, M., Nazarenko, G., Nivison-Smith, I. & Smerdley, P. (2001) Prevalence of malnutrition and 12-month incidence of mortality in two Sydney teaching hospitals. *Medical Journal of Australia*, **31**, 455–461.

Thomas, B. (2001) *A Manual of Dietetic Practice*. Blackwell Science, Oxford, pp. 86–87.

14b Diabetes and cancer

14.6 Key points

- Management depends on the prognosis.
- Provide psychological support.
- Use aseptic techniques.
- Monitor nutritional status.
- Control pain, nausea, vomiting.
- Monitor blood glucose.

Cancer occurs in people with diabetes with the same frequency as in the general population, with the exception of cancer of the pancreas. However, there is no evidence that diabetes leads to pancreatic cancer.

The management of the cancer itself is the same for people with diabetes as for other people; however, some extra considerations apply. Cancer cells trap amino acids for their own use, limiting the protein available for normal functions. This sets the scene for weight loss, especially where the appetite is poor, and the senses of smell and taste are diminished. Weight loss is further exacerbated by malabsorption, nausea and vomiting and radiation treatment. Glucose enters cancer cells down a concentration gradient rather than through insulin-mediated entry and metabolism favours lactate production that is transported to the liver, increasing gluconeogenesis. Hypoalbuminaemia also occurs.

For the person with diabetes this can lead to hyperglycaemia and decreased insulin production, with consequent effects on blood glucose control, and may lead to delayed wound healing.

Diabetic management should be considered in relation to the prognosis and the anti-cancer therapy. Preventing the long-term complications of diabetes may be irrelevant in these people, therefore striving for very good control may not be recommended.

Specific treatment will vary according to the type of cancer the patient has. Diagnosis of some types of cancer (e.g. endocrine tumours) can involve prolonged fasting and radiological imaging and/or other radiological procedures. The appropriate care should be given in these circumstances (see Chapter 13).

Steroid therapy is frequently used in the treatment of cancers, and to relieve cerebral oedema. The steroids may be given over a prolonged time or in large doses for a short period. Steroids are antagonistic to insulin and their use can lead to high blood glucose levels, even in people without diabetes. Therefore urine and blood glucose will be monitored regularly in patients on steroid medications (see Section 14d).

14.7 Objectives of care

In addition to the specific management of the cancer indicated by the cancer type and prognosis, diabetes management aims are:

(1) To achieve as good a lifestyle as possible for as long as possible.
(2) To achieve an acceptable blood glucose range in order to avoid the distressing symptoms associated with hyperglycaemia.
(3) To prevent malnutrition, dehydration with possible consequent hypoglycaemia, delayed healing and decreased resistance to infection. Diet should be appropriate for

the presenting cancer symptom and in some cases is part of the treatment of some cancers. Sufficient protein and carbohydrate are needed for hormone synthesis and to maintain stores that are being depleted by the cancer. Small frequent feeds; enteral or parenteral feeds may be needed, see Section 14a. High fibre diets can cause diarrhoea, vomiting and bloating if the cancer involves the bowel.

(4) To control pain.
(5) To prevent trauma.
(6) To monitor renal and hepatic function during administration of cytotoxic drugs.
(7) To provide education and psychological support.

14.8 Nursing responsibilities

(1) To provide a safe environment.
(2) To consider the psychological aspects of having cancer and diabetes (fear of death, body image changes, denial).
(3) To ensure appropriate diabetic education if diabetes develops as a consequence of the altered metabolism of cancer.
(4) To attend to pressure areas, including the feet and around nasogastric tubes.
(5) To provide oral care, and ensure a dental consultation occurs.
(6) To control nausea, vomiting and pain.
(7) To monitor blood glucose levels as frequently as necessary.
(8) To chart accurately fluid balance, blood glucose, TPR, weight.
(9) To ensure referral to the dietitian, psychologist, diabetes nurse specialist/educator.
(10) To be aware of the possibility of hypoglycaemia if the patient is not eating, is vomiting or has a poor appetite. Where the appetite is poor and food intake is inadequate hypoglycaemia is a significant risk. QID insulin regimes using rapid-acting insulin such as Novorapid or Humalog may reduce the hypoglycaemia risk. Oral hypoglycaemic agents may need to be stopped because of their duration of action which increases the risk of hypoglycaemia. In addition, if hypoglycaemia does occur it can be more profound and the energy reserves may be insufficient to correct it.
(11) To be aware of the possibility of hyperglycaemia as a result of medications such as steroids, and pain and stress.
(12) Short-acting sulphonylureas or insulin may be indicated in Type 2 diabetes. Biguanides may be contraindicated if renal or hepatic failure is present because of the risk of lactic acidosis.
(13) To monitor biochemistry results and report abnormal results.
(14) To provide appropriate care during investigative and surgical procedures, see Chapters 12 and 13.
(15) To consider the possibility that people with cancer often try complementary therapies in an attempt to cure their cancer. It is important to ask about the use of complementary therapies and provide or refer the person for appropriate information about the risks and benefits of such therapies (see Chapter 26).
(16) To maintain skin integrity by appropriate skin care especially where steroid medications are used. They cause the skin to become thin and fragile and it is easily damaged during shaving and routine nursing care, and brittle hair can exacerbate the effects of chemotherapy and bone loss. Steroids are also associated with mood changes which can cause distress to the patient and their relatives. Careful explanations and reassurance are required.

Clinical observations

(1) Narcotic pain medication can mask the signs of hypoglycaemia.
(2) Insulin/oral agents may need to be adjusted frequently to meet the changing metabolic needs. In the late stages of cancer they may be withheld, so long as the patient is comfortable and not subject to excursions in blood glucose that can lead to discomfort.

Practice point

Since the introduction of serotonin inhibitors, e.g. Ondansetron, to control nausea and vomiting, these effects of anticancer therapy have decreased. Consequently there is less disruption of normal eating patterns.

Reference

Jung, R.T. & Sikora, K. (1984) *Endocrine Problems in Cancer*. Heinemann Medical Books, London.

14c: Autonomic neuropathy

14.9 Key Points

- Often several organs are involved.
- Signs and symptoms are often non-specific.
- Autonomic neuropathy is often undiagnosed.
- Postural hypotension is the most significant sign of autonomic neuropathy.
- People with postural hypotension and nocturnal diarrhoea should be investigated for autonomic neuropathy.
- The progression to autonomic neuropathy is related to poor metabolic control.
- It is more common in people over 65 but it can occur in the first year after diagnosis.

Rationale

Autonomic neuropathy is a distressing condition for people with diabetes. It can cause erratic blood glucose readings. People are often accused of manipulating their food and/or diabetic medications, which causes stress and anxiety. The symptoms associated with the various manifestations of autonomic neuropathy can be uncomfortable, painful and have an adverse impact on the individual's quality of life.

14.10 Introduction

The autonomic nervous system plays an important role in the regulation of carbohydrate metabolism. Many processes are affected by it, e.g. it both facilitates and inhibits insulin secretion.

(1) Stimulation of the right vagus nerve, which innervates the pancreatic islet cells, or the beta-adrenergic receptors in the islet cells, stimulates insulin secretion.
(2) Stimulation of the alpha-adrenergic receptors in the islet cells decreases insulin secretion.

This is an aspect of blood glucose regulation essential to maintaining glucose homeostasis.

The autonomic nervous system also has a role in the conversion of glycogen to glucose in the liver where free fatty acids undergo further metabolism to ketones. Neurogenic stimulation of the hypo-pituitary axis results in cortisol secretion, one of the counter-regulatory hormones that have a role in correcting hypoglycaemia. In stress situations, especially prolonged stress, hyperglycaemia results (Feinglos & Surwit 1988).

Diabetes is the commonest cause of autonomic neuropathy but it also occurs in association with other diseases such as advanced Parkinson's disease and Guillain-Barre syndrome.

Autonomic neuropathy is a common, under-diagnosed condition associated with a range of signs and symptoms, depending on the specific nerves and organs affected (Vinik *et al.* 2000, Aly & Weston 2002). It has a slow onset and affects up to 30–40% of people with diabetes, and although many people only have mild, often subclinical features, significant functional abnormalities can be present.

Rarely, in <5% of cases, overt clinical features develop. Autonomic neuropathy can involve any system, but commonly affects the heart, GIT and genitourinary systems (Spallone & Menzinger 1997). The GIT is one of the most frequently affected systems but GIT problems, not associated with autonomic neuropathy, occur in 50% of the general population and are more common in people with diabetes (Lock *et al.* 2000). Older people are at risk of having many neuropathic GIT changes but some GIT changes are age-related or associated with the use of vasoconstrictive drugs (Aly & Weston 2002). Therefore many factors can be involved in an individual.

Practice points

(1) Autonomic neuropathy is physically uncomfortable and treatment options are limited. Where the GIT is involved, frequent adjustment to the food and medication regime is often needed. Blood glucose monitoring is important to allow such changes to be made appropriately.
(2) Psychological distress is common. Support and understanding are important aspects of management.

The commonly affected systems and associated clinical manifestations are shown in Table 14.1.

14.11 Diagnosis and management

Special tests are required to make a definitive diagnosis. The particular test depends on which organs are being tested, e.g. gastric emptying times for the GIT, Valsalva manoeuvre for the cardiovascular system and voiding cystourethrogram to determine the effects on the bladder. In many cases specific treatment is commenced on the basis of the clinical history and assessment.

Management consists of:

(1) Adopting preventative strategies early by:
   - improving blood glucose control and lipid levels.
   - treating hypertension.
   - regular complication screening.
   - adequate self-care.
   - being aware that antioxidants may have a role in preventing oxidative tissue damage.
(2) Direction when present.

Treatment is often by trial and error and is aimed at alleviating the unpleasant symptoms. Preventative measures should be continued. Treatment for specific autonomic neuropathic conditions consists of:

(1) Gastrointestinal tract
   Small, light, frequent meals that are low in fat. Fat delays gastric emptying and exacerbates the already slow gastric emptying time.
   - Using gluten free foods could help some people.
   - Medications such as Metoclopramide and Cisapride may give some relief but should not be used continuously.

Table 14.1 Organs commonly affected by diabetic autonomic neuropathy and the resultant clinical features.

Affected organ	*Main clinical features*	*Consequences*
Gastrointestinal tract (gastroparesis)	Decreased peristalsis Abdominal distension and feeling of fullness Early satiety Postprandial nausea Vomiting undigested food Diarrhoea, especially at night Depression	Weight loss Erratic blood glucose control Stomach may not be empty even after fasting, e.g. for procedures
Urinary tract	Distended bladder Urine overflow Feeling of incomplete bladder emptying Stress incontinence Nocturia Vaginal mucous membrane excoriation in women	Silent urinary tract infection Falls in elderly people Sleep disturbance Uncomfortable sexual intercourse
Genitals	Erectile dysfunction in men Indeterminate, if any effect in women Possibly vaginal dryness in older women	Psychological sequelae including depression Negative impact on sexual health
Cardiovascular system	Blood pressure: Postural hypotension Loss of diurnal variation Dizziness when standing Resting tachycardia Reduced sympathetic tone Decreased beta-adrenergic responsiveness	Silent myocardial infarction Stroke Falls
Lower limbs	Reduced sweating Reduced blood flow Reduced pain Redness Defective thermoregulation	Foot ulcers and infection Sleep disturbance
Brain	Cognitive impairment	Reduced self-care ability
General	Excessive sweating, especially of the upper body, resembling a hot flush and sometimes mistaken for hypoglycaemia Slow pupillary reaction Heat intolerance	Trauma Depression

Note: Many of these conditions predispose elderly people to falls (see Chapter 18).

- Antibiotics such as Tetracycline or Trimethoprim, may be required to treat bacterial overgrowth that occurs as a consequence of gastric stasis.
- Cholestyramine can be used to chelate bile salts, which immobilise the gut.
- Treating constipation, nausea and vomiting as they occur.
- Elevating the head of the bed to use gravity to assist gastric emptying.
- Jejunostomy is a last resort.

(2) Cardiovascular system
- Support garments such as stockings or a body stocking to support venous return and relieve stress on the heart. They should be put on while the person is lying down.
- Managing postural hypotension – finding a balance between increasing the pressure on standing and preventing hypertension when lying. Fludrocortisone or Midodrine can be used. Medications should be reviewed to exclude drugs that precipitate postural hypotension.

(3) Genitourinary
- Urinary catheterisation and self-catheterisation. Sometimes parasympathomimetic drugs are also used.
- Managing erectile dysfunction with drugs such as Sildenafil, intracavernosal injections or mechanical and implanted devices and counselling (see Chapter 17).

(4) General measures
- Adjusting insulin or OHAs and diet to cater for the erratic blood glucose profile.
- Topical glycopyrrolate to alleviate gustatory sweating.
- Stopping smoking.
- Careful explanations about autonomic neuropathy and counselling to address the psychological consequences and treatment options.
- Encouraging activity.

14.12 Nursing care

Nursing care is palliative and supportive in nature. Providing a safe environment and reducing the risk of falls is essential, especially in older people, to prevent trauma, e.g. fractures. This could involve ensuring the home environment is safe before discharging patients.

Nurses can have a role in the early identification of autonomic neuropathy by having a level of suspicion and taking a careful history.

Important nursing responsibilities are:

(1) The prevention, early recognition and management of hypoglycaemia.
(2) Taking care when moving the patient from a lying to a sitting position, and from sitting to standing. Give them time for the blood pressure to adjust. Ensure their footwear will not contribute to the risk of falling.
(3) Providing adequate foot care and appropriate advice to minimise the risk of ulcers, including advice about footwear.
(4) Arranging counselling if indicated.
(5) Using aseptic technique.
(6) Being alert to the possibility of silent pathology – myocardial infarction, urinary tract infection.
(7) Encouraging people to remain physically active within their individual limits. Physical activity aids many body systems and improves mental outlook.

Clinical observation

Gentle abdominal massage and warm compresses can help alleviate the discomfort of gastroparesis. Aromatherapy essential oils can be added to the compress. The abdomen is a vulnerable part of the body and this needs to be taken into consideration when offering an abdominal massage (see Chapter 26).

References

Aly, N. & Weston, P. (2002) Autonomic neuropathy in older people with diabetes. *Journal of Diabetes Nursing*, **6** (1), 10–14.

Locke, D., Ill, G. & Camileri, M. (2000) Gastrointestinal symptoms among persons with diabetes in the community. *Archives of Internal Medicine*, **160**, 2808–2816.

Spallone, V. & Menzinger, G. (1997) Autonomic neuropathy: clinical and instrumental findings. *Clinical Neuroscience*, **4** (96), 346–358.

Surwit, R. & Feinglos, M. (1988) Stress and autonomic nervous system in Type 2 diabetes. A hypothesis. *Diabetes Care*, **11**, 83–85.

Vinik, A., Stansberry, K. & Pittenger, G. (2000) Diabetic neuropathies. *Diabetalogia*, **43**, 957–973.

14.4d Diabetes and corticosteroid medications

14.13 Key points

- Corticosteroid medications predispose the person to insulin resistance, dose-related hyperglycaemia, and hyperinsulinaemia.
- They are used to control disease processes or are given as hormone replacement therapy for some endocrine diseases, e.g. pituitary tumours. In the latter case corticosteroid doses are usually small or physiological levels and are less likely to cause hyperglycaemia.
- People on high doses, long-term or intermittent corticosteroids should be monitored and should test their blood glucose.

Rationale

Steroid medications are very effective for a range of conditions. They predispose the individual to hyperglycaemia in both the short and long term.

14.14 Introduction

Steroids are naturally occurring hormones produced by the adrenal glands under the control of the pituitary hormone ACTH. There are three major classes of steroids:

(1) Glucocorticoids
(2) Mineralocorticoids
(3) Androgen and oestrogen.

Glucocorticoids affect blood glucose.

Corticosteroid drugs are an essential part of the management of inflammatory disease processes, haematologic malignancies, allergic reactions and shock. The long-term use, especially in high doses, predisposes the individual to steroid-induced diabetes or to hyperglycaemia in people with established diabetes.

Corticosteroids have the propensity to cause insulin resistance, increased hepatic glucose output, reduced glucose transport and to inhibit insulin secretion resulting in hyperglycaemia.

14.15 Effect on blood glucose

The effect on blood glucose depends to some extent on the duration of the biological action of the steroid preparation used. Hyperglycaemia usually occurs with doses of Prednisolone (or equivalent) > 7.5 mg/day.

Specific short courses of corticosteroids usually affect the blood glucose temporarily or not at all, but hyperglycaemia occurs if the dose is increased or the medication is needed intermittently or in the long term (Williams & Pickup 1992). If given for less than one week, even large doses do not usually present problems, although impaired glucose tolerance can be present and can occur in 48 hours. IV steroids usually have a shorter duration of action than steroids given by other routes and do not increase the blood glucose if only 1–2 doses are given (Jackson & Bowman 1995).

14.16 Predisposing factors

People with existing risk factors for diabetes run the greatest risk of developing steroid-induced diabetes. These risks are described in Chapter 1. They include the following conditions:

- Old age.
- Existing impaired glucose tolerance.
- Current or previous GDM.
- Cardiac disease.
- Psychosis.

The presence of one or more of these risk factors may influence the decision to use steroids and the dose. In many cases steroids are the drugs of choice and management strategies seek to minimise the risk of developing diabetes.

14.17 Management

- Screen for the risk factors for diabetes before commencing steroids.
- Where diabetes is present, diabetic medications need to be reviewed and may require adjustment according to the blood glucose profile. In many cases the blood glucose increases towards the end of the day.
- Over 50% of people with Type 2 diabetes treated with OHAs require insulin if they require corticosteroids, sometimes permanently (Williams & Pickup 1992).
- Select the optimal route of administration for the particular problem: oral, IV, inhaled, cream.
- Use the lowest effective dose for the shortest possible time.
- Monitor blood glucose 4-hourly if the person has diabetes and at least weekly if they do not.
- Monitor for ketones, especially in Type 1 diabetes because steroids predispose them to DKA.
- Explain to the patient the reasons for the blood glucose monitoring, especially if they do not have diabetes. Reassure them that steroids are the best drug choice for their condition and that hyperglycaemia can be controlled.
- Steroids required on a temporary basis must be withdrawn gradually to allow the pituitary–adrenal axis to return to normal activity (Jackson & Bowman 1995).
- If OHAs/insulin doses were commenced or increased they will need to be reduced as the steroid dose is reduced to avoid hypoglycaemia.
- Prolonged steroid use depresses the immune system. Aseptic technique is important if any invasive procedures are required and the immune system should be supported with a healthy diet and regular activity within the individual's tolerance level.

  Steroids can mask some of the signs and symptoms of infection, as can diabetes. Common infection sites should be closely monitored, e.g. injection sites, feet, mouth and gums and the urinary tract.
- The skin can become thin and fragile and easily damaged if steroids are required in the

long term, predisposing the individual to bruising, skin tears, ulcers and other trauma, especially in the elderly. A skin care regime that protects the skin is important.

- Protecting the elderly from falls that predispose to trauma is essential where long-term steroids are required because of the effects on bone and the increased risk of fractures.
- Alternate-day steroid regimes show greater effects on the blood glucose on the day steroid medications are taken. OHA/insulin regimes for steroid and non-steroid days may be needed.
- Insulin is often required for people on OHAs if long-term steroids are required or if hyperglycaemia persists despite compliance with their OHAs, and an appropriate diet.
- Where permanent steroid therapy is required, e.g. after surgery for a pituitary tumour, the steroid dose usually needs to be increased during illness or surgery. Careful, *written* instructions detailing how to manage steroid dose reductions in these circumstances and close liaison with their endocrinologist is essential. OHAs/insulin will also need to be adjusted in these circumstances.
- Achieving acceptable growth and development in children on permanent steroids is important and should be closely monitored. Growth hormone may be required.
- Body image changes can occur when the steroid affects such as weight gain, moon face, thinning hair and acne develop.
- Steroids can cause mental changes ranging from mild changes to psychosis, which can affect the person's self-care. If psychosis occurs it will need to be managed appropriately. The help of a psychiatrist may be necessary.

References

Dunning, T. (1996) Corticosteroids medications and diabetes mellitus. *Practical Diabetes International*, **13**, 186–188.

Jackson, R. & Bowman, R. (1995) Corticosteroids. *Medical Journal of Australia*, **162**, 663–665.

Williams, G. & Pickup, J. (1992) *Handbook of Diabetes*. Blackwell Science, Oxford.

14e Brittle diabetes

14.18 Key points

- A careful holistic history is essential.
- Wide fluctuations in blood glucose are characteristic.
- DKA and hypoglycaemia are significant risks.
- Frequent hospital admissions are common.
- Management takes a long time and requires patience, support and a non-judgemental attitude.

Rationale

Brittle diabetes is a contentious issue. Understanding and time are required to manage the condition, and frequent hospital admissions are common.

14.19 Introduction

There is no easy way to define brittle diabetes. Some experts consider it to be a psychological condition; others regard it as having a physical basis. Brittle diabetes usually refers to wide fluctuations in the blood glucose level despite optimal medical management. Whichever definition is used, brittle diabetes is difficult to manage and requires an holistic approach. Repeated admissions to hospital for bouts of DKA or severe hypoglycaemia are common.

The causes of brittle diabetes are multifactorial. It is easy to ascribe the problem to social/psychological factors alone but this is often not the case. However, there is a subset of people with diabetes, usually young women with Type 1 who have psychosocial problems who manipulate their insulin and have frequent hospital admissions.

14.20 Management

Management is protracted and requires a great deal of patience and support for the person with diabetes and their family. Taking a careful holistic history and a thorough physical assessment can identify physical causes. Physical causes include:

- Impaired insulin response. This could be due to rare conditions such as degradation of insulin at the injection site. In these cases an insulin pump can improve insulin absorption. In other cases there can be reduced insulin absorption from specific injection sites. Changing sites may help (Martin 1995).
- Communication problems such as dyslexia that can make education and therefore self-care difficult. People frequently hide their difficulty, and tactful questioning is needed to identify it.
- Drug addiction.
- Gastroparesis leading to erratic food absorption, see Section 14c. Other gastrointestinal problems can also be present, e.g. coeliac disease, and should be excluded.
- Seizure disorders.

- Inappropriate management regime.
- Presence of other endocrine disorders, e.g. thyrotoxicosis. Of people with Type 1 diabetes, 2 to 3% have Hashimoto's thyroiditis.
- Eating disorders, either under- or overeating.
- Unrecognised hypoglycaemia and inappropriate insulin dose increases that lead to further hypoglycaemia, rebound hyperglycaemia and DKA.

Psychological causes include:

- Anger and non-acceptance of diabetes.
- Difficult relationships where diabetes is used to escape from the situation or to manipulate it, or gain attention.
- Sexual abuse.

A long-term management strategy is required that involves an agreed coordinated care plan that is communicated to all relevant health professionals and the patient and their family/carers. Regular case conferencing with the relevant health professionals is important. Liaison with a psychiatrist is desirable if the underlying cause is psychological, and may help the individual come to terms with their diabetes by going back to the time of diagnosis and exploring the issues in operation at the time. The focus should be taken off 'diabetic control' and placed on quality of life initially. If other issues are addressed metabolic control is easier to achieve. A basal bolus regime using rapid-acting insulin can be commenced if it is not already being used.

14.20.1 Role of the ward nurse

Support and patience are required to manage people with brittle diabetes. Ward nurses need to be aware that it exists and that it can have a physiological basis as well as an underlying psychological component.

Ward nurses can play a key role in organising case conferences, supporting diabetes education and identifying barriers to learning. This might include inspecting injection sites and observing the person administering an injection and monitoring their blood glucose.

Follow agreed management protocols and/or identify strategies to enhance management and ensure the person has follow-up appointments with appropriate health professionals on discharge.

Regular blood glucose monitoring in hospital can help identify excursions in blood glucose levels and identify unrecognised hypoglycaemia, which will assist with appropriate care planning.

Reference

Martin, F. (1995) Brittle diabetes. *Diabetes Communication*, **July**, 7–8.

14f Teeth, gums and diabetes

14.21 Key points

- Dental care is often overlooked and is not part of regular diabetic complication screening programmes.
- Dental disease can affect metabolic control and nutrition status.
- Infected teeth and gums should be considered as a potential source of infection.
- Dentists may be the first practitioners to recognise diabetes when a patient presents with oral cavity disease.

14.22 Introduction

People with diabetes are at increased risk of periodontal disease, a deep infection that affects bone caused by bacteria (plaque), which destroys the fibrosis attachment that anchors the teeth to the jaw (Peridontal Position Paper 1996; Holmes & Alexander 1997). Increased glucose levels in saliva and reduced buffering power of saliva because of reduced saliva flow rates has been demonstrated (Connor *et al.* 1970). The pattern of dental decay and the decay rates vary between young and older people with diabetes but are largely unknown.

People with diabetes also have increased rates of oral candidiasis and a range of other oral cavity diseases, e.g. lichen planus, painless swelling of the salivary gland (sialosis) that could be due to disordered fat metabolism and changed taste sensation (Lamey *et al.* 1992).

14.22.1 Symptoms of oral cavity disease

- Bleeding gums.
- Halitosis.
- Inflamed receding gums.
- Loose teeth.
- Painful abscesses are a late symptom and indicate permanent damage.

Of people over 65, 67% have few or no natural teeth. This affects their overall food intake and the type of food selected. There is a propensity towards low fibre, low protein foods. This can represent a significant risk of hypoglycaemia and nutritional deficiencies, which in turn affect mental and physical functioning and quality of life, see Chapters 8 and 18.

Ageing also leads to submucosal changes and increasing prevalence of gum disease due to hyperglycaemia and the resultant dry mouth as well as the effect on tissue and high sugar diets. Saliva production can be reduced (xerostomia) and is often exacerbated by medications that cause dry mouth (NHMRC 1999). The degree of metabolic control, duration, age and dental hygiene influence the likelihood of gum disease occurring.

Younger people with diabetes are also at risk of tooth and gum disease primarily as a result of inappropriate diet and inadequate dental care.

14.23 Causal mechanisms

- Uncontrolled diabetes.
- Microangiopathy.
- Increased collagen breakdown.
- Defective neutrophil function, decreased chemotaxis and phagocytosis, during hyperglycaemia.
- Depressed immune response during hyperglycaemia.

Insulin resistance and deterioration of control can occur as a result of oral infection and require adjustment to the diabetic medication regime.

14.24 Management

- Consider the possibility of oral problems where signs of infection or deteriorating control are present.
- Include in nursing history and assessment.
- Nurses have a responsibility to educate their patients about preventative oral hygiene. This includes:
  - dental checks and education.
  - regular teeth checks.
  - good blood glucose control.
  - eating a healthy well-balanced diet.
  - seek dental advice early for any pain, bleeding, redness, and persistent bad breath so infection can be treated early.
  - correct method of brushing teeth, not gums, to reduce bleeding risk.
  - mouth rinses and mouth toilets in hospital.
- Refer for dental assessment if existing disease is identified.
- Check dentures regularly to ensure they fit.
- Assist in educating dental practitioners about diabetes. Dental practitioners should also be aware of the possibility of hypoglycaemia occurring during dental procedures and how to manage it, see Chapters 12 and 13.

References

Connor, S., Iranpour, B. & Mills, J. (1970) Alteration in the parotid salivary flow in diabetes mellitus. *Oral Surgery*, **30**, 15.

Holmes, S. & Alexander, W. (1997) Diabetes in dentistry. *Practical Diabetes International*, **14** (4), 107–110.

Lamey, P., Darwazeh, A. & Frier, B. (1992) Oral disorders associated with diabetes mellitus. *Diabetic Medicine*, **9** (5), 410–416.

National Health Medical Research Council (NHMRC) (1999) *Dietary Guidelines for Older Australians*. Commonwealth of Australia, Canberra.

Position Paper (1996) Diabetes and peridontal disease. *Journal of Peridontology*, **67**, 166–176.

14g Haemochromatosis and hepatic iron overload

14.25 Key points

- Haemochromatosis is rare.
- Diabetes is common in people with haemochromatosis.
- Depression and suicidal tendencies are common in people with haemochromatosis.
- Blood glucose control is often difficult.

14.26 Haemochromatosis

Heamochromatosis is an inherited disease and occurs secondary to thalassaemia, some types of anaemia and excess alcohol consumption. It is characterised by increased iron absorption. The excess iron is deposited in the liver, pancreas, heart and pituitary gland causing tissue damage that disrupts the normal function of these organs and glands. The liver is usually the first organ to be affected.

Sixty-five per cent of people with haemochromatosis have a family history of impaired glucose tolerance or a diagnosis of diabetes (Mender *et al.* 1999). Men are ten times more likely than women to develop haemochromatosis. This could be due, in part, to iron loss with menstruation in women. Haemochromatosis is rarely seen before the age of 20 and the peak incidence occurs in people aged between 40 and 60 years.

Other diabetic complications such as nephropathy, neuropathy and peripheral vascular disease are often also present. Xarthropathy occurs in two-thirds of patients with acute crystal synovitis which can make self-care tasks, e.g. insulin administration, difficult (Sherlock 1981).

14.27 Iron overload

Iron overload is associated with various metabolic conditions besides diabetes. Steatohepatitis is an iron overload condition distinct form haemochromatosis. It is characterised by hyperferritinaemia and transferrin saturation. Liver damage includes steatosis and non-alcoholic fatty liver disease (NASH). Type 2 diabetes is often associated with NASH (Mendler *et al.* 1999). Obesity and hyperlipidaemia that can lead to fibrosis and cirrhosis of the liver are common. The excess iron can increase the risk of cancer, and most probably stroke. Diagnosis is by MRI, liver biopsy and blood glucose and lipid levels.

14.28 Management

Management consists of:

- Venesection to remove excess iron. Hypoglycaemia can occur after venesection and the nurse needs to be aware of the possibility and know how to prevent and manage hypoglycaemia. The patient should be informed of the possibility of hypoglycaemia and how to manage their diet and medications on venesection days to reduce the hypoglycaemia risk.
- Blood glucose can be easy to control or the patient might require large doses of insulin

because of insulin resistance. Oral hypoglycaemic agents often do not lead to acceptable blood glucose control and insulin is needed.
- Blood glucose monitoring to enable changes to medication and diet to be made early.
- Regular blood tests to monitor ferritin, iron levels and metabolic control.
- Counselling and medication to manage depression, if indicated.
- Care during tests and procedures such as liver biopsy (see Chapter 13).

References

Mendler, M.-H., Turlin, B., Moirrand, R. *et al.* (1999) Insulin resistance-associated iron overload. *Gastroenterology*, **117**, 1155–1163.

Sherlock, S. (1981) *Diseases of the Liver and Biliary System*. Blackwell Science, Oxford.

14h Diabetic mastopathy

14.29 Key points

- Diabetic mastopathy is uncommon.
- It causes fear, body image changes and can affect relationships and psychological well-being.

14.30 Diabetic mastopathy

Diabetic mastopathy is a rare disease that usually occurs in women with long-standing Type 1 diabetes around the time of the menopause. Most women with diabetic mastopathy also have microvascular disease and often other concomitant diseases such as autoimmune thyroid disease and cheiroarthropathy. There is relatively little information available about the causes of the disease but it is likely that it occurs as a result of an immune reaction to deposits in the breast as a result of hyperglycaemia.

The breast masses are usually firm-to-hard, poorly defined, freely movable and not fixed to the skin. It is important to exclude cancer to allay fear and anxiety and avoid unnecessary surgical intervention (Wilmshurst 2002).

14.31 Diagnosis

Investigations include:

- Mammogram or ultrasound.
- Fine needle aspiration biopsy. This is often difficult to perform in people with diabetic mastopathy because the fibrous tissue is difficult to aspirate into the needle. Frequently core or excision biopsy is required. The tissue is usually fibrous with lymphocyte infiltration but no glandular changes.

14.32 Management

(1) Single lesions can be removed. However, 63% of lesions are bilateral and often recur after excision.
(2) Regular annual follow-up is necessary with repeat mammogram and ultrasound on a regular basis.
(3) Supportive bras may help relieve breast discomfort.
(4) Regular breast self-examination and early help-seeking should be routine practice.
(5) Counselling and reassurance is important.

Reference

Wilmshurst, E. (2002) Facts about diabetic breast disease all women should know. *Diabetes Conquest*, **Autumn**, 13.

Chapter 15
Diabetes and Eye Disease

15.1 Key points

- Encourage independence. People with visual loss are capable of caring for themselves if they are provided with appropriate tools and information. However, visual impairment has a profound impact on an individual's ability to learn diabetes self-care tasks and on their psychological wellbeing.
- Maintain a safe environment.
- Orient patient to the environment and staff.
- Explain procedures fully.
- Return belongings to the same place.

Rationale

Retinopathy is a significant complication of diabetes. Prevention and early identification of people at risk are essential. Nurses need to be aware of the impact of visual loss on the self-care and psychological wellbeing of people with diabetes and their role in preventative care.

15.2 Introduction

Visual impairment and blindness are significant complications of diabetes. They occur as a result of:

- Maculopathy
- Retinopathy – stages of retinopathy have been described based on a system of photographic grading that requires comparison with a standard set of photographs showing different features and stages of retinopathy (DRS 1981; EDTRS 1991)
- Generalised ocular oedema
- Lens opacity – cataract
- Papillopathy – optic disc swelling that occurs in Type 1 diabetes.

Retinopathy occurs in almost all people with Type 1 diabetes after 20 years duration of diabetes and 70% of people with Type 2 diabetes (DRS 1981; DCCT 1993). Retinopathy occurs as a result of microvascular disease that manifests as increased capillary permeability and closure of the retinal capillaries, which causes vascular leakage, retinal oedema and accumulation of lipids that is seen as hard exudates in the retina and retinal ischaemia.

15.3 Risk factors for retinopathy

The factors which lead to an increased risk of retinopathy include:

- Long duration of diabetes.
- Poor metabolic control.
- Renal disease.
- Pregnancy in people with diagnosed diabetes (but it does not develop in women with gestational diabetes).
- Smoking.
- Hypertension.

People with diabetic eye disease are at greater risk of developing other diabetic complications unless they are screened regularly, take appropriate preventative action and treatment is commenced early.

Visual impairment from non-diabetic causes can coexist with diabetes. People with diabetes also have an increased incidence of glaucoma and cataracts and there is an increasing correlation with age-related macular degeneration. This can be a significant disadvantage during diabetes education and general living because most diabetic and general health information contains essential visual components (IDF-DECS 2000).

15.4 Eye problems associated with diabetes

Practice points

(1) The shape of the lens changes with blood glucose concentrations, leading to refractive changes and blurred vision. This usually corrects as the blood glucose is normalised, but may take some time if the blood glucose has been high for a long time.
(2) Vision can worsen in the short term when blood glucose control begins to improve, e.g. when commencing insulin. It can also worsen during pregnancy.

---

(1) One-third of people with diabetes have retinopathy as a result of microvascular disease. The incidence is related to the duration of diabetes. Sixty per cent of people with diabetes and a duration of more than 15 years have some degree of retinopathy, this applies especially to women. There is increasing evidence that ACE inhibitors can reduce the incidence of microvascular disease (see Chapter 16).
(2) People can have severe eye damage without being aware of it. Vision is not always affected and there is usually no pain or discomfort.
(3) Cataracts are more common in people with diabetes.
(4) Maculopathy is the most common cause of visual loss in people with diabetes.
(5) Sudden loss of vision is normally an emergency. It may be due to:

- vitreous haemorrhage;
- retinal detachment;
- retinal artery occlusion.

Reassurance, avoidance of stress and sudden movement, and urgent ophthalmological assessment are required.

(6) Prevention and early detection are important aspects in the management of visual impairment. It involves:
- good blood glucose control can slow the rate of progression in Type 1 diabetes (DCCT 1993);
- regular eye examinations (commencing at diagnosis in Type 2 and within 5 years in Type 1);
- non-mydriatic fundus photography, as the name suggests, does not require mydriatic eye drops to be used. This means people do not have to wait long periods to have their eyes examined and can drive themselves home after the procedure. The procedure is not painful but the patient should be warned that the flash of light is very bright. Retinopathy screening committees in both Australia and the UK recommend indirect fundoscopy and digital photography to screen for retinopathy;
- retinal photography;
- fluorescein angiography.

(7) Laser treatment is very effective in preventing further visual loss (see Chapter 13).

Clinical observation

Eye drops occasionally cause pain and increased pressure in the eye some hours after they were instilled. If this occurs the patient should be advised to call the doctor.

15.5 Resources for people with visual impairment

People with significant visual loss often require assistance to perform blood glucose monitoring and to administer their own insulin. It is important to encourage independence as far as possible. Careful assessment is important and should include assessment of the home situation.

Vision Australia and the Royal National Institute for the Blind in the UK offer a variety of services for people who have degrees of visual loss. These services include:

- Assessment of the home situation to determine if modifications are necessary to ensure safety at home.
- Low vision clinics.
- Talking library and books in braille.
- Training on how to cope in the community with deteriorating vision.

Other help includes:

- Services such as pensions which may be available from the government.
- Seeing eye dogs (guide dogs for the blind).
- A range of diabetes products are available that can help visually impaired people remain independent (see next section).

The nursing community and home-based services play a major role in maintaining visually impaired people in their own homes.

15.6 Aids for people with low vision

Various magnifying devices are available to help people continue to care for themselves. They can be obtained from diabetes associations and some pharmacies specialising in diabetic products. Other aids include:

(1) Insulin administration:
- clicking syringes, Instaject devices, clicking insulin pens
- chest magnifying glass (available from some opticians); Magniguide – fits both 50 and 100 unit syringes and enlarges the markings
- location tray for drawing up insulin if syringes are used.

(2) Blood glucose monitoring:
- strip guides for accurate placement of the blood onto the strips
- talking blood glucose meters, blood pressure monitors and talking weight scales
- meters with large result display areas.

(3) Medications:
- dosette boxes which can be prefilled with the correct medication.

Practice point

People with visual problems and/or red/green colour blindness may have difficulty interpreting the colours on visual test strips where they are still used.

15.7 Nursing care of visually impaired patients

15.7.1 Aims of care

- To encourage independence as far as possible.
- To ensure the environment is safe when the patient is mobile.

15.7.2 Patients confined to bed

(1) Introduce yourself and address the patient by name, so the patient is aware that you are talking to them.

(2) Ascertain how much the patient is able to see. (Few patients are totally blind.) Assess if the blood glucose fluctuates at certain times. High and low levels can interfere with clear vision. Plan education to avoid these times and determine measures that can avoid such fluctuations, e.g. appropriate timing of meals and medications. Dexterity and cognitive function may also be impaired especially in the elderly and hamper diabetes education. Visual impairment increases the risk of falls in elderly patients (see Chapter 18).

(3) Some patients prefer a corner bed because it makes location easier, avoids confusion with equipment belonging to other patients and enables greater ease in setting up personal belongings.

(4) Introduce the patient to other people in their ward or close by.
(5) If you move the patient's belongings they must be returned to the same place.
(6) Explain all procedures carefully and fully before commencing. (An injection when you can't see it and don't expect it can be very unnerving.)
(7) If eye bandages are required, make sure the ears and other sensory organs are not covered as well.
(8) Consider extra adjustable lighting for those patients with useful residual vision.
(9) Mark the patient's medication with large print labels or use a dosette.
(10) A radio, talking clock, talking watch, braille watch, or a large figured watch, helps the patient keep orientated to time and place.
(11) Indicate when you are leaving the room and concluding a conversation.

15.7.3 Patients who are mobile

(1) A central point (like the patient's bed) assists with orientating a patient to a room.
(2) When orientating a patient to a new area, walk with them until they become familiar with the route.
(3) Keep obstacles (trolleys, etc.) clear of pathways where possible.

15.7.4 Meal times

(1) Describe the menu and let the patient make a choice.
(2) Ensure the patient knows their meal has been delivered.
(3) Ask 'Do you need assistance with your meal?' rather than say, 'I will cut your meat for you.'
(4) Colour contrast is important for some patients. A white plate on a red tray-cloth may assist with location of place setting.

References

DCCT (1993) The effect of intensive treatment of diabetes on the development and progression of long-term complications in insulin-dependent diabetes mellitus. *New England Journal of Medicine*, **329**, 977–986.

DRS (1981) Photocoagulation treatment of proliferative diabetic retinopathy: clinical implications of DRS findings. DRS Report No. 8. *Ophthalmology*, **88**, 583–600.

EDTRS (1991) Early photocoagulation for diabetic retinopathy: EDTRS Report No. 9, *Ophthalmology*, **98** Suppl, 767–785.

International Diabetes Federation Consultative Section on Diabetes (2000) Position Statement *Diabetes Education for People who are Blind or Visually Impaired*. International Diabetes Federation, Brussells, pp. 62–72.

Ponchilla, S., Richardson, K. & Turner-Barry, M. (1990) The effectiveness of six insulin measurement devices for blind persons. *Journal of Visual Impairment and Blindness*, **84**, 364–370.

Chapter 16

Diabetes and Renal Disease

16.1 Key points

- Diabetes may be the underlying cause of renal disease.
- Measurement of microalbuminuria and overt proteinuria is the most useful method of detecting abnormal renal function.
- Elevated blood pressure is an early indicator of renal disease.
- There is a strong association between retinopathy and renal disease.
- Microalbuminuria indicates early renal disease and predicts cardiovascular disease in people with diabetes.

16.2 Introduction

Diabetic nephropathy is a significant microvascular complication of diabetes and diabetes is the second most common cause of end stage renal disease in Australia and the UK (ANZDATA 2000; Department of Health 2001). There is a similar initial disease progression in both Type 1 and Type 2 diabetes. Eventually microalbuminuria occurs in up to 20% of people with Type 1 diabetes and in a similar percentage of people with Type 2. Some cultural groups are at significant risk, e.g. Aboriginal and Torres Strait Islander peoples and Afrocaribbeans.

16.3 Risk factors for renal disease

There is a strong link between hypertension and the progression of renal disease. The risk of end stage renal failure increases as the diastolic blood pressure increases to >90–120 mmHg (Klag *et al.* 1996). Other risk factors include:

- Smoking, which represents a significant and dose-dependent risk.
- Hyperglycaemia, predialysis control is an independent predictor of the outcome in people with Type 2 diabetes on haemodialysis (Wu *et al.* 1997). The Diabetes Control and Complications Trial (DCCT) demonstrated that good control of blood glucose delayed the rate and progression of microvascular disease including renal disease (DCCT 1993).
- The presence of microalbuminuria and proteinuria are independent risk factors for the development and progression of renal disease in people with diabetes (Keane 2001). Incipient renal disease is present when the albumin excretion rate reaches 20–200 μg/

minute and becomes overt when it exceeds 200 μg/minute. Once macroproteinuria is present the decline in renal function is regarded as irreversible. In addition, proteinuria is an important marker for cardiovascular disease in Type 2 diabetes. Tests for microalbuminuria include timed urine collections (12- or 24-hour collections) usually on an outpatient basis, but compliance is poor. Initial screening can be achieved by testing the first early morning specimen voided (50 ml). The third method is to use dipsticks such as Micral test (Gilbert *et al.* 1998) (see Chapter 4).
- Presence of retinopathy (Gilbert *et al.* 1998).
- Long duration of diabetes.
- Male sex.
- Increasing age.

16.4 Renal failure

Renal failure, often requiring dialysis, occurs in 25% of people diagnosed with diabetes before the age of 30. The presence of mild renal disease increases the risk of cardiovascular disease even with only small elevations of urinary protein, but the relationship is not clear. The presence of other cardiovascular risk factors increases the risk, and endothelial cell dysfunction may play a part. Angiotensin converting enzyme (ACE) inhibitors have been shown to delay or stabilise the rate of progression of renal disease and to decrease cardiac events (Keane 2001).

The development of renal problems is insidious and frank proteinuria may not be present for 7–10 years after the onset of renal disease. Microalbuminuria, on the other hand, is detectable up to 5–10 years before protein is found in the urine. Regular urine collections to screen for microalbuminuria controlling blood glucose and blood pressure, the use of ACE inhibitors (Type 1) and angiotensin receptor blockers (Type 2) and avoiding nephrotoxic agents can attenuate renal and cardiac disease (Gilbert & Kelly 2001).

ACE inhibitors have been shown to be more effective than other antihypertensive agents in reducing the time-related increase in urinary albumin excretion and plasma creatinine in Type 2 diabetes and in people with other cardiovascular risk factors, heart failure and myocardial infarction (Ravid *et al.* 1993). Likewise the HOPE and MICRO-HOPE studies demonstrated that ACE inhibitors reduced cardiovascular events and overt nephropathy whether or not microalbuminuria was present (HOPE 2000).

Great care should be taken if IV contrast media are required for diagnostic purposes, see Chapter 13.

Over 50% of patients on OHAs with significant renal disease require insulin therapy. Insulin requirements often decrease in people already on insulin because insulin, like many other drugs, is degraded and excreted by the kidney. Kidney damage can delay degradation and excretion of many drugs and prolong their half-life, increasing the risk of unwanted side effects and drug interactions. The dose, or dose interval, of drugs may need to be altered.

16.5 Renal disease and anaemia

Anaemia occurs as a consequence of chronic renal insufficiency. Renal anaemia occurs earlier in people with diabetes than in people without diabetes. It is more severe and is associated with other factors such as erythrocyte abnormalities and increased osmotic stress that are associated with decreased erythropoietin production (Bosman *et al.* 2001; Ritz 2001). As renal function declines the anaemia becomes more marked.

Anaemia is associated with fatigue, decreased quality of life, depression, left ventricular hypertrophy, decreased exercise capacity, malaise and malnutrition. It is treated with recombinant human erythropoietin (rhEPO) in conjunction with intravenous iron.

Clinical observation

To date there has been little, if any, focus on monitoring haemoglobin as part of routine biochemical monitoring or diabetes complication screening in patients with renal impairment.

16.6 Diet and renal disease

Improving nutritional status can delay end stage renal failure (Chan 2001). Nutritional needs are individual and depend on the stage and type of renal disease. The aim is to maintain homeostasis and electrolyte balance, decrease uraemic symptoms and regularly reassess dietary requirements to ensure changing needs are addressed (National Kidney Foundation 2002).

Protein and energy malnutrition are common and need to be corrected to prevent catabolism lipid metabolism and anaemia. Sodium restriction is often recommended, but salt substitutes should not be used because they are usually high in potassium and can increase the serum potassium, usually already elevated in renal disease. Water-soluble vitamin supplementation may be required when dialysis commences, e.g. B group and vitamin C.

Anorexia is often a feature of renal disease and food smells can further reduce appetite and predispose the patient to malnutrition. Small frequent meals may be more appealing. Malnutrition has implications for the individual's immune status and phagocyte function and increases the risk of infection (Churchill 1996). Referral to a dietitian is essential.

16.7 Renal disease and the elderly patient

Elderly people with renal disease are at increased risk of adverse drug events. A wide range of drugs are used in the elderly and some may need dose adjustments especially digoxin, ACE inhibitors, narcotics, antimicrobials and OHAs (Howes 2001). Long-acting agents are contraindicated because of the risk of hypoglycaemia (see Chapter 6).

Drug therapy needs to be closely monitored along with the monitoring of renal function and nutritional status and non-drug alternatives used where possible.

Practice points

(1) Lower rates of creatinine are produced by older people and creatinine clearance rates can be misleading especially in people with low muscle mass.
(2) Renal disease is an important cause of drug toxicity necessitating a hospital admission.

16.8 Kidney biopsy

See Chapter 13. Extra care is required for people with renal disease undergoing renal biopsy. A pressure dressing should be applied to the site and the patient should lie supine after the procedure for six hours. The blood pressures should be monitored and fluids encouraged to maintain urine output unless fluid is restricted. Activity should be reduced for two weeks.

16.9 Renal dialysis

Dialysis can be used in the management of diabetic kidney disease. Dialysis is a filtering process which removes excess fluid and accumulated waste products from the blood. It may be required on a temporary basis or for extended periods of time. Some patients may eventually receive a kidney transplant.

There are several forms of dialysis in use:

Haemodialysis (artificial kidney)
Blood is pumped through an artificial membrane then returned to the circulation. Good venous access is required and special training in management.

Hypotension is common when heamodialysis therapy is commenced for the first time. Management consists of:

- An appropriate haemodialysis prescription
- Minimising interdialytic fluid gains by setting limits on fluid intake
- Elevating the foot of the bed
- Differentiating between disequilibrium syndrome and hypoglycaemia
- Advising the patient to sit on the edge of the bed or chair to allow the blood pressure to stabilise before standing (Terrill 2002).

Strict aseptic technique and careful patient education are essential when managing dialysis therapies.

Peritoneal dialysis
The filtering occurs across the peritoneum. This form of dialysis is an excellent method of treating kidney failure, in people without diabetes as well. The uraemia, hypertension and blood glucose can be well controlled without increasing the risk of infection, if aseptic techniques are adhered to.

Continuous ambulatory peritoneal dialysis (CAPD)
CAPD is a form of peritoneal dialysis in which dialysate is continually present in the abdominal cavity. The fluid is drained and replaced 4–5 times each day or overnight if the patient is on automated peritoneal dialysis (APD). The patient can be managed at home, which has psychological advantages, once the care of equipment is understood and the patient is metabolically stable.

CAPD can also be used postoperatively to control uraemia related to acute tubular necrosis or early transplant rejection.

Insulin added to the dialysate bags achieves smoother blood glucose control because the insulin is delivered directly into the portal circulation and is absorbed in the dwell phase, which is closer to the way insulin is normally secreted after a glucose load.

The usual insulin dose may need to be increased because of glucose absorption from the dialysate fluid, and to account for insulin binding to the plastic of the dialysate bags and tubing. The continuous supply of glucose and lactate in the dialysate fluid are calorie-rich energy sources and can lead to weight gain and hyperglycaemia. The art is to calculate insulin requirements to avoid hyperinsulinaemia, which carries its own complication risks. The recent availability of glucose-free solutions such as Nutrimeal and glucose polymers may help reduce complications associated with high insulin and glucose levels (Rutecki & Whittier 1993).

16.9.1 Priorities of dialysis treatment

(1) Remove waste products and excess fluids from the blood (urea and creatinine).
(2) To provide adequate nutrition and safe serum electrolytes, and to prevent acidosis.
(3) Patient comfort.
(4) To prevent complications of treatment.
(5) To provide information and support to the patient.
(6) To ensure privacy.

16.10 Objectives of care

The individual's ability to carry out self-care tasks needs to be assessed early when considering renal replacement therapies. Changed joint structure due to oedema and tissue glycosylation (e.g. carpel tunnel syndrome) can limit the fine motor skills required to manage CAPD. Visual impairment due to retinopathy frequently accompanies renal disease and if present, can limit self-care abilities.

(1) To assess the patient carefully in relation to:
  - knowledge of diabetes
  - preventative healthcare practices
  - ability to use aseptic technique
  - usual diabetic control
  - presence of other diabetic complications
  - support available (family, relatives)
  - motivation for self-care
  - uraemic state.
(2) To ensure thorough instruction about administration of dialysate and intraperitoneal medication (insulin).
(3) To ensure a regular meal pattern with appropriate carbohydrate in relation to dialysate fluid.
(4) To maintain skin integrity by ensuring technique is aseptic especially in relation to catheter exit site and skin care.
(5) To monitor urea, creatinine and electrolytes carefully.
(6) To provide psychological support.
(7) To encourage simple appropriate exercise.
(8) To ensure adequate dental care and regular dental assessments.
(9) To prevent pain and discomfort, especially associated with the weight of the dialysate.
(10) To ensure the patient reports illness or high temperatures immediately.

16.11 Nursing responsibilities

(1) Meticulous skin care.
(2) Inspect catheter exit site daily, report any redness, swelling, pain or discharge.
(3) Monitor fluid balance carefully:
- measure all drainage
- maintain progressive total of input and output
- report a positive balance of more than 1 litre – the aim generally is to achieve a negative balance to maintain the dry weight.

(4) Monitor blood glucose.
(5) Monitor temperature, pulse and respiration, and report abnormalities.
(6) Monitor nutritional status – intake and biochemistry results.
(7) Weigh daily to monitor fluid intake and nutritional status.
(8) Ensure patency of tubes and monitor colour of outflow. Report if:
- cloudy
- faecal contamination
- very little outflow (tube blocked).

(9) Report lethargy and malaise that can be due to uraemia or high blood glucose levels.
(10) Warm dialysate before the addition of prescribed drugs and before administration to decrease the possibility of abdominal cramps.
(11) Oral fluid intake may be restricted – provide mouth care and ice to suck.
(12) Assess self-care potential:
- blood glucose testing
- adding medication to bags
- aseptic technique
- psychological ability to cope.

(13) Protect the kidney during routine tests and procedures by avoiding dehydration and infection (Chapter 13).

Practice point

Overestimation of blood glucose levels can occur using some blood glucose meters and hypoglycaemia can be missed in patients using Icodextrin for dialysis. It is recommended that meters which use glucose oxidase reagent strips be used in these patients (Oyibo *et al.* 2002).

16.12 Commencing CAPD in patients on insulin

Prior to commencing intraperitoneal insulin, most patients require a 24-hour blood glucose profile to assess the degree of glycaemia in order to calculate insulin requirements accurately. The glucose profile should be carried out following catheter implantation, with the patient stabilised on a CAPD regime.

16.12.1 Suggested method

(1) Obtain venous access for drawing blood samples.
(2) Obtain hourly blood glucose levels for 24 hours.

(3) At each bag exchange send:
- 10 ml new dianeal fluid for glucose analysis
- 10 ml drained dianeal fluid for glucose and insulin analysis to the appropriate laboratory.

16.13 Protocol for insulin administration in people with diabetes on CAPD – based on four bag changes each day

(1) Calculate usual daily requirement of insulin and double it.
(2) Divide this amount between the four bags.

Note: The overnight bag should contain half of the daytime dose. Some centres add only 10% to the overnight bags.

Example

usual total insulin units	= 60 units
multiply this amount by 2	= 120 units
divide 120 units by 4 exchanges	= 30 units/bag
3 daily exchanges	= 30 units/bag
overnight exchange	= 15 units/bag

Adjustments for the dextrose concentration of the dialysate may be necessary. Intraperitoneal insulin requirements are usually one-third higher than the amount needed before CAPD.

16.14 Education of patient about CAPD

The patient should be instructed to:

(1) Not have a shower or bath for the first 5 days after the catheter is inserted.
(2) Always carefully wash hands prior to changing the bags.
(3) Wear loose fitting clothes over exit site.
(4) Examine feet daily for signs of bruising, blisters, cuts or swelling.
(5) Wear gloves when gardening or using caustic cleaners.
(6) Avoid hot water bottles and electric blankets because sensory neuropathy can diminish pain perception and result in burns.
(7) Avoid constrictive stockings or wearing new shoes for a long period of time.
(8) Wash cuts or scratches immediately with soap and water and apply a mild antiseptic (for example betadine ointment). Any wound that does not improve within 24 to 36 hours or shows signs of infection (redness, pain, tenderness) must be reported promptly.
(9) Bag exchanges should be carried out 4–6 hours apart. The person may be on APD having overnight exchanges.
(10) Only short-acting clear insulin must be used in bags.
(11) Adjust insulin doses according to diet, activity and blood glucose levels and at the physician's discretion.
(12) Accurately monitor blood glucose 4-hourly. A blood glucose meter may be required.
(13) Provide written information.

Immediate help should be sought if any of the following occur:

- Decreased appetite.
- Bad breath/taste in mouth.
- Muscle cramps.
- Generalised itch.
- Nausea and vomiting, especially in the morning.
- Decreased urine output.
- Signs of urinary infection such as burning or scalding.

16.15 Renal disease and herbal medicine (see also Chapter 23)

People with end stage renal failure often try complementary therapies to alleviate the unpleasant symptoms of their disease. Some therapies, for example aromatherapy to reduce stress and maintain skin condition, or counselling for depression, are beneficial and usually safe. Herbal medicines are popular with the general public but they may not be appropriate for people with renal disease (Myhre 2000).

The kidneys play a key role in eliminating drugs and herbal products from the system. Some of these drugs and herbs can cause kidney damage that may be irreversible and put already compromised renal function at great risk. In addition some herbal products, particularly those used in traditional Chinese medicine (TCM) are often contaminated with drugs, heavy metals and other potentially nephrotoxic products (Ko 1998). Frequently these contaminants are not recorded in the list of ingredients for the product. As well as the direct effect of the herbs on the kidney, the intended action of particular herbs can complicate conventional treatment.

A herb, *Taxus celebica*, used in TCM to treat diabetes, contains a potentially harmful flavonoid and has been associated with acute renal failure and other vascular and hepatic effects (Ernst 1998). Kidney damage can be present with few specific overt renal symptoms; therefore, it is vital that kidney and liver function is closely monitored in people taking herbs, especially if kidney function is already compromised by diabetes.

Practice point

Nurses must know when their renal patients are taking herbal medicines so that their kidney function can be closely monitored. Patients should be asked about the use of complementary therapies periodically.

The potentially adverse renal-effects are:

- electrolyte imbalances, e.g. *Aloe barbardinesis*
- fluid imbalances, e.g. *Liquorice root*
- hypokalaemia, e.g. *Aloe, Senna*
- kidney damage, e.g. *Aristolochia*

References

ANZDATA Registry (2000) Australian and New Zealand Dialysis Transplant Registry, Adelaide, South Australia.

Bosman, D., Winkler, A., Marsden, J., MacDougall, I. & Watkins, P. (2001) Anemia with erythropoietin deficiency occurs early in diabetic nephropathy. *Diabetes Care*, **24** (3), 495–499.

Chan, M. (2001) Nutritional management in progressive renal failure. *Current Therapeutics*, **42** (7), 23–27.

Churchill, D. (1996) Results and limitations of peritoneal dialysis. In: *Replacement of Renal Function by Dialysis* (eds C. Jacobs, C. Kjellstrand, K. Koch & F. Winchester). Kluwer Academic Publishers, Boston.

DCCT (Diabetes Control and Complications Trial Research Group) (1993) Effects of intensive insulin therapy on the development and progression of long-term complications in IDDM. *New England Journal of Medicine*, **329**, 977–986.

Department of Health (2001) *Diabetes National Service Framework: Standards for Diabetes Services*. Department of Health, London.

Ernst, E. (1998) Harmless herbs? A review of the recent literature. *American Journal of Medicine*, **104** (2), 170–178.

Gilbert, R. & Kelly, D. (2001) Nephropathy in Type 2 diabetes: current therapeutic strategies. *Current Therapeutics*, **6**, 266–269.

Gilbert, R., Akdeniz, A. & Jerums, G. (1992) Semi-quantitative determination of microalbuminuria by urinary dipstick. *Australian New Zealand Journal Medicine*, **22**, 334–337.

Gilbert, R., Akdeniz, A. & Jerums, G. (1997) Detection of microalbuminuria in diabetic patients by urinary dipstick. *Diabetes Research in Clinical Practice*, **35**, 57–60.

Gilbert, R., Tsalamandris, C., Allen, T., Colville, D. & Jerums, G. (1998) Early nephropathy predicts vision-threatening retinal disease in patients with Type I diabetes mellitus. *Journal of the American Society of Nephrology*, **9**, 85–89.

HOPE (Heart Outcomes Prevention Evaluation Study Investigators) (2000) Effects of ramipril on cardiovascular and microvascular outcomes in people with diabetes mellitus: results of the HOPE study and MICRO-HOPE substudy. *Lancet*, **355**, 253–259.

Howes, L. (2001) Dosage alterations in the elderly: importance of mild renal impairment. *Current Therapeutics*, **42** (7), 33–35.

Keane, W. (2001) Metabolic pathogenesis of cardiorenal disease. *American Journal of Kidney Disease*, **38** (6), 1372–1375.

Ko, R. (1998) Adulterants in Asian patent medicines. *New England Journal of Medicine*, **339**, 847.

Myhre, M. (2000) Herbal remedies, nephropathies and renal disease. *Nephrology Nursing Journal*, **27** (5), 473–480.

National Kidney Foundation (2002) Clinical Practice Guidelines for Nutrition in Chronic Renal Failure. Kidney Outcome Quality Initiative, *American Journal of Kidney Disease*, **35** (6), Supp. 2.

Oyibo, S., Prichard, G., Mclay, L. *et al.* (2002) Blood glucose overestimation in diabetic patients on continuous ambulatory peritoneal dialysis for end-stage renal disease. *Diabetic Medicine*, **19**, 693–696.

Ravid, M., Savin, H. & Jutrin, I. (1993) Long-term stabilising effect of angiotensin-converting enzyme on plasma creatinine and on proteinuria in normotensive Type II diabetic patients. *Annals of Internal Medicine*, **118**, 577–581.

Ritz, E. (2001) Advances in nephrology: success and lessons learnt from diabetes. *Nephrology Dialysis Transplant*, **16** (Suppl. 7), 46–50.

Rutecki, G. & Whittier, F. (1993) Intraperitoneal insulin in diabetic patients on peritoneal dialysis. In: *Dialysis Therapy* (eds A. Nissenson & R. Fine). Hanley & Belfus, Philadelphia.

Terrill, B. (2002) *Renal Nursing: A Practical Approach*. Ausmed Publications, Melbourne.

Wu, M., Yu, C. & Yang, C. (1997) Poor pre-dialysis glycaemic control is a predictor of mortality in Type II diabetic patients on maintenance haemodialysis. *Nephrology Dialysis Transplant*, **12**, 2105–2110.

Chapter 17
Diabetes and Sexual Health

17.1 Key points

- Sexual problems are common.
- The presence of a sexual problem and diabetes does not mean one led to the other.
- Physical, psychological and social factors should be considered.
- Sex education is part of preventative diabetes care.
- There is a fine line between taking a sexual history and voyeurism.
- Put the focus on what is normal and achievable rather than dysfunction.
- Health professionals need to be comfortable with their own sexuality to advise effectively.

Rationale

Nurses are often the person's first point of contact. People with diabetes expect them to have some knowledge about the impact of diabetes on their sexual health. Nurses are ideally placed to be able to emphasise the need for primary prevention and early identification of sexual difficulties and to dispel sexual mythology.

17.2 Sexual health

Sexual health is a core aspect of the general wellbeing of an individual. Sexual functioning is an integration of many components into a unified complex system – endocrine hormonal regulators and the vascular, nervous and psychological systems. Diabetes can profoundly affect the individual's sexual identity and the physical ability to engage in sexual activity. The sexual aspects of an individual's life should be an integral part of an holistic management plan for people with diabetes. Sexual issues are highly sensitive and must be approached with tact and consideration of the person's privacy and confidentiality.

The World Health Organisation (WHO) (1975) stressed the importance of sexuality as an integral component of health and defined sexual health as:

> The capacity to control and enjoy sexual and reproductive behaviour, freedom from shame, guilt and false beliefs which inhibit sexual responsiveness and relationships.

Freedom from medical disorders that interfere with sexual responsiveness and reproduction.

(WHO 1975)

Masters and Johnson first described the human sexual response in 1970. They described four phases: arousal, plateau, orgasm and resolution (Masters & Johnson 1970). These phases blend into each other and sexual difficulties can occur in one or all of them. Kaplan (1979) described a biphasic response that involved parasympathetic nerve activity – vasocongestion, vaginal lubrication and erection; and sympathetic nerve activity – reflex muscle contraction, orgasm and ejaculation. Kaplan's description makes it easier to see how diabetes can affect physical sex given that autonomic neuropathy causes nerve damage, see Section 14c.

Sex counsellors continue to utilise many of the sexual counselling techniques developed by Masters and Johnson. Sexual difficulties do not occur in isolation from other aspects of an individual's life and relationships and a thorough assessment and history is necessary to identify the causal factors. Masters and Johnson found that age and chronic disease processes do not affect female sexual responsiveness as severely as they affect male sexuality. In addition, the sexual response is more varied in women than in men.

17.3 Sexual development

Sexual development occurs across the lifespan:

- Chromosomal sex is determined at fertilisation.
- 3–5 years – diffuse sexual pleasure, fantasies and sex play. Often form a close relationship with a parent of the opposite sex.
- 5–8 years – interest in sexual differences, sex play is common.
- 8–9 years – begin to evaluate attractiveness and are curious about sex.
- 10–12 years – preoccupation with changing body and puberty.
- 13–20 years – puberty, development of self-image and sexual identity.
- Late 30–early 40 – peak sexual responsiveness.
- Menopause – variable onset and highly individual effect on sexuality.
- Old age – physical difficulties and limited opportunity.

Effective sex and diabetes education should be part of the diabetes management plan so that issues can be identified early. Health professionals and people with diabetes often have limited information about the impact that diabetes can have on their sexuality. Sex education, good metabolic control, early identification and management of sexual problems are important, but often neglected aspects of the diabetes care plan. The focus is often on dysfunction and performance rather than on what is normal, which can have a negative psychological impact on sexuality. Changing the focus to what can be achieved and focusing on feelings, intimacy, love and warmth have a big impact on sexual well-being.

17.4 Sexual problems

Sexual satisfaction is a combination of physical and emotional factors. Sexual problems can be:

- Primary – usually defined as never having an orgasm.
- Secondary – difficulties occur after a period of normal functioning. Most sexual difficulties fit into this category.
- Situational – where the situation itself inhibits sexual activity, other sexual problems may also be involved.

17.5 Possible causes of sexual difficulties and dysfunction

Sexual difficulties usually involve two people. It may be a shared problem or each person may have individual issues that need to be considered. Interpersonal factors, the relationship and environmental and disease factors need to be explored with the couple involved.

(1) Individual factors
  - Ignorance and misinformation, which are common despite the sexually permissive society of today. A great deal of readily available literature in magazines and on television with an overemphasis on performance sets up unreal expectations.
  - Guilt, shame and fear, which may be fear of getting pregnant, contracting a sexually transmitted disease, not pleasing their partner or being rejected by them.
  - Gender insecurity/uncertainty and sexual preference.
  - Non-sexual concerns, e.g. about finances, children, job.
  - Past sexual abuse.
  - Physical condition, e.g. presence of diabetes.

(2) Interpersonal factors
  Sexual relationships are one of the most complex undertakings two people ever make, yet most people prepare for it casually.
  - Communication problems – the most common sexual difficulty.
  - Lack of trust.
  - Different sexual preferences and desires, e.g. frequency of intercourse.
  - Relationship difficulties that can include difficulties associated with alcohol and violence or be related to disease process, including diabetes.
  - Changes in lifestyle, e.g. having children, retrenchment, retirement and illness.

(3) Chronic disease sequelae
  (a) Psychological.
    - Depression, anger, guilt, anxiety, fear, feelings of helplessness, changed body image and self-identification as a victim, lowered self-image and self-esteem may or may not accompany the disease. Loss of libido is one of the classic signs of depression.

  (b) Physical changes, e.g. arthritis and diabetic neuropathy.
    - Pain, debilitation associated with changed mobility, e.g. arthritis, bad odour associated with infections, cardiac and respiratory problems and sleep apnoeas and snoring.
    - Disease processes and hormonal imbalance, including diabetes, as well as other endocrine and reproductive conditions.
    - Medications, e.g. antihypertensive and antidepressive agents.

  (c) Diabetes-related
    - Hypoglycaemia during intercourse can be frightening and off-putting, especially for the partner, and decrease spontaneity and enjoyment in future encounters.

- Tiredness and decreased arousal and libido are associated with hyperglycaemia.
- Mood disorders such as depression and other psychological problems may be present but mood can change with hypo- and hyperglycaemia and can cause temporary sexual problems.

(d) Autonomic neuropathy leading to erectile dysfunction in men and possibly decreased vaginal lubrication in older women. Vaginal dryness is also associated with normal ageing, not being aroused and painful intercourse and has not been definitively linked to diabetes as a cause.

(e) Infections, e.g. vaginal/penile thrush.

(4) Environmental factors
- Lack of privacy.
- Limited opportunity, e.g. elderly people in elderly care facilities.
- Uncomfortable, noisy surroundings.

17.6 Sexuality and the elderly

Elderly people are capable of having fulfilling sexual relationships but often lack the opportunity or are constrained by environmental factors, ageist attitudes, sexual stereotypes and disease processes (see Chapter 18). Sensory impairment can change the individual's response to sexual stimulation and the multiplicity of medications required by many older people can inhibit sexual functioning.

Touch is important throughout life and caring touch as distinct from providing nursing care is often lacking.

17.7 Women

The biological effect of diabetes on male sexual functioning has been well documented. The effects of diabetes on sexual function in women are poorly understood and the evidence for any effect is less conclusive than the evidence for the effects on male sexual functioning (Leedom *et al.* 1991). Physicians regularly ask men about their sexual functioning but not women (House & Pendleton 1986). Although this is an old study there is no indication that things have changed. There is no real evidence that physical function is impaired by diabetes in the same way as it is in men, except decreased vaginal lubrication in older women with Type 2 diabetes. This could be due to normal ageing, related to diabetic neuropathy or other causes such as inadequate arousal. More women achieve orgasm from foreplay than from intercourse (Clarke & Clarke 1985) and this may also be a factor.

Women who have difficulty accepting that they have diabetes report higher levels of sexual dysfunction than those who accept their diabetes. Type 2 diabetes has a pervasively negative effect on women's sexuality (Schriener-Engel *et al.* 1991). There appears to be little or no effect in women with Type 1 diabetes but they often have concerns about pregnancy, childbirth and hypoglycaemia during sex (Dunning 1994). There is a positive correlation between the degree of sexual dysfunction and the severity of depression that illustrates the connection between physical and psychological factors and the need for an holistic approach.

Changing blood glucose levels can have a negative transient effect on desire and sexual responsiveness and women often report slow arousal, decreased libido and inadequate lubrication during hyperglycaemia. Desire can fluctuate with stages of the menstrual cycle but this also occurs in women without diabetes. However, there is no correlation between the presence of complications and sexual difficulties in women with diabetes (Campbell *et al.* 1989; Dunning 1993). Polycystic disease of the ovaries and its effects could have adverse psychological effects (see Chapter 21).

The developmental stage of the individual should also be considered when assessing sexual health and the impact of diabetes when planning sex education and counselling (see Section 17.2).

- Children and adolescents – diabetes can affect normal growth and development if it is not well controlled and menarche and puberty can be delayed. This could impact negatively on body image and the development of sexual identity and self-esteem. Eating disorders and insulin manipulation can compound the problem.
- Young adulthood – attracting a partner, successful pregnancy and birth can be areas of fear and concern that affect sexual health (Dunning 1994). Hyperglycaemia can occur during menstruation with tiredness, decreased arousal and libido. Vaginal thrush is common and causes itch and discomfort during sexual intercourse. It is also frequently associated with taking oral contraceptives. Thrush-induced balanitis can inhibit male sexual activity.
- Older age group – hormonal changes due to menopause and associated fatigue and depression inhibit sexual enjoyment. Often a long-term partner's life course is different and this affects their sexual relationship. There are fewer partners and opportunities for sexual activity for older women, especially those in care facilities.

Specific problems should be investigated depending on their presentation. Preventative sexual health care such as breast self-examination, mammograms and cervical (pap) smears should be part of the care plan.

17.8 Men

Diabetes does have physical effects that cause erectile dysfunction (ED). Other causes include:

- Vascular damage, both systemic atherosclerosis and microvascular disease.
- Neurological diseases such as spinal cord damage, multiple sclerosis and diabetic neuropathy.
- Psychological causes such as performance anxiety, depression and mood changes may be associated with hypo- or hyperglycaemia.
- Endocrine diseases that result in lowered sex hormones: testosterone, SHBG, prolactin, FSH, LH. Hypogonadism can occur in chronic disease.
- Surgery and trauma to genitalia or its nerve and vascular supply.
- Anatomical abnormalities, e.g. Peyronie's contracture which is often associated with Dupuypten's contracture and other glycosylation diseases including diabetes.
- Drugs such as thiazide diuretics, beta blockers, lipid lowering agents, antidepressants, NSSRI, smoking, alcohol and illicit drug use.
- Normal ageing.

Age-associated ED is defined as the inability to achieve or maintain an erection sufficient for satisfactory sexual performance – penetration and ejaculation. It is common in men with diabetes especially if other diabetic complications are present. It occurs in 50% of men 10 years after the diagnosis of diabetes especially those who smoke. ED is gradual, insidious and progressive (Krane 1991). ED may be a predictor of cardiovascular risk and there is a higher incidence of undiagnosed coronary disease in men with ED. Elevated blood fats and hypertension and antihypertensive agents also play a part in the development of ED. Lowered sperm counts are associated with obesity, smoking and poor diet.

ED significantly reduces the man's quality of life especially in the emotional domain and has a negative effect on self-esteem. When sexual functioning improves, improvement in mental and social status follows. Other sexual issues for men are fatigue, fear of performance failure, and concern about not satisfying their partners.

17.9 Investigation and management

A thorough history and physical examination are required. This includes assessing diabetic status and blood glucose control, identifying the cause and determining the extent of the dysfunction, e.g. using rigiscan and snap gauge to determine if nocturnal erections occur and sleep apnoea studies. There is an association between poor sleep, sleep apnoea and ED. Doppler studies are carried out to determine local blood flow. Testosterone, FSH, LH, SHBG and prolactin levels are assessed.

Management consists of:

- Good metabolic control to prevent ED.
- Early intervention if ED occurs.
- Assessing fitness for sex and modifying risk factors, e.g. lose weight, stop smoking and drinking alcohol.
- Appropriate diet and exercise programme.
- Sex education that includes setting realistic expectations and planning for regular sexual health checks, e.g. prostate disease.
- Diabetes education.
- Counselling, which should include partners and inform them about treatment options and help them find fulfilling sexual alternatives.

Specific options are medications such as Sildenafil (Viagra), a vasodilator that enhances the natural sexual response. It can cause transient hypotension and unmask cardiac ischaemia. It is contraindicated if nitrates are used and if cardiovascular disease is present. Cimetidine and Ketoconozale can increase Viagra levels and Rifampicin decreases them. Intracavernosal injections such as Caverject and a range of surgical implants are also available. Urethurally introduced drugs such as MUSE are helpful for some men.

Clinical observations

Improving sexual functioning can lead to changes in the relationship that result in conflict and disharmony.

Women have reported acute cystitis when their partners begin Viagra due to the increased sexual activity, so-called 'honeymoon cystitis'.

Sex education is part of the management for both men and women, and needs to include:

- Revision of diabetes knowledge and self-care and the importance of blood and lipid control.
- Knowledge about sex and sexuality and what 'normal' functioning is.
- Contraception options.
- Sexual health and the need for protected intercourse and regular monitoring of sexual health, e.g. cervical smears, mammogram, and prostate checks.
- Menopause and control of symptoms.
- Planning pregnancies, breast feeding.

17.10 Sexual counselling

Good communication and trust is essential. Knowledge of the human sexual response, normal ageing and the potential effects of diabetes is needed to counsel effectively. Sexual questions can be included when taking a nursing history. Including sexual questions in the nursing history can be simple and identify sexual problems that require specific questions to obtain a more detailed history or referral to a sex specialist. Respect and regard for the person and empathetic understanding and privacy are essential (Ross & Channon-Little 1991). The main areas to be covered when taking a sexual history are:

(1) Social aspects
  - Childhood experiences.
  - Marital status.
  - Family relationships.
  - Number and sex of any children.
  - Interests, activities.
  - Job demands/unemployment.
  - Religious and cultural beliefs.

(2) Sexual aspects
  - Sexual knowledge, education, fears, fantasies.
  - Previous sexual experiences
  - Contraception method
  - If there is a current problem:
    - Whose problem does the person believe it to be?
    - Description of the problem in the person's own words.
    - Is the partner aware of the problem?
    - Does the problem follow a period of poor diabetic control or illness?
    - Have there been any previous sexual problems?
    - What were those problems?
    - How were they resolved?

(3) Psychological aspects
  - Acceptance of diabetes by self and partner.
  - Body-image concepts.
  - Presence of depression or other psychological problem.

(4) Diabetes knowledge
  - Self-care skills and knowledge of effects of poor diabetic control.

17.11 The PLISSIT model

PLISSIT is an acronym for Permission–Limited Information–Specific Suggestions–Intensive Therapy. It is a model which uses four phases to address sexual problems and moves from simple to complex issues. It can be used in a variety of settings and adapted to the individual's needs (Annon 1975).

(1) Permission-giving
Being open and non-judgemental allows the person to discuss their problem by offering:
- reassurance.
- acceptance of the person's concerns.
- a non-judgemental attitude.
- establishing acceptable terminology.

Questions about the person's sexuality can be asked or the nurse can respond to sexual questions the person asks. These actions establish that it is appropriate and acceptable to discuss sexual issues.

(2) Provision of limited information
This involves giving limited information and general suggestions that might include practising safe sex, diabetes and sex education and giving:
- accurate, limited information.
- some references information for home reading.

(3) Specific suggestions
These are usually made by a qualified sex therapist and often include sensate focus exercises and the squeeze technique for premature ejaculation (Clarke & Clarke 1985).
- involve the partner.
- provide sex education.

(4) Intensive therapy
Therapy at this stage requires referral to a sex psychologist/psychiatrist. Techniques include a range of counselling techniques based on Master's and Johnson's work, behavioural therapy and a range of other therapies.

Practice points

(1) The nurse must have adequate knowledge to undertake this and subsequent steps or refer the person appropriately.
(2) Examples of information to give at this stage is limited information about the differences between typical men and women, e.g. women take longer to become aroused than men and need sufficient quality foreplay to be able to orgasm; the effects of medications, smoking, alcohol and diabetes on sexual responsiveness.

17.12 Role of the nurse

The nurse has an important role in the early identification of sexual problems and helping the individual or couple develop a health plan that includes sexual health. Some sexually transmitted diseases must be notified to government health authorities in some countries. Some specific nursing actions include:

- Being aware of the possibility that a sex problem may exist and allowing people to discuss their concerns.
- Debunking sexual myths, e.g. old people who have sex are 'dirty old men/women'.
- Identifying sexual problems and addressing them or referring appropriately.
- Providing relevant care and information during investigative procedures and surgery.
- Medication advice and management.
- Advice about safe sex and contraception.
- Advice about monitoring quality sexual health.
- Advice about self-care and when it is safe to resume sex after hospitalisation, e.g. after a myocardial infarct or cardiac surgery.
- In care homes for the elderly and rehabilitation settings, providing an appropriate environment and opportunities for couples to enjoy a sexual relationship might be possible.

References

Annon, J. (1975) *The Behavioural Treatment of Sexual Problems*. Enabling Systems, Honolulu.

Campbell, L., Redelman, M., Borkman, M., McLay, S. & Chisholm, D. (1989) Factors in sexual dysfunction in diabetic female volunteer subjects. *Medical Journal of Australia*, **151** (10), 550–552.

Clarke, M. & Clarke, D. (1985) *Sexual Joy in Marriage. An Illustrated Guide to Sexual Communication*. Adis Health Science, Sydney.

Dunning, P. (1993). Sexuality and women with diabetes. *Patient Education and Counselling*, **21**, 5–14.

Dunning, P. (1994) Having diabetes: young adult's perspectives. *The Diabetes Educator*, **21** (1), 58–65.

ED–Alliance Group (2000) *Practical Diabetes International*, **17** (5), 139–140.

House, W. & Pendelton, L. (1986) Sexual dysfunction in diabetics. *Postgraduate Medicine*, **79**, 227–235.

Kaplan, H. (1979) *Making Sense of Sex*. Simon & Schuster, New York.

Krane, R. (1991) Commentary on erectile dysfunction. *Diabetes Spectrum*, **4** (1), 29–30.

Leedom, L., Feldman, M., Procci, W. & Zeidler, A. (1991) Severity of sexual dysfunction and depression in diabetic women. *Journal of Diabetic Complications*, **5** (1), 38–41.

Masters, W. & Johnson, V. (1970) *Human Sexual Inadequacy*. Little Brown Company, Boston.

Ross, M. & Channon-Little, L. (1991) *Discussing Sexuality. A Guide for Health Practitioners*. MacLennan & Pretty, Sydney.

Schriener-Engel, P., Schiavi, P., Vietorisz, D. & Smith, H. (1991) The differential impact of diabetes type on female sexuality. *Diabetes Spectrum*, **4** (1), 16–20.

World Health Organisation (1975) *Education and Treatment of Human Sexuality – The Training of Health Professionals*. Technical Report Series, 572, Geneva.

Chapter 18
Diabetes in the Older Person

18.1 Key points

- Integrated care is essential.
- Increasing age is associated with insulin resistance that predisposes elderly people to diabetes.
- Fat, carbohydrate and lipid metabolism is different in the elderly.
- Diabetes is common in people over 65. Most have Type 2 diabetes but Type 1 also occurs.
- The onset of diabetes in the elderly is often insidious with non-specific symptoms.
- Presentation of hypoglycaemia is often atypical. Many older people have diabetes complications.
- Drug pharmacokinetics is different in the elderly.
- Older people may have outdated knowledge about diabetes management or have had no opportunity to learn about diabetes management.
- Older people often have limited choices when accessing mainstream diabetes services.

Rationale

Management of diabetes in the elderly is an increasingly important aspect of nursing care as the population ages and the incidence and prevalence of diabetes increases with increasing age. Diabetes manifests differently in elderly people and their healthcare needs are different.

18.2 Introduction

Elderly people with diabetes often have multiple health problems, some of which are a result of diabetes-related complications. Elderly people in hospital and facilities for the elderly are a vulnerable group and the latter often receive suboptimal care (Kirkland 2000). Sinclair *et al.* (1997) found 40% of residents in elderly care facilities were on long-acting sulphonylureas, fewer than 1 in 10 had any regular diabetes follow-up, they had more hospital admissions than people without diabetes, stayed in hospital longer and had more complications. In addition, staff and resident knowledge about diabetes was deficient.

The need to improve healthcare services for the elderly was recognised in the UK with the development of practice guidelines (British Diabetic Association 1999) and standards for care homes for older people (Department of Health 2001). Standards for homes for the elderly have been in place in Australia for a number of years (Australian Quality Council 1998) and in 2001 a national committee was established to develop management guidelines for diabetes in the elderly.

In addition to diabetes, many elderly people have some degree of depression, mostly undiagnosed, and the depression frequently precedes placement in a home for the elderly. Depression assessed using the Geriatric Depression Scale was linked in most cases to grief over loss of ability and independence (Fleming 2002). The particular problems encountered in elderly people with diabetes and the resultant risks are shown in Table 18.1.

Table 18.1 Particular problems encountered in the elderly person with diabetes and the resultant risks associated with the problem.

Problem	*Associated risk*
Hyperglycaemia leading to:	Constipation Postural hypotension Dehydration and electrolyte imbalance Polyuria presenting as urinary incontinence Hyperosmolar coma and ketoacidosis Impaired cognition Thrombosis Infection, e.g. UTI Impaired wound healing Postural hypotension Decreased pain threshold Exacerbated neuropathic pain Decreased mood, lethargy, compromised self-care Falls
Poor food intake	Hypoglycaemia Nutritional deficiencies: • impaired immune response • infection risk • decreased plasma albumin • impaired wound healing Energy deficits Increased morbidity Falls
Cerebral insufficiency	Stroke Non-recognition of hypoglycaemia Trauma Impaired cognition TIAs being confused with hypoglycaemia Increased prevalence of vascular dementia and Alzheimer's disease Falls

Cont'd

Table 18.1 *Cont'd*

Problem	*Associated risk*
Cardiac insufficiency	Myocardial infarction Confusion Poor wound healing Poor peripheral circulation Foot ulcers Falls
Autonomic neuropathy	Postural hypotension Gustatory sweating Urinary tract infections and incontinence Unrecognised hypoglycaemia Silent myocardial infarction Decreased/delayed food absorption Poor nutrition Infections, pain Decreased motor skills Erectile dysfunction Falls
Peripheral insufficiency	Trauma Foot/leg ulcers Claudication Falls
Peripheral neuropathy	Unstable gait Foot ulcers Depression Falls
Other neuropathies such as Bell's palsy and carpel tunnel syndrome	Reduced self-care Loss of independence Body image changes
Visual impairment Changed colour perception (blue, green, violet)	Self-care deficits Depression Loss of independence Social isolation Education difficulties with types of materials used: visual blood glucose test strips, differentiating medications
Skin atrophy	Pressure ulcers, skin tears
Communication problems	Misunderstanding Confusion Inaccurate self-care Stress Social isolation
Stress and depression	Inadequate self-care Hypertension Hyperglycaemia Hypoglycaemia Falls

Cont'd

Table 18.1 *Cont'd*

Problem	*Associated risk*
Renal disease associated with diabetes and as a normal part of ageing	Decreased drug clearance and toxicity Reduced renal function risk of dialysis Malnutrition Reduced choice of OHA Dehydration Hyperosmolar coma Lactic acidosis Falls
Failure to recognise thirst (normal ageing process)	Dehydration Hyperglycaemia Confusion Falls
Cognitive impairment	Self-care deficits Education difficulties Reduced quality of life Falls

18.3 Metabolic changes

Glucose metabolism changes progressively as people get older. There are differences between lean and obese elderly people. The fasting hepatic glucose production is normal in both groups but the lean elderly have profound impairment of insulin secretion and minimal resistance to insulin-mediated glucose disposal. The obese elderly have a relatively intact glucose-induced insulin response but marked resistance to insulin-mediated glucose disposal. Hyperglycaemia results in both cases.

Insulin improves vasodilation and accounts for up to 30% of normal glucose disposal. This action is impaired in obese elderly people with diabetes. ACE inhibitors have been shown to improve insulin sensitivity in elderly people with diabetes and hypertension (Paolisso *et al.* 1992). Therefore, drugs that enhance muscle blood flow may be valuable adjunct therapy for the elderly.

Age, life expectancy, other health problems and the person's social situation should be taken into account when planning their care. Achieving near normal blood glucose levels and preventing long-term complications may not be priority management aims, although it is important to control uncomfortable symptoms (polyuria, polydipsia, lethargy) and minimise the risk of hypoglycaemia and the attendant risk of falling.

Suboptimal metabolic control is associated with urinary incontinence, leg/foot ulcers, infections, nutritional deficiencies, exacerbation of neuropathic pain, decreased ability to communicate and confusion and aggression (Kirkland 2000). Although the principles for managing diabetes are the same as for younger patients, strategies and priorities need to be implemented cautiously using a stepwise approach and non-pharmacological measures where possible.

18.4 Aims of treatment

- Prevent hypo- and hyperglycaemia.
- Screen for and prevent and/or manage diabetic complications.
- Manage coexisting illnesses to improve functional ability and improve quality of life.
- Exude a positive attitude.
- Maintain a safe environment to limit adverse events such as falls.
- In terminal cases ensure a comfortable and peaceful death.

18.4.1 Factors affecting treatment decisions

- Age; but age alone may not give an accurate picture of an individual's ability to cope with self-care tasks and activities of daily living. Functional level should be assessed using appropriate tools in an appropriate familiar setting.
- Current diabetes control and complication status including the presence of liver and kidney disease.
- Presence and severity of comorbidities.
- Life expectancy.
- Mental and physical capacity to comply.
- Nutritional status. Inadequate nutrition predisposes the person to hypoglycaemia, falls, decreased immunity, delayed wound healing and infections.
- Education potential, which is influenced by the individual's sight, hearing and cognitive ability.
- Social support from family and the community.
- Financial status.

18.5 Education approaches

A suitable environment, appropriate time and consideration of the duration of the session and the type of education aids used need to be carefully considered. Where appropriate, patients should have their glasses (spectacles) and hearing aid with them during diabetes education sessions (Jennings 1997; Rosenstock 2001).

Spouses and/or carers should be included in diabetes education sessions. Support groups have long-term benefits for knowledge retention, psychosocial functioning and metabolic control (Gilden *et al.* 1992). In the absence of dementia, the main or underlying factor that most affects an older person's ability to learn, retain and recall new information and skills and problem solve is dependent on whether they are actively involved in their community. For example, the older person who attends church, plays lawn bowls and other social activities is far more likely to learn about their diabetes management compared with an older person who is socially isolated and whose only contact is with the 'meals-on-wheels' visitor each day.

Education for diabetes management is rarely age-specific and often occurs in groups that make it difficult for hearing and vision impaired people to participate. Computer-generated learning packages are also difficult to see, access and use for older people. In addition, many older people have poor literacy skills. Small font sizes and/or text printed on shiny or coloured paper with insufficient contrast between the text and the background also compromises comprehension.

Education can provide mental stimulus and help protect mental functioning as well as reduce hospital admissions and improve quality of life. Some memory learning, retrieval and cognitive deficits have been demonstrated in people with Type 2 diabetes particularly when metabolic control is poor (Gilden *et al.* 1993). Several factors affect memory and learning besides cognitive function and vision changes. These include:

- Degree of wellness.
- Physical, psychological and biological capacity.
- Social situation and available support.
- Adjustments to being older and age-related changes, e.g. wearing glasses.
- Sensory loss, tiredness and incontinence can be barriers to effective education.

Poor blood glucose control is associated with decreased cognitive functioning and planning skills. Cognition improves when the blood glucose improves (Gradman *et al.* 1993). Simple tools to screen for cognitive impairment can be used as adjuncts to the diabetes management plan (Sinclair 1995). These include the Mini Mental State Examination and the results can inform diabetes education strategies.

Diabetes education strategies must include ways to increase concentration and enhance attention especially when vision and hearing are impaired. Incorporating relaxation techniques and other complementary therapies into the education session can relieve stress and enhance learning.

18.6 Access and equity to diabetes services

Elderly people are often unable to attend mainstream diabetes services especially where they are fragmented and essential services are offered on different days. Appointments scheduled to allow a 'one stop' approach to diabetes management enhance attendance rates. People are often are required to attend different sites to have their eyes, kidneys and feet checked for diabetic complications. Therefore integrated care involving the general practitioners (GPs) is essential. In Australia the GP incentive schemes and integrated care strategies have done much to improve diabetes care in general practice. The diabetes National Service Framework in the UK promises to improve diabetes care in primary settings, which are often more convenient and accessible for elderly people.

18.7 Factors that can affect metabolic control

'Barriers to good control are often in the minds of physicians rather than the capacity of the elderly person with diabetes' (Halter 2001), for example many GPs are reluctant to commence insulin in elderly people when metabolic control deteriorates, even when the patient and their family/carers are willing. It is important to consider the health professional's influence on an individual's healthcare, especially when the individual is old. Health professionals often judge elderly people in general by the elderly people they manage in elderly care facilities who may not accurately represent the majority of self-caring elderly people living in the community. Some of the factors that can affect diabetes control in the elderly are shown in Table 18.2.

Table 18.2 Factors that can affect diabetes control and management in elderly patients.

Health professionals	Attitudes and beliefs Inadequate knowledge about diabetes Ageist approaches to services and diabetes management choices
Altered senses	Diminished vision and smell, altered taste, decreased proprioception
Food difficulties	Purchasing, preparing and consuming food, understanding of nutritional requirements, poor appetite, early satiety, gastrointestinal problems
Disease processes/effects	Tremor, arthritis, poor dentition, gastrointestinal abnormalities, altered thirst sensation, altered renal and hepatic function, infection (acute and chronic)
Mobility	Decreased ability to exercise
Drugs	Alcohol, medications such as corticosteroids, interactions, self-prescribed medications
Complementary therapies	Hypo- or hyperglycaemia, drug/herb interactions, herb/herb interactions
Malabsorption	Due to diabetes medications, disease processes, drug interactions, diabetes complications
Psychological issues	Bereavement, depression, cognitive deficits
Social factors	Social isolation, living alone or in care facilities, family expectations
Financial status	Purchasing of recommended foods, monitoring equipment, diabetes complication screening, podiatry services

18.8 Infection

The presence of infection can have a big impact on the older patient. Any sudden increase in blood glucose that cannot be accounted for by dietary changes or stress should be investigated for infection. The temperature should be recorded. Foot inspection is important to exclude occult infection. Urinary tract infections are common in older people. A urine dipstick test for white cells and nitrate should be performed. There is growing evidence that consuming cranberry juice on a daily basis can prevent UTI in older people with diabetes. Annual influenza vaccination should be part of the individual's routine health management plan.

18.9 Quality of life

Quality of life is concerned with maximising an individual's enjoyment of life rather than prolonging life, see Chapter 22. Prolonged hyperglycaemia directly affects the quality of life and leads to dehydration and often to thirst, polyuria, nocturia and sleep deprivation. Insulin improves metabolic control in elderly people with Type 2 diabetes but their sense of wellbeing does not improve and is often associated with stress and fear.

Hyperglycaemia and dehydration can present as:

- Constipation
- Dry skin and mucous membranes
- Postural hypotension
- Confusion
- Polyuria – urinary incontinence, which is often not discussed and can be missed in primary care settings
- Increased risk of UTI and URTI
- Poor wound healing
- Receding gums – leading to ill-fitting dentures (see Section 14f)
- Increased risk of pressure ulcers
- Increased incidence of skin rashes and pressure sores
- High risk of falling.

Sexual health is often overlooked in elderly people but is an important aspect of quality of life that can be compromised by health professional and societal attitudes, age-related changes and diabetes, see Chapter 17.

18.10 Safety

Diabetes management in the elderly must address safety issues. The single most important safety issue is the risk of falling. Falls can be attributed to the following diabetes-specific factors (also see Table 18.1):

- Decreased vision
- Peripheral neuropathy
- Limb amputation
- Hypoglycaemia
- Postural and postprandial hypotension
- Postural instability, and gait and balance problems
- Slower responses.

Fall prevention strategies should be incorporated in the diabetes management plan for elderly people with diabetes whether they live at home or in elderly care facilities.

18.11 Medications

Age-related changes in pharmacokinetics must be considered when deciding on medications. Deterioration in renal function is a normal consequence of ageing. Long-acting insulin and oral hypoglycaemic agents are best avoided because of their reduced clearance and longer half-life and the risk of severe hypoglycaemia and falls. When liver and kidney damage is present and food intake is erratic or low in carbohydrate, these risks increase substantially.

18.11.1 Oral agents

Older age and comorbidities limit the choice of OHA. Metformin generally should not be used for people over 80 and serum urea and creatinine should be monitored if it is used.

The dose of Metformin should not be increased if the serum creatinine is >0.15 mg and should be ceased if serum creatinine is >0.2 mg because of the risk of lactic acidosis (see Chapters 6 and 10). Metformin is most effective in overweight people. Elderly people are often malnourished and in particular can be protein deficient.

Normal liver function must be established before commencing some of the newer OHAs, e.g. Thiazolidinediones such as Rosiglitazone. Regular liver function tests must be performed while the patient is on this drug. Cardiac failure is a contraindication to Rosiglitazone. The Glitinides, e.g. Repaglinide, may prove to be very useful for elderly people, particularly those with erratic eating habits. Repaglinide has a similar action to the sulphonylureas but acts faster for a shorter time. This means it can be given with or just after meals.

There is a move to limit the number of medications prescribed for individuals, i.e. reduce polypharmacy particularly in elderly care services. However, several medications are often necessary to achieve blood glucose and lipids targets and to treat the metabolic short- and long-term consequences of hyperglycaemia. To minimise the adverse effects of polypharmacy, drugs should be commenced at low doses and the dose increased slowly, if necessary, and the effects carefully monitored (Howes 2001). Dose intervals may need to be modified for elderly patients.

Often disease processes occur that require drug therapy. Often these drugs tend to increase blood glucose levels, e.g. corticosteroids. Blood glucose monitoring frequency may need to be increased in these circumstances. Other medication issues to be aware of include the propensity for ACE inhibitors to cause postural hypotension when autonomic neuropathy is present (see Section 14c). Beta blockers can reduce the peripheral circulation and impair healing of the foot and lower limb ulcers.

Polypharmacy can result in changed mentation and confusion as well as undesirable drug interactions. Taking medications at the same time or inappropriately increases the risk of undesirable drug interactions. Drug incompatibility, side effects and uncoordinated prescribing by several practitioners are also implicated. Elderly people often become confused and do not take their medications or take them inappropriately and at the incorrect dose. Combining herbal and self-prescribed medications can also lead to unwanted drug interactions. See Chapter 26 for a discussion of drug/herb and herb/herb interaction. Elderly people with diabetes, those over 65 years, are likely to use complementary therapies including herbal medicines and this should be considered when reviewing their medications (Egede *et al.* 2002) (see Chapter 26).

18.11.2 Insulin

There are a number of insulins to choose from and a regime suitable for elderly people can be achieved (see Chapter 7). The key to commencing and maintaining successful insulin therapy in elderly people is to be flexible, and identify and address barriers before insulin is commenced. Often older people can remain on an OHA and insulin can be added before breakfast or at night.

Insulin can be drawn up into syringes and left in a refrigerator for up to seven days (see Chapters 7 and 25). This practice enables older people with impaired vision, hemiplegia or severe arthritis to remain independent and improves their quality of life. There is a range of new insulin devices that also help people remain independent (see Chapter 7). Rapid-acting insulins now available enable insulin to be administered after a meal and tailored to the individual with impaired cognition and erratic food intake.

18.12 Nutrition

Elderly people are often malnourished. In hospital, malnourishment is associated with longer length of stay and increased mortality (Middleton *et al.* 2001). The causes of poor nutrition are shown in Table 18.3. Sometimes it is difficult to distinguish between the effects of malnutrition and disease processes because they are closely related (World Health Organisation 1999). However, the cycle is difficult to break unless both are addressed, for example renal disease (see Chapters 8 and 16).

Table 18.3 Risk factors for inadequate nutrition and malnutrition in the elderly.

Risk factor	*Potential outcome*
Living in an institution	Forced food choices, loss of control over environment
Malabsorption	Bacterial infections, coeliac disease, drugs, disease processes and diabetes complications
Neurological	Stroke, dementia
Drugs	Digitalis, alcohol, sedatives
Sensory deficit	Impaired sight and/or hearing, taste and smell
Dentition	Ill-fitting dentures, caries, missing teeth, gum disease
Social circumstances	Isolation, poverty, inability to shop or prepare food
Medical problems	Chronic disease, pneumonia, heart failure, chronic infection, thyroid disease

18.12.1 Enteral therapy

Many older people, particularly those residing in residential care, have impaired swallowing reflexes, severe malnutrition or other disease processes that require the insertion of a PEG tube (see Section 14a). In the past, these feeds led to hyperglycaemia. Several nutritional feeds now exist that have a low-to-medium glycaemic index and a smaller impact on blood glucose.

Practice point

Diabetes management tasks must reflect enteral therapy routines and *not* oral meal time routines. For example, if a person has an enteral feed five times a day, e.g. at 6 AM, 10 AM, 2 PM, 6 PM and 10 PM, the diabetes medication administration times and blood glucose testing must relate to these feed times.

This means that many diabetes medications should be administered at 6 AM with the first feed and not at 8 AM when breakfast is served. Capillary blood glucose testing should be performed before an enteral feed and not for example at 11.30 AM, which may be the time other residents are tested because it is too soon after their 10 AM feed to be able to determine postprandial glucose clearance.

18.12.2 Nutrition in dementia

Inadequate nutritional intake is common in dementia. People with dementia accept or refuse meals on a day-to-day basis and may be anorexic. The glycaemic index can be a useful tool to improve the nutritional intake, e.g. most dairy-based drinks and foods have a low GI score. When a person with diabetes and cognitive impairment refuses meals they can be encouraged to take drinks and light foods such as hot chocolate, milkshakes, ice cream, fruit yoghurt, custard and rice dessert. A favourite meal can be repeated, e.g. if the person likes breakfast and refuses dinner, breakfast food can be repeated at dinnertime. Familiar foods, made at home may be preferred.

Nutritional supplements in medication form are also useful, for example 60 ml Two-Cal® administered with normal prescribed medications four times a day will increase protein intake.

18.13 Hypoglycaemia

Hypoglycaemia occurring in elderly patients managed with OHAs can be difficult to recognise. The usual signs and symptoms can be masked or absent and can present as chronic confusion, and not be recognised and is potentially more dangerous, see Chapter 8. The presentation of hypoglycaemia may resemble a cerebrovascular accident or mental confusion leading to an incorrect diagnosis of impaired mental function and delayed treatment or failure to treat the hypoglycaemia. This has decreased since the introduction of capillary blood glucose testing on all unconscious patients presenting to emergency departments.

Hypoglycaemia caused by OHAs, that artificially increase blood insulin levels, is often more profound and prolonged and can become chronic or fatal, and if protracted can lead to brain damage or provoke a myocardial infarction (Tiengo 1999). If a person on insulin and a sulphonylurea or Glitinide starts to feel unwell, test their blood glucose to exclude/confirm hypoglycaemia as a cause.

The risk of hypoglycaemia in the elderly is increased by:

- Treatment with oral hypoglycaemic agents, especially long-acting agents such as Glibenclamide and Amaryl, see Chapter 6.
- Renal and/or hepatic disease that leads to impaired metabolism and excretion of medications and accumulation of drugs with long half-lives (Jennings 1997; Howes 2001).
- Patients on multiple drugs where the risk of drug interactions is high.
- Impaired cognitive function where the individual fails to recognise hypoglycaemia and the signs can be confusing for family, carers and health professionals.
- Patients who are sedated.
- Inadequate nutrition and malnutrition where glucose stores are inadequate to respond to the counter-regulatory hormone response to hypoglycaemia.
- Autonomic neuropathy, which can mask the symptoms of hypoglycaemia so the patient is unaware that their blood glucose is low. These asymptomatic hypoglycaemic episodes are not recognised and therefore not treated early enough to avoid a severe episode. Alternatively, autonomic neuropathy can cause upper body sweating that can be mistaken for hypoglycaemia, see Section 14c.
- Patients who are fasting for medical procedures or investigations.
- Excessive consumption of alcohol.

- Inadequate communication between health professionals caring for the patient and between health professionals and the patient, leading to confusion and management mistakes.

It is important to monitor the blood glucose of elderly patients presenting with these risk factors and to be aware that usually more than one risk factor is operating in the individual. The more risk factors present the greater the likelihood of hypoglycaemia occurring.

18.13.2 Management of hypoglycaemia

The method of treating the hypoglycaemia must reflect the functional level of the individual:

- People on a normal oral diet:
  - Treat with a high glycemic index food such as 10 g of glucose powder dissolved in water *or* 1 glass glucozade *or* 5 glucose jelly beans.
- People having thickened fluids/vitamised diets:
  - 15 g tube glucose gel.
- People fed through a PEG tube:
  - 10 g of glucose powder dissolved in water and inserted into the PEG tube.

Practice point

Hypoglycaemia leading to unconsciousness is rare in older people. However, such an event is very stressful to an elderly person; myocardial infarction often occurs as a result of an unconscious hypoglycaemic episode and a 12 lead ECG should be taken.

18.14 Diabetes and falls

Falls are the sixth leading cause of death in older people with and without diabetes, but having diabetes significantly increases the risk. People who fall do so repeatedly and falls are a common cause of placement in a home for the elderly. Falls are a result of a combination of accumulated effects of disease processes, impairment and medications (Quayle 2001). It can be seen from Table 18.1 that a significant number of diabetes-related problems significantly increase the likelihood that an elderly person with diabetes will fall.

People at risk of falling:

- Fell in the last year.
- Have difficulty with mobility and sensory deficits.
- Are on four or more medications particularly oral agents, insulin, antihypotensives, antidepressive agents.
- Have an acute illness.
- Were recently discharged from hospital.
- Have decreased strength and require a walking stick or frame.
- Wear inappropriate footwear.
- Are subject to environmental hazards.

- Have balance problems.
- Diabetes complications such as autonomic neuropathy and visual loss. Postural hypotension is a significant risk factor. Postprandial hypotension is described as a blood pressure fall of 20 mmHg, an hour after eating. In aged care facilities post-prandial hypotension is associated with an increased incidence of falls, syncope, stroke and new coronary events (Aronow & Ahn 1997).

Additional risks are patients who are sedated, especially in an unfamiliar environment such as hospital or aged care facility. They can become disorientated and fall going to the toilet at night.

18.15 Nursing care

- Careful assessment of the individual from an holistic approach that incorporates physical, psychological, social and relationship functioning.
- Strategies need to be in place to assess the risk of falls and to minimise the risk of falling. These include providing a safe environment, orientating the patient to the ward, considering the place of hip protectors, careful discharge planning and early referral to the social worker, domiciliary or aged care team for home assessment.
- Timing meals, PEG and enteral feeds and drug rounds to reduce the risk of hypoglycaemia.
- Adequate preparation of the patient for surgical and investigative procedures, see Chapters 12 and 13.
- Reminding the person to drink, especially in hot weather.
- Monitoring blood glucose and taking steps to correct persistent levels outside the target range.
- Clear, careful explanations to the patient.
- Identifying stress and depression.
- Identifying the barriers to control, recognising and changing those things that can be changed and those that cannot.

References

Aronow, W. & Ahn, C. (1997) Association of post prandial hypotension with incidence of falls, syncope, coronary events, stroke, and total mortality at 29 months follow-up in 499 older nursing home residents. *Journal of the American Geriatrics Society*, **45**, 1051–1053.

Australian Quality Council (1998) *Accreditation Standards for Aged Care*. Canberra.

British Diabetic Association (1999) *Guidelines for Residents with Diabetes in Care Homes*. British Diabetic Association, London.

Department of Health (2001) Care Homes for Older People: National Minimal Standards. Care Standards Act 2000. HMSO, London.

Egede, L., Xiaobou, Y., Zheng D. & Silverstein, M. (2002) The prevalence and pattern of complementary and alternative medicine use in individuals with diabetes. *Diabetes Care*, **25**, 324–329.

Fleming, R. (2002) Report of Federal Department of Health survey into depression in the elderly. *Australian Doctor*, March 14.

Gilden, J., Hendryx, M., Clar, S., Casia, C. & Singh, S. (1992) Diabetes Support Groups improve health care of older diabetic patients, *Journal of the American Geriatrics Society*, **40**, 145–150.

Gradman, T., Laes, A., Thompson, L. & Reaven, G. (1993) Verbal learning and/or memory improves with glycaemic control in older subjects with non insulin-dependent diabetes mellitus. *Journal of the American Geriatrics Society*, **41**, 1305–1312.

Halter, J. (2001) Report of the American Diabetes Association Meeting, *Practical Diabetes International.*

Howes, L. (2001) Dosage alteration in the elderly – importance of mild renal impairment. *Current Therapeutics*, **42** (7), 33–35.

Jennings, P. (1997) Oral antihypoglycaemics: considerations in older patient with non insulin-dependent diabetes mellitus. *Drugs and Aging*, **10** (5), 323–331.

Kirkland, F. (2000) Improvements in diabetes care for elderly people in care homes. *Journal of Diabetes Nursing*, **4** (5), 150–155.

Middleton, M., Nazarenko, G., Nivison-Smith, I. & Smerdely, P. (2001) Prevalance of malnutrition and 12-month incidence of mortality in two Sydney teaching hospitals. *International Medicine Journal*, **31**, 455–461.

Paolisso, G., Gambardella, A., Verza, M. D'Amora, A., Sgambato, S. & Varrichio, M. (1992) ACE-inhibition improves insulin-sensitivity in age insulin-resistant hypertensive patients. *Journal of Human Hypertension*, **6**, 175–179.

Quayle, S. (2001) Gains of minimising falls: managing the older patient. *Australian Doctor*, **July**, 43–44.

Rosenstock, J. (2001) Management of Type 2 diabetes in the elderly: special considerations. *Pulsebeat*, **Oct–Nov**, 5.

Schwartz, M., Woods, S., Porte, D., Seeley, R. & Baskin, D. (2000) Central nervous system control of food intake. *Nature*, **404**, 661–671.

Sinclair, A. (1995) Initial management of NIDDM in the elderly. In: *Diabetes in Old Age* (eds P. Funacane, A. Sinclair). John Wiley & Sons, pp. 181–201.

Sinclair, A., Allard, I. & Bayes, A. (1997) Observation of diabetes care in long-term institutional settings with measures of cognitive function and dependency. *Diabetes Care*, 778–786.

Tiengo, A. (1999) Burden of treatment in the elderly patient: reducing the burden of diabetes. *Diabetes Care*, **11**, 6–8.

World Health Organisation (1999) *Guidelines for Older Australians.* Commonwealth of Australia, Canberra.

Zhao, W., Chen, H., Xu, H. *et al.* (1999) Brain insulin receptors and spatial memory. *Journal of Biological Chemistry*, **274**, 34893–34901.

Chapter 19
Foot Care

19.1 Key points

- Lower limb problems represent a significant physical, psychological, social and economic burden for people with diabetes and the health system.
- Forty to seventy per cent of lower limb amputations occur in people with diabetes.
- Peripheral neuropathy, vascular disease, infection, foot deformity and inappropriate footwear predispose people to foot disease.
- Screening for foot disease and preventative self-care practices are essential.
- Foot complications are common in the elderly.
- Although people with Type 2 diabetes are the main focus of many foot-care guidelines, people with Type 1 diabetes also develop foot problems.
- A multidisciplinary team approach and good communication are essential.

Rationale

Foot disease is a significant cause of hospitalisation for people with diabetes. Careful assessment, consideration of the causative factors and management of existing problems can limit further exacerbation of diabetic foot disease. Appropriate nursing care can prevent foot problems occurring as a result of hospitalisation or aged care placement.

Diabetic foot disease is a common cause of hospital admissions and is associated with significant morbidity and mortality. It is a heterogeneous disease entity, defined as a group of syndromes that lead to tissue breakdown. Infection, neuropathy and ischaemia are usually present and increase the risk of infection (Apelqvist & Larsson 2000).

Forty to seventy per cent of lower limb amputations occur in people with diabetes and most begin with an ulcer. The amputation rate can be reduced by preventative foot care. The spectrum of diabetic foot disease varies globally depending on socioeconomic circumstances, but the basic underlying pathophysiology is the same (Bakker 2000). Charcot deformity is a severe form of diabetic foot disease that is often missed through misdiagnosis in the early stages and delay in appropriate management. The possibility of Charcot's deformity should be considered in any person with long-standing diabetes, neuropathy and foot disease.

Foot disease and its management, have an adverse impact on the wellbeing and quality of life of people with diabetes (Brod 1998). The disease itself and some management practices, e.g. non-weight-bearing regimes, restrict physical activity and social interaction and often result in non-compliance.

Foot care is an extremely important aspect of the nursing care of people with diabetes in any setting and is often neglected in acute care settings. The combination of mechanical factors and vascular and nerve damage as a complication of diabetes leads to an increased risk of ulceration, infection and amputation.

It is estimated that 40% of diabetics have peripheral neuropathy and 20% of hospital admissions are for foot-related problems.

19.2 Vascular changes

People with diabetes and peripheral vascular disease are predisposed to atherosclerosis, which is exacerbated by chronic hyperglycaemia, endothelial damage, non-enzymatic tissue glycosylation and polyneuropathy. These conditions impair vascular remodelling.

(1) *Macrovascular* (major vessel) disease may lead to:
- intermittent claudication and rest pain
- poor circulation to the lower limbs which leads to decreased nutrition, tissue hypoxia and delayed healing if any trauma occurs in this area. The injured tissue is prone to infection and gangrene can result.

(2) *Microvascular* (small vessel) disease leads to thickening of capillary basement membranes, poor blood supply to the skin and tissue hypoxia, predisposing the feet to infection and slow healing.

19.3 Infection

Foot infections are a common and serious problem in people with diabetes. They occur as a result of skin ulceration or deep penetrating injuries, e.g. standing on a drawing pin. These injuries can go unnoticed for days because the person does not feel pain if they have peripheral neuropathy. Aerobic gram-positive cocci are the most frequently encountered pathogens and in complex, previously treated wounds gram-negative bacilli and anaerobic organisms can be present (Lipsky & Berendt 2000).

Antibiotic regimes are usually commenced on clinical grounds and modified on the basis of the culture and sensitivity results from a wound swab, and the patient's response.

Management includes:

- Broad spectrum antibiotics that may need to be given IV for severe infections. Antibiotic therapy may be required for 1–2 weeks and up to 6 weeks if osteomyelitis is present.
- X-ray and MRI bone scans to determine the extent of the infection.
- Surgical débridement and/or revascularisation, e.g. femoral/popliteal bypass, or amputation if indicated.
- Selection and application of appropriate wound dressings (Edmonds *et al.* 2000; Harding *et al.* 2000).
- Biomechanical measures such as total contact casts to relieve pressure in high-pressure ulcers and Charcot's foot deformity. Casts allow the person to remain mobile thus improving their social and psychological wellbeing. Infection and subsequent oedema must be managed because they aggravate the pressure on muscles and can lead to muscle necrosis.

Practice point

Swabs need to be taken from deep in the ulcer cavity. This can be painful and analgesia may be required. Superficial swabs often do not identify all the organisms present, particularly anaerobes.

19.4 Neuropathy

Diabetic neuropathy is defined as the presence of clinical or subclinical evidence of peripheral nerve damage which cannot be attributed to any other disease process. Neuropathy can affect the sensory nerves resulting in pain, tingling, pins and needles or numbness. These symptoms are often worse at night. The sensory loss results in insensitivity to pain, cold, heat, touch and vibration. Trauma, pressure areas, sores, blisters, cuts and burns may not be detected by the patient. Callous formation, ulceration and bone involvement can occur.

The motor nerves can also be affected, resulting in weakness, loss of muscle fibres and diminished reflexes. Both types of nerves can be affected at the same time. Medications may not be effective in the treatment of neuropathic pain, but some commonly used drugs employed to manage the discomfort are:

- Simple measures such as aspirin, codeine, topical capsaicin cream (wear gloves to apply) and massage.
- Opsite applied to the affected areas (Foster *et al.* 1994).
- Tricyclic antidepressive medications which may have secondary benefits where the person is depressed.
- Anticonvulsants such as Phenytoin.
- Gabapentin for people who are unable to tolerate other traditionally used agents has been shown to be effective in the short term but long-term use has not been evaluated (Hemstreet & Lapointe 2001).
- Nerve blocks using lignocaine can give relief for 3–21 days and IV lignocaine has been used (Boulton & Jervell 1998).
- Diazepam, especially where cramps are present.
- Physiotherapy to maintain muscle tone.

Differentiating between the different types of nerve fibres involved allows a more targeted approach to pain management. Where unmyelinated c fibres are affected, characterised by burning, dysthetic pain, capsaicin or Clonidine may be effective. Where the alpha fibres are involved the pain is often deep and boring and insulin infusion, lignocaine or gabapentin may be effective (Vinik *et al.* 2000). Often both types of fibres are affected.

Other drugs include the aldose reductase inhibitors such as Tolrestat that aim to prevent conversion of glucose to sorbitol in the polyol pathway.

Other non-drug measures include improving blood glucose control, stopping smoking, reducing alcohol intake and eating a healthy diet.

The autonomic nervous system may also be affected by diabetes. Autonomic nervous system involvement may lead to an absence of sweating, which causes dry, cracked skin and increases the risk of infection. Other effects of autonomic neuropathy include gastric stasis, impotence, hypoglycaemic unawareness and incontinence (see Section 14c).

The small muscle wasting secondary to longstanding neuropathy can lead to abnormal foot shapes, e.g. clawing of the toes, making the purchase of well fitting shoes difficult.

Vascular disease, neuropathy and infection are more likely to develop if there is longstanding hyperglycaemia, which contributes to the accumulation of sorbitol through the polyol pathway, leading to damage to the nerves and small blood vessels. Figure 19.1 illustrates the interaction of factors leading to foot problems in people with diabetes.

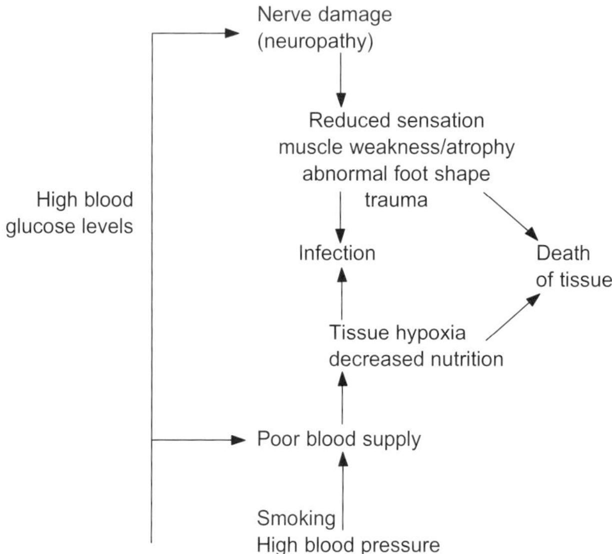

Figure 19.1 Diagrammatic representation of the factors leading to foot problems in people with diabetes.

Table 19.1 lists changes in feet due to the normal ageing process, and Table 19.2 lists the risk factors for the development of foot problems in people with diabetes. These factors should all be incorporated in the nursing assessment to ensure that appropriate foot care is part of the overall management of the patient.

Table 19.1 Changes in feet due to normal ageing.

(1) Skin becomes thin, fragile
(2) Nails thick and often deformed
(3) Blood supply is reduced
(4) Nerve function often impaired
(5) Muscle weakness and wasting
(6) Arthritis, may lead to pain and deformity

19.4.1 Stages of peripheral neuropathy

Chronic and painful – improve metabolic control.
Acute and painful – analgesia.
Painless – education, orthoses, regular assessment.
Late complications (Vinik *et al.* 2000).

Table 19.2 Risk factors for the development of foot problems in people with diabetes.

(1)	Diabetes, especially if blood glucose is continually high
(2)	Smoking
(3)	Obesity
(4)	High blood pressure
(5)	Cardiac disease
(6)	Lack of or inadequate foot care
(7)	Visual impairment
(8)	Inappropriate footwear
(9)	Delay in seeking help
(10)	Previous foot problems
(11)	Depression

Note: These factors should be part of the nursing assessment. The more risk factors present the greater the likelihood of amputation (Pecorara 1990).

19.5 Objectives of care

(1) To identify feet most at risk of trauma, ulceration and infection in aged care, rehabilitation and hospital settings by assessing vascular, nerve and diabetic status:
sensation using 10 g Semmes-Weinstein monofilaments, 128 Hz tuning forks and disposable pin prickers (Apelqvist *et al.* 2000);
presence of vascular insufficiency by checking capillary return and the presence of foot and peripheral pulses; and
foot deformity.
(2) To assess patient knowledge of foot care.
(3) To reinforce appropriate preventative foot care.
(4) To prevent trauma, infection and pressure ulcers.
(5) To treat any problem detected.
(6) To refer to podiatry, orthotics, physiotherapy, rehabilitation, diabetes nurse specialist/diabetes educator or specialist foot clinic as necessary.
(7) To control or eliminate any factors which predispose the patient to the risk of foot problems in hospital.
(8) Risk of falls in the elderly (see Chapter 18).
(9) Pain management.

19.6 Nursing responsibilities

(1) To assess the feet carefully on admission. Assess self-care potential (can the patient reach the feet, see clearly?). When assessing the feet, obtain information about:
   (a) Past medical history:
      - glycaemic control
      - previous foot-related problems/deformities
      - smoking habits
      - nerve and vascular related risk factors

- claudication, rest pain
- previous foot ulcer/amputation
- alcohol intake.

(b) Type of footwear (socks, shoes):
- hygiene
- activity level.

(c) Social factors:
- living alone
- elderly.

(2) When examining the feet:
Check both feet
- check pulses, dorsalis pedis, posterior tibial
- assess toenails: thick, layered, curved, ingrowing toenails will need attention
- note foot structure; overlapping toes, prominent metatarsal heads on the sole of the foot
- check for callus, cracks and fungal infections that can indicate inadequate foot care and poor hygiene.

(3) Note also:
- pallor on elevation of leg
- capillary return (normally 1–2 seconds)
- any discoloration of legs
- hair loss.

(4) To ensure appropriate foot hygiene:
- wash in lukewarm water – use pH neutral soap products that do not dry the skin especially in elderly people or people on steroid medications and those with atopic skin
- check water temperature with wrist before putting the patient into a bath
- dry thoroughly, including between toes
- apply cream to prevent dryness and cracks (urea cream, sorbelene).

(5) Ensure Elastoplast/Band Aids, bandages do *not* encircle toes as they can act like tourniquets and reduce the circulation which could result in gangrene. Apply elastic support stockings correctly.

(6) Maintain a safe environment:
- use a bed cradle
- ensure shoes are worn if walking around the ward
- strict bed rest may be necessary while the ulcer is healing
- maintain aseptic technique.

(7) Check feet daily and report any changes or the development of any callus, abrasion or trauma.

(8) Monitor blood glucose control.

(9) Attend to dressings and administer antibiotics according to treatment order. Antibiotics are often given intravenously if foot infection is present.

(10) Take the opportunity to ensure self-care knowledge is current and that complication screening has been attended to. Ensure preventative foot care education is provided, to give the patient with diabetes:
- an understanding of effects of diabetes on the feet
- a knowledge of appropriate footwear
- the ability to identify foot risk factors
- an understanding of the principal effects of poor control (continual hyperglycaemia) on foot health

- knowledge about the services available for assistance with their diabetes care and how to obtain advice about foot care
- knowledge about appropriate foot care practices, in particular that they must inspect their feet daily and seek help early if any problems are found
- odour control can be an issue when infection and gangrene are present. Some wound dressings have an absorbent layer that eliminates odour by absorbing bacteria. Good foot hygiene helps reduce the odour.

19.7 Classification of foot ulcers

A number of ulcer classification systems are in existence and nurses are advised to follow the system in their place of employment. In 2002 an international working party was established to develop an international consensus foot ulcer classification system. Foot ulcers can be loosely classified as:

(1) Clean, superficial ulcer.
(2) Deeper ulcer, possibly infected, but no bone involvement.
(3) Deep ulcer, tracking infection and bone involvement.
(4) Localised gangrene and necrosis (usually forefoot, heel).
(5) Extensive gangrene of foot.

The depth and width of the ulcer should be recorded regularly; a plastic template, dated and filed in the patient's history, aids in the assessment of changes in ulcer size. The presence, amount and type of exudate must be recorded.

Clinical observation

Aromatherapy essential oils on the *surface of the secondary dressing* can help. They should not be applied directly to the wound. They can be used in a vapouriser for environmental fragrancing. Some essential oils can help improve mood.

Practice point

Painting the area with a betadine or other skin antiseptic is of little value. Coloured antiseptics can obscure some of the signs of infection.

19.8 Wound management

Dressings may be needed to absorb the exudate and protect the foot. No dressing is appropriate for all wound types. Surgical débridement, amputation or an occlusive dressing may be required. It is important to keep the temperature at 37°C, the dressing moist and the pH acidic to promote healing. Choose a dressing that does not cause tissue damage when it is removed, i.e. does not stick to the wound and protects the wound from infection. The moisture aids in pain relief, decreases the healing time and gives a better cosmetic result. An acidic environment promotes granulation tissue. The management of ulcers in hospital and other specific foot problems are listed in Table 19.3.

Table 19.3 Management of specific foot problems while the person is in hospital.

Problem	*Treatment*
Burning, paraesthesia, aching	Encourage person to walk Maintain euglycaemia
Pain	Foot cradle, sheepskin, medications as ordered
Dry skin, cracks	Clean, dry carefully, apply moisturiser, e.g. urea cream, sorbelene
Claudication	Medications as ordered Rest Elevate feet Vascular assessment Angiography
Foot deformity	Consult podiatrist Physiotherapy Orthotist
Ulcers, infection	Refer to specific medical order Assess daily Make template to note change in size of ulcer Antibiotics See classification of foot ulcers, Section 19.7 Débridement, amputation

Diabetic foot ulcers heal slowly and bed rest is important. The patient may be otherwise well. Encourage independence with blood glucose testing and insulin administration. Refer for occupational therapy. The person may benefit from counselling if they are depressed.

Careful discharge planning is imperative:

- To ensure mobilisation and rehabilitation and that there is a safe environment at home.
- Interim placement in an extended care facility may be necessary.
- Assess the physical and social support available after discharge.

Practice point

Orthopaedic patients with diabetes and foot or leg plasters should be encouraged *not* to scratch under the plaster, especially if they have 'at risk' feet. Damage can occur and remain undetected until the plaster is removed.

19.8.1 Wound management techniques under study

Several new wound management products for hard-to-heal ulcers are under study:

- Platelet-derived growth factor applied topically to increase granulation;
- Hyaff;

- Dermagraft;
- Apilgraf;
- Granulocyte-colony stimulating factor (Edmonds *et al.* 2000).

Hyperbaric oxygen may be beneficial in some serious ulcers. Oxygen is necessary for wound healing and hyperbaric oxygen can increase tissue oxygen levels and improves the killing power of phagocytes (Bakker 2000).

19.9 Rehabilitation

Despite the best care, amputations are sometimes required. A rehabilitation process is necessary once the acute stage has settled. Below-knee amputations give a favourable result even if the popliteal pulses are diminished (Steinberg 1991). The goals of rehabilitation are:

- Appropriate stump care. In the early stages this may involve bandaging to reduce oedema. Circular bandages should be avoided because they tend to act like tourniquets and reduce the blood supply to the stump. Analgesia should be available. Later, correctly fitting the stump into the socket of the prothesis and regular inspection for the presence of infection or pressure areas.
- Prevent muscle contracture with regular physiotherapy.
- Independence.
- Ambulation with a prothesis or wheelchair depending on the individual assessment, e.g. people who have advanced neurological disease such as stroke or Parkinson's disease, CCF and unstable angina may not be suitable for a prothesis.
- Early mobilisation is usually desirable.

Practice points

(1) Amputation should not always be seen as treatment failure. It can relieve pain, allow the person to return home and enjoy an improved quality of life. Amputation is distressing for the person with diabetes and their family and careful explanation, support and counselling are essential. The patient should be included in the decision-making process and make the final decision. Their social and psychological situation should be considered as well as their physical needs.

(2) Amputation does increase the risk of a second amputation.

References

Apelqvist, J. & Larsson, J. (2000) What is the most effective way to reduce incidence of amputation in the diabetic foot? *Diabetes/Metabolism Research and Reviews*, **16**, suppl 1, s75–s83.

Apelqvist, J., Bakker, K., Van Houtum, W., Nabuurs-Franssen, M. & Schaper, N. (2000) The International Consensus and Practical Guidelines on the Management and Prevention of the Diabetic Foot. *Diabetes/Metabolism Research and Reviews*, **16**, suppl 1, s84–s92.

Bakker, D. (2000) Hyperbaric oxygen therapy and the diabetic foot. *Diabetes/Metabolism Research and Reviews*, **16**, suppl 1, s55–s58.

Boulton, A. (2000) The diabetic foot: a global view. *Diabetes/Metabolism Research and Reviews*, **16**, suppl 1, s2–s5.

Boulton, A. & Jervell, J. (1998) International Guidelines for the Management of Diabetic Peripheral Neuropathy. *Diabetic Medicine*, **15** (6), 508–514.
Brod, M. (1998) Quality of life issues in patients with diabetes and lower limb extremity ulcers: patients and caregivers. *Quality Life Research*, **7**, 365–372.
Edmonds, M., Bates, M., Doxford, M., Gough, A. & Foster, A. (2000) New treatments in ulcer healing and wound infection. *Diabetes/Metabolism Research and Reviews*, **16**, suppl 1, s51–s54.
Foster, A., Eaton, C., McConville, D. & Edmonds, M. (1994) Application of Op-cite film: a new effective treatment for painful diabetic neuropathy. *Diabetic Medicine*, **11**, 768–772.
Harding, K., Jones, V. & Price, P. (2000) Topical treatment: which dressing to choose. *Diabetes/Metabolism Research and Reviews*, **16**, suppl 1, s47–s50.
Hemstreet, B. & Lapointe, M. (2001) Evidence for the use of gabapentin in the treatment of diabetic peripheral neuropathy. *Clinical Therapeutics*, **23** (4), 520–531.
Lipsky, B. & Berendt, A. (2000) Principles and practice of antibiotic therapy of diabetic foot infections. *Diabetes/Metabolism Research and Reviews*, **16** suppl 1, s42–s46.
Pecorara, R. (1990) Pathways to diabetic limb amputation. *Diabetes Care*, **13** (5), 513–530.
Steinberg, F. (1991) Rehabilitation after amputation. *Diabetes Spectrum*, **4** (1), 5–9.
Sutton, M., McGrath, C., Brady, L., Wood, J. (2000) Diabetic foot care: assessing the impact of foot care on the whole patient. *Practical Diabetes International*, **17** (5), 365–372.
Vinik, A., Park, T., Stansberry, K. & Henger, P. (2000) Diabetic neuropathy. *Diabetologia*, **43**, 957–973.

Chapter 20
Diabetes in Children and Adolescents

20.1 Key points

- A supportive family is an important aspect of diabetes management.
- Family stress and marital disharmony affect the child's metabolic control.
- Clinicians dealing with children with diabetes must spend time assessing the family structure and help the family to support their child.
- Most children have Type 1 diabetes and insulin should never be withheld.
- There is an increasing incidence of Type 2 diabetes occurring in children.

Rationale

Diabetes in children and adolescents impacts on the family dynamics. Family support is essential if the child is to achieve euglycaemia and psychological wellbeing. Management plans need to incorporate normal growth and development.

20.2 Introduction

At least 60 000 children worldwide are diagnosed with diabetes annually and the incidence continues to rise by 3–5% per year. Type 2 diabetes, once rare in children, is increasing (IDF Consultative Section on Diabetes Education 2002; Sinha *et al.* 2002). Insulin resistance and impaired glucose tolerance was present in 25% of obese children in Sinha *et al.*'s study.

Children and adolescents have changing needs as they grow and develop. Therefore regular assessment of their diabetes management is essential because there are major physical, psychological and social differences between the growth and development stages. Assessment of maturity, sensitive supervision and allowing the child to gradually take over diabetes self-care tasks should be factored into a holistic diabetes plan.

Educating teachers and other carers is important and the child should be involved in these activities as appropriate. Diabetes should not preclude the child from attending school excursions and camps but extra precautions will need to be taken, e.g. being able to eat on time. Diabetes camps provide an important learning experience and many children who attended camps when they were young help out on camps as they grow older. This kind of peer support contributes to psychological wellbeing.

20.3 Diabetes in children and adolescents

Type 1 usually present with a sudden onset of symptoms and insulin injections are needed for survival. Insulin and dietary requirements can change rapidly, especially in children, due to rapid changes in activity levels and growth. Therefore consistent acceptable blood glucose levels may be difficult to achieve.

A supportive and encouraging family is important if the child is to accept diabetes and eventually take over diabetic self-management. The family in turn needs support, advice and encouragement. Good control is associated with a structured supportive family (Johnson *et al*. 1990; Thompson *et al*. 2001). Families need to provide appropriate supervision and discipline and maintain a family structure that meets the needs of the child and other family members.

Hypoglycaemia can be unpredictable in children whose activity level and intake can vary enormously from day-to-day and within the day. Hypoglycaemia can be difficult to deal with in young children and can manifest as:

- Unaccustomed naughtiness
- Noisy behaviour
- Aggression
- Crying
- Tremulousness

If it is not recognised and treated promptly the child can become unconscious, which is frightening for the child and those around them (see Chapter 8). Parents often feel safer if they have glucagon available and some also like it available at school.

During adolescence the hormonal surge at puberty can make blood glucose control difficult. Dietary restrictions and the diabetic regime can be seen as obstacles to fitting in with peer activities and may be neglected. Achieving independence from the family can be difficult if diabetes is diagnosed at this time.

Social pressure and the emphasis on food that is part of the diabetes management regime can increase the likelihood of eating disorders. Young people with diabetes fear putting on weight and skip meals and run their blood glucose levels high to avoid weight gain (Dunning 1994). Eating disorders are widespread among adolescent girls and diabetic-specific concerns may contribute to their development. The full range of sub-clinical and clinical eating disorders may be more prevalent in women with diabetes (Levine & Marcus 1997).

The menarche affects control in girls and the blood glucose profile often reflects the stages of the menstrual cycle (see Chapter 17). When the child becomes an adolescent contraceptive and pregnancy counselling are vital.

Polycystic disease of the ovaries (PCOS) is associated with insulin resistance syndromes and diabetes and has a typically menarchal onset. The effects of unpredictable and heavy menstrual bleeding are disabling and place the young woman at risk of iron deficiency anaemia (Legro & Dunaif 1997). Chronic anovulation increases the risk of endometrial hyperplasia and endometrial cancer. Infertility is a consequence and has a negative impact on the young person's self-concept. Early diagnosis and management is important. PCOS often manifests as excess facial hair and irregular periods.

The transfer from paediatric care to adult specialist care can be very stressful. Neglect of the diabetes, failure to attend appointments and poor control are not uncommon (Court 1991). Tact and understanding are very important if these young people are not to be lost to adequate medical supervision (Dunning 1993).

Children from single parent families and families with marital conflict are at increased risk of poor metabolic control (Thompson *et al.* 2001). Family dysfunction, inadequate treatment adherence and unacceptable glycaemic control often go hand-in-hand (Lorenz & Wysocki 1991). Unacceptable glycaemic control carries the risk of admissions to hospital in ketoacidosis and the development of long-term diabetic complications (see Chapter 10).

20.3.1 Management goals

(1) To achieve normal growth and physical and psychological development. A basal bolus insulin regime is preferred.
(2) To prevent or delay the onset of diabetes-related complications including short-term complications such as hypoglycaemia and ketoacidosis. Long-term complications are extremely rare before puberty but some adolescent centres are beginning to screen for complications from about the age of 10 to establish complication screening as a routine part of diabetes care.
(3) To ensure a balanced diet.
(4) To promote acceptance of the diabetes by the child and the family.
(5) To assist the child to gradually take over the self-care tasks.
(6) To develop an integrated health plan that includes sexual health, responsible contraception and planned pregnancy as suitable to the age and development stage of the young person.
(7) To transfer to adult care.
(8) The child should be involved in developing their diabetes management plan within their capabilities. Disagreements between mothers and their children about who is assuming responsibility and adherence levels are predictors of HbA1c (Anderson *et al.* 1991). Their child's involvement in their self-care gradually increases as they mature and develop fine motor skills.
(9) The availability of acute care should the need arise.

20.4 Strategies to enhance compliance in adolescence

Establishing a therapeutic relationship with the young person is essential so that they feel comfortable about discussing issues with health professionals.

Young people with and without diabetes engage in risk-taking behaviour including not following medical advice, but no more so than adults (Johnson *et al.* 1990). A management approach that seeks concordance between health professional advice and the young person's behaviour is more likely to be successful (Fleming & Watson 2002).

There is a range of issues that has an impact on development and some issues have a greater priority than health status for the young person. It is normal adolescent behaviour to think in the short term and want to learn from their experience. This means that short-term goals are more likely to be effective and can be modified progressively. Young people should be encouraged to discuss their experiences, which can be used as experiential teaching and learning strategies.

Many young people feel vulnerable and this can be exacerbated by diabetes and the need to take on the responsibility for adult roles and diabetes management. Exploring these concerns can help young people acknowledge and deal with them.

Many young people feel frustrated when they 'do all the right things' and their metabolic control is inadequate. This can lead to decreased motivation and feelings of helplessness and hopelessness especially if they do not have a supportive family (Kyngas 2000). Focusing on the positive aspects and small gains and not on 'good' and 'bad' control can take the focus off failure. Striving for diabetes balance is more important than control. Metabolic control will be achieved if the individual's life is in balance.

The lack of a consistent and accessible health service and dealing with new health professionals when moving to adult care can be stressful. Collaboration between paediatric and adult services and a planned transition process can overcome some of these problems (Department of Health 2001; Dunning 1993).

Using multiple strategies and consultation techniques that encourage young people to ask questions is more likely to uncover accurate and meaningful information than is the consultation where the young person tells the health professional 'what they want to hear'. Compliance issues should be discussed in the context of what the young person's goals are. Compliance can be enhanced by:

- Organising a youth appropriate service.
- Seeing the young person separately from their parents as they mature and begin to take responsibility for their diabetes management.
- Addressing the broader issues and life priorities and put diabetes into that context.
- Giving clear simple instructions and supporting verbal information with written instructions and the availability of telephone advice.
- Utilising family/carers as appropriate.
- Considering the type of questions likely to get honest answers, e.g. instead of asking 'do you always take your correct dose of insulin?' try 'what dose of insulin suits you best?' (Fleming & Watson 2002).

20.4.1 Nursing responsibilities

In addition to those nursing tasks outlined in specific chapters it is important to:

- Document height and weight on percentile charts.
- Encourage independence and allow the child to inject and test if already doing so.
- Monitor dietary intake and ensure appropriate dietary review by dietitian.
- Ensure diabetic knowledge is assessed.
- Ensure privacy during procedures.
- Avoid admitting adolescents and children to wards with elderly people, if possible.

Clinical observation

Enuresis is an unusual presentation of diabetes in children.

20.5 Ketoacidosis in children

The management of ketoacidosis is described in Chapter 10. Additional issues specific to children are:

- Cerebral oedema is a very serious medical emergency in children. Monitoring mental status and strict fluid calculations are essential.
- Headache and/or altered behaviour may indicate impending cerebral oedema.

Management includes bolus IV mannitol, nursing with the head of the bed elevated and fluid restriction.

- Sodium bicarbonate is not usually given in childhood DKA because of the risk of hypokalaemia, cerebral acidosis and changed oxygen affinity of haemoglobin.
- Monitor sodium levels and adjust IV fluid appropriately as the blood glucose falls. Hyponatraemia can herald impending cerebral oedema.

References

Anderson, B., Auslander, W., Jung, K., Miller, P. & Santiago, J. (1991) Assessing family sharing of diabetes responsibilities. *Diabetes Spectrum*, **4** (5), 263–268.

Court, J. (1991) *Modern Living with Diabetes*. Diabetes Australia, Victoria.

Department of Health (2001) *Diabetes National Service Framework: Standards for Diabetes Services*. Department of Health, London.

Dunning, P. (1993) Moving to adult care. *Practical Diabetes*, **10** (6), 226–228.

Dunning, P. (1994) Having diabetes: young adult perspectives. *The Diabetes Educator*, **21** (1), 58–65.

Fleming, T. & Watson, P. (2002) Enhancing compliance in adolescents. *Current Therapeutics*, **43** (3), 14–18.

International Diabetes Federation Consultative Section on Diabetes Education (2002) *International Diabetes Curriculum: Paediatric and Adolescent Module*, International Diabetes Federation, Brussels.

Johnson, S., Freund, A. & Silverstein, J. (1990) Adherence–health status relationships in childhood diabetes. *Health Psychology*, **9**, 606–631.

Kyngas, H. (2000) Compliance of adolescents with diabetes. *Journal of Paediatric Nursing*, **15** (4), 260–267.

Legro, R. & Dunaif, A. (1997) Menstrual disorders in insulin resistant states. *Diabetes Spectrum*, **10** (3), 185–190.

Levine, M. & Marcus, M. (1997) Women, diabetes and disordered eating. *Diabetes Spectrum*, **4** (5), 191–195.

Lorenz, R. & Wysocki, T. (1991) Conclusions: Family and childhood diabetes. *Diabetes Spectrum*, **4** (5), 290–292.

Sinha, R., Fisch, G., Teague, B. *et al.* (2002) Prevalence of impaired glucose intolerance among children and adolescents with marked obesity. *New England Journal of Medicine*, **346**, 802–810.

Thompson, S., Auslander, W. & White, N. (2001) Comparison of single-mother families on metabolic control of children with diabetes. *Diabetes Care*, **24** (2), 234–238.

Chapter 21
Diabetes in Pregnancy and Gestational Diabetes

21.1 Key points

- Good control before and during pregnancy reduces the risks to mother and baby.
- Planned pregnancies have better outcomes.
- Insulin is required in Type 2 diabetes during pregnancy and breastfeeding.
- Existing renal disease and retinopathy may deteriorate during pregnancy.

Rationale

Coordinated care and prepregnancy planning is necessary to ensure optimal outcomes for mother and baby. Planning for an optimal delivery begins in adolescence with diabetes education and sexual counselling.

Diabetes can develop during pregnancy, gestational diabetes, see Chapter 1. Most women are screened for diabetes during pregnancy so that blood glucose levels can be controlled to avoid the risks that having diabetes places on both mother and baby. Women particularly at risk are those with a history of diabetes in the family, diabetes during a previous pregnancy or previous delivery of a large baby.

21.2 Introduction

Hormones released by the placenta predispose the mother to hyperglycaemia and increase the burden of fuel use by the fetus. Insulin sensitivity increases in the first trimester but insulin resistance develops in the second and third trimesters. The placental glucose transporter, GLUT-1, increases the transplacental glucose flux. The activity of GLUT-4 at the maternal cellular level decreases, which means glucose is not utilised by the mother and high levels cross the placenta where they are utilised by the fetus. This sets the scene for macrosomia and fetal abnormalities and makes vaginal delivery difficult (Hollingsworth 1992). Prepregnancy counselling is essential to limit risks to mother and baby (Coustan 1997).

21.2.1 Gestational diabetes

Gestational diabetes (GDM) refers to carbohydrate intolerance of variable severity that first appears during pregnancy (Metzger 1998). GDM is the most common metabolic complication of pregnancy.

An international workshop held in 1997 made temporary recommendations about the diagnostic criteria and the degree of glucose intolerance that is a threat to the pregnancy (Metzger 1998). Generally, a screening test is performed between 24 and 28 weeks using either 50 or 75 g of glucose. Fasting is not required. A formal oral glucose tolerance test is performed if the blood glucose is ≥7.8 mmol/L–50 gram load or >8 mmol/L–75 gram load (see Chapter 1). GDM is present if the fasting level is ≥5.5 mmol/L and the 2-hour postprandial level is ≥8 mmol/L.

Blood glucose levels may return to normal after delivery; however, the possibility of diabetes manifesting again in later life is increased, as are the risks of developing long-term diabetic complications. Prepregnancy counselling and achieving good control is important for the women with existing diabetes, contemplating pregnancy.

Regular appointments with the obstetrician and diabetologist and close fetal monitoring are very important. Care of the mother and baby during labour and delivery are specialty areas and outside the scope of this Manual.

21.2.1 Management goals

A management plan should be developed that aims for a vaginal delivery at term unless there are contraindications. A multidisciplinary team consisting of an endocrinologist, diabetes nurse specialists/diabetes educators or midwife, obstetrician, paediatrician and dietitian is required.

(1) To achieve good blood glucose control before becoming pregnant to decrease the possibility of:
- Stillbirth;
- Prematurity;
- Fetal abnormalities – abnormalities and poor metabolic control increase the risk of miscarriage, macrosomia, prematurity, respiratory distress, death in utero and fetal metabolic complications such as hypo- or hyperglycaemia at birth. Fetal adipocytes develop in the third trimester predisposing the baby to obesity and Type 2 diabetes in later life. Regular fetal monitoring including scans, if indicated, and good maternal blood glucose control are essential;
- Macrosomia;
- Respiratory distress;
- Caesarian section.

(2) Manage existing complications. The presence of autonomic neuropathy (Section 14c) may predispose the mother to intractable vomiting and precipitate metabolic disturbances such as ketoacidosis (see Chapter 10). Existing renal disease and retinopathy often deteriorate during pregnancy and should be closely monitored each trimester. Renal disease increases the risk of pre-eclampsia and hydramnios. Blood pressure control is essential. Some authorities cite existing renal and cardiovascular disease as contraindications to pregnancy.

(3) Revise home management of emergencies such as sick days/hyperglycaemia and morning sickness.

(4) To maintain good blood glucose control during pregnancy (4–5 mmol/L, i.e.

normal) but avoid hypoglycaemia. Women with Type 2 diabetes will require insulin. The insulin dose may decrease in the first trimester in women with Type 1 diabetes but requirements gradually increase between 22 and 32 weeks as insulin resistance develops until it stabilises from 34 weeks to term. After delivery, insulin requirements drop dramatically.

(5) To provide adequate carbohydrate intake to avoid ketonaemia, especially during the second trimester.
(6) To provide adequate nutrient intake to allow normal growth and development of the baby without compromising the mother's health. This requires the advice of a dietitian so that weight gain is appropriate and the diet is tailored to the individual. Folate supplements are usual to prevent fetal neural tube defects.
(7) To monitor kidney function and screen for pre-eclampsia and hydramnios.
(8) To monitor maternal weight.
(9) To encourage no smoking and limited alcohol consumption.
(10) To deliver the baby. Insulin is given as required during labour. Some units use insulin infusions to avoid hyperglycaemia (see Chapter 7). Frequent blood glucose monitoring is required because insulin requirements fall dramatically after delivery and maternal hypoglycaemia is possible. The baby is prone to hypoglycaemia after delivery and should be monitored closely for 24 hours or as indicated.
(11) Encourage breast-feeding. Breast-feeding provides essential nutrition and immunity for the baby. It decreases the risk of obesity and Type 2 diabetes in later life in babies of women who develop GDM.

Practice point

OHAs should not be used during pregnancy. People with Type 2 diabetes often require insulin during pregnancy and continue to need it during breast-feeding.

Important points concerning pregnancy in a patient with existing diabetes:

- The risk of the child developing diabetes is relatively low.
- Babies of diabetic mothers who maintain normal blood glucose levels throughout pregnancy are less likely to develop congenital abnormalities.
- If the woman has Type 2 diabetes and is taking OHAs prior to pregnancy, the doctor will change the treatment to insulin during pregnancy.
- OHAs prior to pregnancy do not prevent the mother breast-feeding her baby as long as she remains on insulin.

References

Coustan, D. (1997) Is preconception counselling for women with diabetes cost-effective? *Diabetes Spectrum*, **10** (3), 195–2000.

Hollingsworth, D. (1992) *Pregnancy, Diabetes and Birth*. Williams & Wilkins, USA.

Metzger, B.E. (1998) International Hyperglycaemia and Adverse Pregnancy Outcomes (HAPO): temporary recommendations. Fourth International Workshop on GDM. *Diabetes*, **40** (Suppl. 2), 197–201.

Ross, G. (2002) How to plan a healthy pregnancy. *Diabetes Conquest*, **Autumn**, 28.

Chapter 22
Psychological and Quality of Life Issues Related to Having Diabetes

22.1 Key points

- Focus on achieving a balanced life rather than control.
- Most quality of life research indicates people with diabetes have worse quality of life than those without diabetes.
- Quality of life is influenced by a complex interplay of many factors.
- Avoid labels such as 'non-compliant' or 'a diabetic'.
- Offer support, respect and encouragement.

Rationale

Achieving a balanced lifestyle and good quality of life is essential to the physical and psychological wellbeing of people with diabetes. Depression is more common in people with diabetes and can impact on their self-care and long-term health outcomes. Health professionals are often preoccupied with metabolic control. Changing the focus to achieving balance is more likely to assist the person to achieve metabolic control.

22.2 Introduction

Psychological adaptation and maintaining a good quality of life is dependent on the individual's resilience. Resilience refers to the ability to overcome adversity and not only to rise above it, but to thrive. It has its foundation in belonging, life meaning and expectations and happiness.

Chronic conditions such as diabetes have a major impact on an individual's life plan, their partner, family and other relationships. Acquiring coping skills and being resilient have positive effects on emotional wellbeing and therefore on physical outcomes. Coping can be an issue for some people. Coping issues for young people with Type 1 diabetes centre around:

- being expected to cope;
- being expected to cope all the time;
- being seen to cope by others;

- having to cope for the rest of their lives;
- no respite from coping (Dunning 1994).

These issues are important across the lifespan as people with diabetes face life's challenges.

This chapter presents a brief outline of the complex psychological and quality of life aspects of having diabetes. Reactions to the diagnosis of diabetes are unique to the individual concerned; however, several common reactions have been documented. They include: anger, guilt, fear, helplessness, confusion, relief and denial. A knowledge of some of the issues involved will enable nursing staff to better understand the difficulties associated with living with diabetes and to plan appropriate care.

Many factors influence how a person accepts the diagnosis of diabetes and assumes responsibility for self-care. These factors include:

- age
- existing knowledge about diabetes
- health beliefs
- locus of control
- family support
- cultural attitudes.

A period of grief and denial is normal. Figure 22.1 is one model of the 'diabetic grief cycle' loosely based on Helen Kubler Ross's work, associated with death and dying. Lack of knowledge, or inaccurate knowledge about diabetes, produces stress and anxiety. The invisible nature of the condition – in Type 2 diabetes there are often no presenting symptoms – can lead to disbelief and denial of the diagnosis. Denial is appropriate early in the course of the disease and enables people to maintain a positive attitude and cope with the altered health status.

Adequate time must be allowed for the person to grieve for the losses they perceive to be associated with diabetes, e.g. loss of spontaneity, lifestyle, and a changed body image. However, prolonged denial can inhibit appropriate self-care, cause people to ignore warning signs of other problems and can lead to failure to attend medical appointments increasing the risk of diabetes complications. Denial can occur $\geq$5 years after the initial diagnosis in people with Type 1 diabetes (Gardiner 1997). This could equate with burnout from the unremitting demands of living with diabetes and accounts for frequent use of health services and inadequate control in a number of young people with diabetes.

Acceptance of diabetes involves dealing with:

- pain
- hospitalisation
- the health system, including health professional's beliefs and attitudes, and often hospitals and emergency services
- lifelong treatment
- body image changes
- friends/family relationships
- fluctuating blood glucose levels
- emotional lability
- loss of independence.

The tasks required to maintain acceptable blood glucose control are tedious and

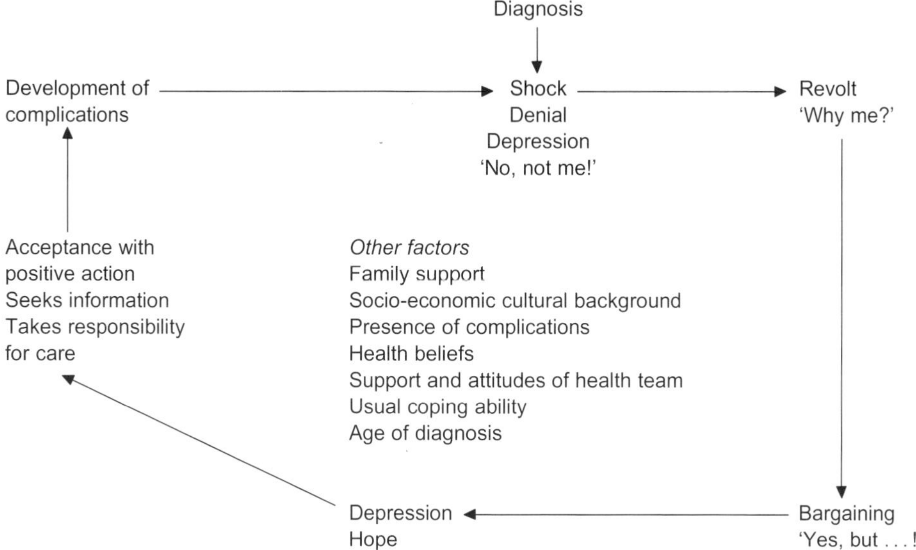

Figure 22.1 Model of the diabetic grief cycle.

sometimes painful. There are financial costs involved which can be a burden for some people (insulin, testing equipment, doctors' visits, increased insurance premiums). They add to the stress associated with having a disease no one wanted in the first place.

Clinical observation

There is no holiday from diabetes for the patient. The individual has to live with diabetes 365 days a year for the rest of their life. 'Diabetes is a designer disease. It was designed for people with routine lives – and that's not me' (young woman with recent diagnosis of Type 1 diabetes).

Managing a chronic illness means straddling two paradigms – the biomedical and the psychosocial. These two paradigms need to be integrated in order to achieve optimal health outcomes. An individual's path through life is influenced by life trajectories and turning points and these include the diagnosis of diabetes, expectations of treatment, and social support. Helping an individual define their life trajectory and identify turning points is part of holistic care.

Diabetes has a 'bad reputation' in the community, with many associated myths, e.g. 'eating sugar causes diabetes', and Type 2 diabetes is a mild form of the disease, which must be discussed and dispelled. Such myths can be associated with self-blame and guilt feelings. In addition, social pressures make denial of the diabetes and failure to follow medical advice easy. 'A little piece of cake won't hurt you.'

22.3 Depression

The World Health Organisation predicts that depression will be the second major health issue by 2020. People with diabetes have a higher incidence of depression than the general public and the depression often precedes the diagnosis of diabetes. Depression could be a component of the insulin resistance syndrome (see Chapter 1). People who are depressed are more likely to have inadequate self-care, present to the emergency department, require specialist intervention and exhibit lowered self-worth and physical functioning (Ciechanowski *et al.* 2000).

Cavan *et al.* (2001) suggested that the reasons for depression in people with diabetes might be:

- The heavy disease burden.
- The strain it places on relationships, especially family relationships.
- The stigma of diabetes in the family and the community.
- Shock and guilt at the diagnosis that are not adequately addressed and resolved.
- The uncertainty of the future.
- Loss of control.
- Past negative experiences with health professionals.

Depression is characterised by:

- Disinterest.
- Decreased confidence.
- Reduced energy.
- Changed sleep and eating patterns.
- Neglect of self-care. However, not all people who neglect their self-care are depressed. Assumptions must always be checked (Lustman *et al.* 1996).

The perceived severity of diabetes also affects the person's mental status. Type 2 diabetes has traditionally been considered to be less serious than Type 1 diabetes especially where it is treated without medications. Health professionals often convey these beliefs (Dunning & Martin 1997, 1999). Such messages convey false hope, and depression and stress occur when insulin is required. Considering the silent, insidious nature of Type 2 diabetes and the frequency with which complications are present at diagnosis, it is hardly a mild disease.

Practice points

(1) Finding ways to help people cope with the diagnosis of diabetes could be as important as diet, medications and education.
(2) Monitoring the individual's mood and ongoing screening for depression should be part of complication screening.

22.4 Type 1 diabetes

Diabetes diagnosed in childhood can produce enormous guilt and anxiety for the child and the parents. Marital strife is not uncommon and is often exacerbated by the diabetes.

The parents must learn how to care for the child at the same time as coping with their own feelings. Inflicting pain on a child (injections, blood tests) is very difficult to do, and such tasks often fall to the mother.

As the child matures and develops they need to take over the care of their diabetes. It can be extremely difficult for the parents to 'let go' and therefore for the child to achieve independence. Other children in the family may feel deprived of attention. Sweets, the traditional reward for good behaviour, are often withdrawn and this may be seen as a punishment.

Some childhood behaviour such as irritability and awkwardness can be difficult to distinguish from hypoglycaemia, making management difficult. Hypoglycaemia itself is feared and hated by children and parents and mostly underrated by healthcare staff. It is not unknown for people to deliberately run their blood glucose levels high to avoid hypoglycaemia (Dunning 1994).

People with diabetes may have concerns about passing diabetes to their own children in the future. Support, encouragement and referral for counselling, if necessary, are vital aspects of diabetes care.

Diabetes is the perfect disease for manipulating others and gaining attention. Withholding insulin can result in ketoacidosis, with the mobilisation of family, friends and health resources. Hypoglycaemia can have the same effect. Repeated admissions for hypoglycaemia or DKA need to be investigated carefully and diplomatically.

An individual's response to the diagnosis of diabetes depends on their overall psychological and social adjustment and the availability of structured family support (Johnson 1980) (see Chapter 20). Fitting diabetes into family life can be difficult and changes with duration of diabetes and the intensity of the treatment regime (Gardiner 1997).

The *Australian National Diabetes Strategy and Implementation Plan* (Diabetes Australia 1998) identified some issues personal to people with Type 1 diabetes. They are:

- Dependency, e.g. during severe hypoglycaemia and fears of being dependent should they develop complications such as blindness.
- Loss of control, either in the short term, e.g. during hypoglycaemia or in the long term.
- Public confusion about the difference between Type 1 and Type 2 diabetes. This confusion extends to health professionals as the following quote from a referral for diabetes education indicates: 'He used to have Type 2 but the doctor started him on insulin yesterday and he is now Type 1. Needs education.'
- Who to tell about their diabetes at work – workmates, friends.
- Restrictions, e.g. some sporting activities and jobs, and hassles getting driver's licences.

22.5 Type 2 diabetes

The diagnosis of diabetes in later life means the person may need to change behaviours developed over years. Eating patterns often have to be modified. Restrictions are often resented with resultant anger, denial or neglect. Alternatively the patient may meticulously follow the management plan.

Knowledge about possible diabetic complications or the development of complications leads to stress, which in turn contributes to elevated blood glucose levels. Relationships may be disrupted as in Type 1 diabetes, with families/spouses becoming overprotective, resulting in overdependence or rebelliousness. People tend to cope better and manage the self-care tasks more easily if the family is supportive yet allows independence.

Over half of the people with Type 2 diabetes on insulin report reduced quality of life. Insulin has a negative impact, which is greater in younger people with a long duration of diabetes from non-English-speaking backgrounds (Rubin 2000; Davis *et al.* 2001). Men with Type 2 diabetes self-report depression, disempowerment and perceived loss of control (Tun *et al.* 1990). This hopelessness and depression may well be the result of the mythology that insulin indicates severe disease. More support and early explanations of the likely progression to insulin are required.

22.6 Compliance/non-compliance

These terms are judgemental, prejudiced and negative in nature. They are labels best avoided in relation to diabetic self-care tasks. Failure to comply with one aspect of care does not necessarily indicate complete neglect of the diabetes. In fact, forgetting and omitting aspects of care are probably 'normal' behaviours and obsessive attention to routine can indicate underlying fear and anxiety.

It is important to establish why a particular task is neglected. Reasons include:

- Unreal expectations of the staff resulting from a lack of knowledge of the person's goals, capabilities and social situation.
- Setting of health professional rather than patient goals.
- Lack of knowledge of what is required.
- Lack of understanding as a result of poor communication.
- Inadequate support from family/friends and the healthcare team (see Chapter 20).
- Health beliefs and attitudes of the patient.
- Physical disabilities such as low vision, and diminished fine motor skills.
- Patient 'burnout'.
- Financial difficulties.

This is the human side of diabetes (Raymond 1992).

22.6.1 Requirements of people with diabetes

- To be treated as normal.
- To be treated as a person, not 'a diabetic'.
- To be trusted and accepted.
- To know how and where to obtain advice.

Support, encouragement and focusing on positive achievements are far more helpful than 'shame and blame'.

Achievable goals should be negotiated with the patient. It is the patient's expectations that will be met rather than those of the health professional. It is important to recognise that diabetes is never easy. 'Good' and 'bad' when referring to blood glucose levels are judgemental terms. Substitute 'high' and 'low'. Some people resent being called 'a diabetic'. It is preferable to say 'a person with diabetes'.

Some patients express concern about being admitted to hospital, over and above the usual reactions to illness/hospitalisation. They feel abnormal by being singled out for special meals and having labels such as 'diabetic diet' attached to the bed. They are sometimes made to feel incompetent when they have often been caring for their diabetes for years. For example, when requesting sugar to avoid hypoglycaemia or not being allowed to test their blood glucose or to give their own injections.

Some people feel that they are blamed if they are admitted with a diabetic complication. They 'should have known better' and taken care of their diabetes better. Patients become frustrated when they are labelled 'non-compliant'. Continuous negative feedback only reinforces that the person is not coping and learned helplessness can result.

22.7 Quality of life

Quality of life is a highly subjective and multidimensional concept concerned with cognitive status, satisfaction and emotional happiness (Cox & Gonder-Frederick 1992). It has become a major issue in behavioural diabetes research. Poor quality of life is associated with neglect of self-care and may predict an individual's capacity for self-care.

There are four categories of determinants of quality of life:

(1) Medical – diabetes type, treatment regime, level of metabolic control and presence of complications. The severity of complications reduces quality of life.
(2) Cognitive – acute and chronic blood glucose control and neuropsychological changes can reduce quality of life for the person with diabetes and their family.
(3) Attitudinal – self-efficacy, locus of control and social support. People with good support have better quality of life and less depression. Empowerment strategies and improving an individual's sense of being in control improve their quality of life.
(4) Demographic – gender, education level, ethnicity and age. Men report better quality of life than women and young people better than old people. Higher education is associated with better quality of life.

22.7.1 Measuring quality of life

Most people understand what is meant by 'quality of life' but it is a difficult concept to measure. A number of tools have been developed that measure the general aspects of quality of life and are widely used. Diabetes-specific quality of life tools are now also available. These tools the include generic Health-Related Quality of Life, Short Form 36 (SF-36), the Diabetes Specific Quality of Life and the Symptoms Check List, and the DCCT tool (Bradley & Gamsu 1994). Sometimes a number of tools are used together.

Some are simple to use and could be incorporated into the routine diabetes assessment undertaken by nurses. Measuring quality of life may be useful to plan holistic nursing care and address issues of empowerment. It is important to consider individual meaning of quality of life and to ask about these individual issues as well as global issues.

22.7.2 Guidelines to encourage wellbeing

- Recognise that psychological issues affect metabolic control and need to be addressed in order to maintain quality of life and effective diabetes self-care.
- Provide supportive education and advice, as it is required and tailor education to the individual's needs. An empowerment model of care and an holistic approach are more appropriate for chronic diseases such as diabetes where frequent visits to health professionals are required. Empowerment models seek to involve the individual in

decisions about their management and to establish a therapeutic relationship with the individual, see Chapter 23.

- Improve communication. Provide an appropriate environment for consultations, plan for continuity of care, ask open questions and give the individual the opportunity to ask questions.
- Address complications honestly but optimistically. Foster self-esteem and coping skills. In hospital this may mean allowing the person with diabetes to perform their own blood glucose tests and administer their own medications.
- Offer options and help with goal setting.
- Give the message that diabetes is a serious disease and focus on the benefits of good control rather than what will happen if control is poor.
- Focus on the person not their diabetes or metabolic control.
- Acknowledge that it is difficult to live with diabetes.
- Monitor psychological wellbeing as well as physical status (Bradley & Gamsu 1994).

References

Bradley, C. & Gamsu, D. (1994) Guidelines for encouraging psychological wellbeing. *Diabetic Medicine*, **11**, 510–516.

Cavan, D., Fosbury, J. & Tigwell, P. (2001) Psychology in diabetes – why bother? *Practical Diabetes International*, **18** (7), 228–229.

Ciechanowski, P., Katon, W. & Russo, W. (2000) Impact of depressive symptoms on adherence, function and costs. *Archives of Internal Medicine*, **160**, 3278–3285.

Cox, D. & Gonder-Frederick, L. (1992) Major developments in behavioural diabetes research. *Journal of Consulting Clinical Psychologists*, **60**, 628–638.

Davis, T., Clifford, R. & Davis, W. (2001) Effect of insulin therapy on quality of life in Type 2 diabetes mellitus – The Fremantle diabetes study. *Diabetes Research and Clinical Practice*, **52**, 63–67.

Diabetes Australia (1998) *Australian National Diabetes Strategy and Implementation Plan*, Diabetes Australia, Canberra.

Diabetes Control and Complications Trial Research Group (1993) Influence of intensive diabetes treatment on quality of life outcomes in the DCCT. *Diabetes Care*, **19**, 195–203.

Dunning, P. (1994) Having diabetes: young adult perspectives. *The Diabetes Educator*, **21** (1), 58–65.

Dunning, P. & Martin, M. (1997) Using a focus group to explore perceptions of diabetes severity. *Practical Diabetes International*, **14** (7), 185–188.

Dunning, P. & Martin, M. (1999) Health professional's perceptions of the seriousness of diabetes. *Practical Diabetes International*, **16** (3), 73–77.

Gardiner, P. (1997) Social and psychological implications of diabetes mellitus for a group of adolescents. *Practical Diabetes International*, **14** (2), 43–46.

Johnson, S. (1980) Psychosocial factors in juvenile diabetes. *Journal of Health Psychology*, **9**, 737–749.

Lustman, P., Griffith, L. & Clouse, R. (1996) Recognising and managing depression in patients with diabetes. In: *Practical Psychology for Clinicians* (eds B. Anderson & R. Rubin). American Diabetes Association, Alexandria, 143–152.

Raymond, M. (1992) *The Human Side of Diabetes: Beyond Doctors, Diet, Drugs*. Noble Press, Chicago.

Rubin, R. (2000) Diabetes and quality of life. From research to practice. *Diabetes Spectrum*, **13** (1).

Tun, P., Nathan, D. & Perlminter, L. (1990) Cognitive and affective disorders in elderly diabetics. *Clinical Geriatric Medicine*, **6**, 731–746.

Useful reading

Dunning, P. (1991) Why counsel the patient and family with Type 2 diabetes? *Treating Diabetes*, 5, Australia.
Horn, B. (1990) *Living with Diabetes*. Houghton, Victoria.
Lubkin, I.M. (1990) *Chronic Illness Impact and Interventions*. Jones & Bartlett, Boston.

Chapter 23
Diabetes Education

23.1 Key points

- Establishing a therapeutic partnership with the person with diabetes is very important. The focus should be on autonomy and empowering the person with diabetes to be in control.
- Written instructions should be provided.
- Information should be supplied in 'chunks' and be culturally relevant.
- Information should be supplied according to individual needs.
- Regular knowledge assessment is important.
- Information must be consistent between all health professionals caring for the person with diabetes.
- Establishing how people learn is as important as how people teach.
- Significant others should be included in the education programme.

Rationale

Diabetes education is the cornerstone of diabetes management and is an ongoing process. Person-centred education that empowers people with diabetes and a balanced therapeutic relationship between the person and the health professional are essential aspects of the diabetes education process.

23.2 Introduction

Diabetes education is an integral part of the management of diabetes. The overall goal of diabetes education is to assist the patient to accept and integrate the diabetes management tasks successfully into their lifestyle and self-concept, in order to achieve and maintain a balanced lifestyle and optimum diabetic control.

There are standardised patient education guidelines, but each patient should be assessed and a teaching plan developed to ensure individual learning needs are addressed. Diabetes education is a lifelong process and is often divided into:

- Survival skills – the initial information necessary to be safe at home.
- Basic knowledge – that information which will enable greater understanding about diabetes and its care.

- Ongoing education – the continued acquisition of new knowledge, including changes in technology and management practices applicable to self-care.

In an education encounter the health professional has specific ideas about what could/should be taught. The person with diabetes knows what they want and it is essential to deal with their issues. People are often well informed and seek to gain some of the health professional's power especially if they have a chronic illness like diabetes (Cox 1992).

An empowering education framework allows clarification of the individual's needs and opportunities for negotiation to take place to ensure essential issues are not overlooked. Education encounters are often emotional as well as cognitive and rational, and involve reflection and action.

The following issues need to be considered when designing an empowering education encounter:

- The individual's feelings and beliefs.
- Psychosocial situation.
- Education level and the level of the information to be used in the session.
- Coping style.
- Learning style.
- Goals for the session and the future.
- Ability to carry out self-care behaviours.
- Satisfaction with the service.

The learning process is much more effective if a partnership relationship is established (Coulter 1997). Health professionals have a powerful influence on the beliefs and attitudes of their patients and must use the relationship with respect and honesty (Dunning & Martin 1998).

23.2.1 Survival skills

Survival skills are taught at diagnosis and should be reviewed regularly. The family should be involved whenever possible. Minimal information for safety is given and written information supplied. However, specific concerns/questions of the patient should be addressed. The patient should be able to:

- Demonstrate correct insulin care and administration techniques.
- Know the effect of medications and food on blood glucose levels.
- Know the names of their insulin/tablets.
- Demonstrate correct monitoring techniques (blood and/or urine ketone testing) and appropriate documentation of the results.
- Know the significance of ketones in the urine (Type 1).
- Recognise the signs and symptoms, causes and appropriate treatment of hypoglycaemia.
- Know that regular meals containing the appropriate amount of carbohydrate are important.
- Have an emergency contact telephone number if help is required.
- Demonstrate safe disposal of sharps.

A sample diabetes education record used to document 'survival information' and plan for further teaching is shown overleaf.

Sample diabetes education record chart

DIABETES EDUCATION RECORD

Date of referral . . . .

Referred by Dr/RN . . . .

Unit . . . .

Ward/Op . . . .

Language spoken at home . . . .

Understanding of English: good/fair/poor . . . .

Other communication issues . . . .

Method used to address issues . . . .

Indicate perceived level of skill and understanding attained . . . .

Follow-up requirements . . . .

Information Supplied

(1) What is diabetes? . . . .

(2) How it is controlled:

- diet . . . .
- tablets/insulin . . . .

(3) Urine ketone testing . . . .

(4) Home glucose monitoring . . . .

(5) Diet and nutrition . . . .

(6) Insulin and tablets:

- care of . . . .
- insulin administration . . . .
- when to take tablets/insulin . . . .
- sharps disposal . . . .

(7) Hypos . . . . (8) Sick days . . . .

(9) Foot care . . . . (10) Sport & exercise . . . .

(11) Dentist . . . . (12) Travel & Driving . . . .

Sample diabetes education record chart *cont'd*

Other information discussed . . . .

Family support: good/fair/poor . . . .

Domiciliary instructions . . . .

. . . .

. . . .

Patient Discharge Checklist

(1) Education material – itemise . . . .

(2) Record book . . . .

(3) Blood testing equipment – type . . . .

(4) Ketone testing . . . . (5) Diet advice . . . .

(6) Diabetic card complete . . . .

(7) Starter pack: syringes/needles/monolets . . . .

(8) Discharged to: diabetic clinic/LMO/specialist . . . .

(9) Referred for further education . . . .

Enrolment in Diabetic Association . . . .

Signature of Registered Nurse . . . . Date . . . .

23.2.2 Ongoing education

Education can be continued on an individual basis or in group programmes. As education is a lifelong process both systems are usually employed. Survival information should be reviewed and further information given. The patient should gradually be able to:

- Demonstrate appropriate insulin adjustment considering the effects of food, activity and medication on blood glucose.
- Know the appropriate management of illnesses at home, especially to continue insulin/diabetes tablets, to continue to drink fluids and to test the urine for ketones, especially Type 1.
- Recognise the signs and symptoms of hypoglycaemia and treat appropriately.
- Cope in special situations, such as eating out, during travel and playing sports, in terms of medication and food intake.
- Know that appropriate foot care will help prevent foot problems and hospital admissions.
- Know that good diabetic control and regular examination of the eyes, feet, blood pressure, cardiovascular system and kidney function can prevent or delay the development of long-term diabetic complications.

- Know that certain jobs and activities are unsuitable for people with diabetes on insulin, e.g. scuba diving, driving heavy vehicles.
- Accept the wisdom of wearing some form of medical alert system identifying them as having diabetes.

Practice points

(1) Education methods that incorporate behavioural strategies, experiential learning, goal setting and reinforcement are more likely to be effective.
(2) Patient satisfaction is a key element of compliance.
(3) Reflection on events and considering future strategies make education more personal.

23.3 Empowerment

There is no doubt that diabetes education is essential, but knowledge alone does not predict health behaviour. Beliefs, attitudes and satisfaction are some of the intervening variables between knowledge, behaviour and disease status. These are not constants and they need to be assessed on a regular basis, for example deciding what is happening at the time, what could/will change and how will the change affect the individual and their significant others.

Empowerment models of diabetes education are based on shared governance and consideration of the whole person. These issues are not a new concept. Hippocrates is credited with saying, 'In order to cure the human body it is necessary to have knowledge of the whole.' Likewise, the psychiatrist in T.S. Elliot's *The Cocktail Party* states that he needed to know a great deal more about the patient than the patient himself could always tell him.

Empowerment models developed with the realisation that people with diabetes must, and mostly want to be responsible for their own care. Empowerment is based on three characteristics of diabetes:

(1) The person with diabetes makes choices affecting their healthcare.
(2) The individual is in control of their care.
(3) The consequences of the choices affect the person with diabetes.

Empowerment then, is a collaborative approach to care where management is designed to help the individual make informed choices and maximise their knowledge, skills and self-awareness. It requires the individual to make deliberate conscious choices on a daily basis.

Empowerment education requires health professionals to accept the legitimacy of an individual's goals even if they result in suboptimal control (Anderson *et al.* 1996). An essential part of empowerment is that the individual accepts responsibility for their decisions. Not everybody is capable of taking control. Some people require specific instructions, e.g. an individual who has an external locus of control. In addition, stress and anxiety at specific times can impair an individual's ability to take control.

An empowerment model of diabetes education seeks to determine what the person with diabetes wants, and to reach agreement between what should be done and what the individual wants done in order to balance the burden of treatment and quality of life (see

Chapter 22). Diabetes is only one aspect of people's lives and affects them on many levels:

- Observable, e.g. signs and symptoms of hyper/hypoglycaemia.
- Not directly observable, e.g. personhood.
- Insights into their disease.
- Relationships.

Practice point

Consistency of information given by various members of the healthcare team is important to avoid confusion.

23.4 Special issues

The individual's questions should be addressed as they arise and planned into teaching programmes as appropriate to the individual. Questions may relate to:

- Pregnancy and diabetes.
- Sexuality and diabetes.
- Exercise.
- Weight control.
- A range of other issues such as diabetes information in media reports.

It is not absolutely necessary for people with diabetes to have a detailed knowledge about the causes and pathophysiology of diabetes in order to achieve good control.

23.5 The role of the bedside nurse in diabetes education

Patient teaching is a recognised independent nursing function and education is a vital part of the diabetic treatment plan. Therefore the teaching of patients in acute, elderly and extended care facilities by the bedside nurse is well within the scope of professional nursing practice. Some key points should be kept in mind when educating people with diabetes:

(1) The aim of diabetes education is autonomy and empowerment.
(2) Consider the psychological and social aspects when discussing diabetes.
(3) Encourage questions and dialogue.
(4) Ask open questions and use active listening.
(5) Teach specific skills and allow the patient time to practise new skills (e.g. insulin administration).
(6) Allow time for patients to discuss difficulties and concerns about diabetes.
(7) Relate new information to the patient's experience.

Practice point

Although there are many disadvantages to bedside teaching, e.g. noise, distractions, illness, other priorities and concerns, lack of privacy, it can allow for teaching at a 'teachable moment' and effective reinforcement of information. It must be consistent with diabetes team teaching and hospital policies/procedures. The nurse must have the appropriate knowledge.

Nurses make a substantial contribution to the health and wellbeing of the patient by allowing them to participate in decision making about their care in hospital and to make appropriate decisions at home.

Teaching in the ward effectively reinforces the information supplied by the diabetes nurse specialist/diabetes educator, doctor, podiatrist and dietitian. However, ward teaching *must* be consistent with that of the diabetes team and procedures such as insulin technique and blood glucose monitoring performed correctly according to the diabetic protocols. Patients are quick to perceive inconsistencies and may become confused or have their faith in the staff undermined. Some examples of relevant instruction sheets will be found at the end of this chapter.

Learning is facilitated when the need/readiness to learn is perceived and immediately applied in a given situation: that is, 'teaching at a teachable moment'. Teachable moments often occur when the ward staff are performing routine nursing care, such as blood glucose tests, or giving injections.

Teaching is non-verbal as well as verbal. In fact >60% of communication is non-verbal. People learn by observation, therefore the nurse is a role model and care should be taken to perform procedures correctly and to refer questions to another person if the answer is not known. In this way, formal and informal ongoing education in the ward is possible and desirable. The nurse's own knowledge about diabetes will influence their willingness and ability to participate in patient teaching. Theories of teaching and learning were not traditionally part of the nurse training. This is changing as empowerment in chronic disease management is recognised and accepted along with a focus on preventative healthcare.

Many factors can influence teaching and learning. Some of these are shown in Table 23.1. It is the responsibility of the teacher to ensure that the environment is not distracting. Noise in a busy ward can make conversation difficult and hinder learning. The patient should be as comfortable as possible and free from pain.

Table 23.1 Factors which influence teaching and learning.

Factor	*Patient*	*Nurse*
Health beliefs	✓	✓
Social support	✓	
Wellbeing/illness	✓	✓
Environment	✓	✓
Knowledge	✓	✓
Skills	✓	✓
Time	✓	✓
Perceived responsibility	✓	✓
Work priority		✓
Perception of teaching role		✓

The following basic principles need to be considered when planning a teaching session, whether it is for an individual or group:

- The aim of the session.
- The patient's needs/goals.
- Objectives should be realistic and achievable.
- The environment must be conducive to learning.
- Ascertain and build on the patient's existing knowledge.
- Relate teaching to patient's own experience.
- Demonstrate skills to be acquired.
- Provide opportunity for the patient to practise the skill.
- Evaluate the skill and knowledge.
- Provide positive reinforcement.
- Review information before commencing next teaching session.

It is usual to begin with the simple concepts and proceed to more complex ones.

The Instruction Sheets at the end of this chapter are examples of information material used in teaching, which is often available in several languages. In some cases the medical terms may need to be replaced with the patient's words. Blood glucose monitoring is discussed in Chapter 4. Specific patient instruction will depend on the testing system being used.

23.6 Insulin administration

Insulin can be administered using a range of insulin delivery systems, see Table 7.1, Chapter 7. Syringes are not used as often as the other devices which offer greater flexibility, portability and are discreet, thus avoiding some of the stigma attached to syringes.

The person should be shown a range of options and helped to choose one that suits them. The short fine needles in use today mean injections are relatively painless – less painful than blood glucose testing.

Insulin should be given subcutaneously (see how to give an injection, p. 241). IM injections, through incorrect technique, cause erratic blood glucose levels because the insulin is absorbed faster than via the subcutaneous route (Vaag *et al.* 1990).

Reuse of needles and syringes causes local trauma, microscopic damage to the needle tip and increases the likelihood that the needle will bend and/or break off in the injection site; it should therefore be discouraged. Needles left on insulin pens form a conduit to the outside allowing air to enter the vial and dose inaccuracies (Ginsberg *et al.* 1994).

23.7 Guidelines for instructing patients about insulin delivery systems

23.6.1 Patient learning requirements

The patient should be familiar with the structure and function of the particular insulin device chosen. They must be able to:

- Assemble the device in the correct sequence.
- Load the insulin correctly if necessary.

- Ensure insulin is expelled from the needle after loading the insulin.
- Know when to replace the insulin cartridge/device.
- Know how to inject the insulin according to the particular device chosen, for example, one depression of the plunger of NovoPen 3 delivers 2 units of insulin.
- Know how to store and transport the device.
- Know the appropriate method of cleaning and maintaining the device.
- Recognise signs that the device may be malfunctioning and know what action to take to remedy the situation.

Note: It is recommended that a supply of insulin syringes and one bottle of insulin be kept for emergencies.

It is important to discuss with and advise the patient about safe disposal of used equipment, especially sharps disposal at home. The guidelines for sharps disposal in the home can be found in Chapter 25.

Examples of patient instruction sheets appear on the following pages (see over).

Example Instruction Sheets

These Instruction Sheets are designed to be used with a practical demonstration of the procedure/s. They should not be handed out without adequate discussion. **They are examples only**.

Example Instruction Sheet 3: How to draw up insulin – one bottle only

HOW TO DRAW UP INSULIN – ONE BOTTLE ONLY

Your insulin is called . . . .

(1) Remove insulin bottle from fridge. Check expiry date – do not use if exceeded.

Cloudy insulin must be mixed before drawing up.

(2) Gently invert insulin bottle or roll between hands until well mixed (**do not shake**). Insulin should be 'milky'; there should be no lumps.

Clear insulin should be clear and colourless.

(3) Clean bottle top with spirit.

(4) Draw back plunger to . . . . units of air.

(5) Inject air into insulin bottle, invert bottle and draw back . . . . units of insulin, ensuring that all air bubbles are removed from the syringe.

(6) Administer insulin.

Example Instruction Sheet 4: How to draw up insulin – two bottles

HOW TO DRAW UP INSULIN – TWO BOTTLES

Your insulins are called . . . . (clear)

. . . . (cloudy)

(1) Remove insulin bottles from fridge. Check expiry date – do not use if exceeded.

(2) Gently invert or roll bottle of 'cloudy' insulin between hands, until 'milky' (**do not shake**).

(3) Clean bottle tops with spirit.

(4) Draw back plunger to . . . . units of air.

(5) Inject air into cloudy insulin and remove needle from the bottle.

(6) Draw back plunger to . . . . units of air.

(7) Inject air into clear insulin.

(8) Invert bottle and draw back . . . . units of clear insulin, ensuring that all air bubbles are removed from syringe.

(9) Put needle into cloudy bottle and withdraw . . . . units of cloudy insulin to the exact required dose of the syringe.

(10) If more cloudy insulin is accidently drawn up, discard contents of the syringe and start again.

(11) Total clear and cloudy insulin equals . . . . units.

Example Instruction Sheet 5: How to give an insulin injection

HOW TO GIVE AN INSULIN INJECTION

(1) Insulin can be injected into the abdomen, thighs, buttock or upper arm. The abdomen is the preferred site.

(2) Inject into a different spot each time.

(3) Pinch up a fold of skin between two fingers.

(4) Quickly push the needle into the skin at right angles.

(5) Gently push the plunger all the way to inject your insulin.

(6) Pull the syringe/device out quickly and apply pressure to the injection site.

Insulin should be stored away from heat and light. The bottle/cartridge in use can be kept at room temperature.

Stores should be kept in the refrigerator.

The same injection technique applies to insulin pens.

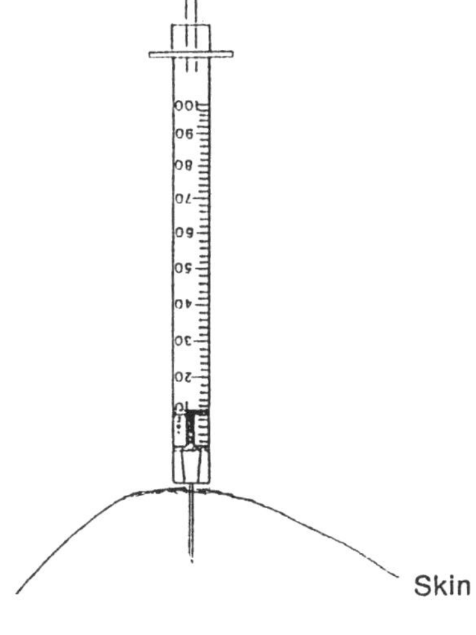

Example Instruction Sheet 6a:
Managing your diabetes when you are ill: patients with Type 1 diabetes

MANAGING YOUR DIABETES WHEN YOU ARE ILL

Illness (such as colds and flu) cause the body to make hormones which help the body fight the illness. These hormones usually also cause the blood glucose to go high. High blood glucose levels can lead to unpleasant symptoms like thirst, tiredness and passing a lot of urine.

By taking some simple precautions the minor illness can usually be treated at home.

What to Do

(1) Continue to take your insulin. You may need to increase the dose during illness to control the blood glucose and prevent ketones from developing.

(2) Test your blood glucose every 2–4 hours. Write down the test results.

(3) Test your urine for ketones. If moderate to heavy ketones are detected consult your doctor.

(4) Continue to drink fluids or eat if possible (see recommended food list).

(5) Read the labels on any medication you take to treat the illness because it may contain sugar, sugar substitutes or other ingredients which cause the blood glucose to go high.

(6) Rest.

(7) Keep the phone number of your doctor, diabetes clinic or diabetes nurse specialist/diabetes educator beside the telephone.

When to Call the Doctor

(1) If you have diarrhoea and/or vomiting.

(2) If ketones develop in your urine.

(3) If the blood glucose continues to rise.

(4) If you develop signs of dehydration (loss of skin tone, sunken eyes, dry mouth).

(5) If the illness does not get better in 2–3 days.

(6) If you feel you need advice.

Example Instruction Sheet 6a *cont'd*

What to Tell the Doctor When You Call

(1) How long you have been sick.

(2) What the blood glucose level is.

(3) How long the blood glucose has been high.

(4) How many ketones are in the urine.

(5) How frequently you are passing urine and how much.

(6) If you are thirsty, tired or have a temperature.

(7) What medications you have taken to treat the illness.

(8) If you have vomiting or diarrhoea, how frequently and how much.

Food for Days When You are Sick

It is important to continue to eat and drink. Small frequent meals may be easier to digest.

Suggested foods

- sweetened jelly (not low cal)
- ice cream (1/2 cup)
- custard with sugar (1/2 cup)
- honey (3 teaspoons)
- sugar (1 tablespoon)
- sweetened ice block (one small or 90 ml)
- egg flip – sweetened (similar to egg nog but less creamy 8 oz)
- tea or coffee + 4 teaspoons sugar
- milk (10 oz)
- Coke, lemonade or other sweetened soft drink (3/4 cup – not low cal)
- unsweetened tinned fruit (3/4 cup)
- orange juice (3/4 cup)
- apple juice (1/2 cup)
- pineapple juice (1/2 cup)
- orange (one medium)
- banana (one small)
- unflavoured yoghurt (100 g or 1/2 carton)
- flavoured (sweetened) yoghurt (200 g or one carton)
- broth or soup

Example Instruction Sheet 6a *cont'd*

Continuing Care

(1) If the doctor prescribes antibiotics to treat the illness it is important to complete the full course.

(2) Continue to test urine for ketones until they show clear for 24 hours.

(3) Continue to test your blood glucose 2–4 hourly and record the results until you recover and then go back to your usual routine.

(4) Go back to your usual food plan when you recover.

(5) If your insulin has been increased during the illness decrease it again when you recover to avoid hypoglycaemia.

(6) Consider writing down a medical history for quick reference in times of illness or in an emergency.

List:

- all the medications you are taking
- past illnesses
- blood group
- date of last tetanus and flu injection
- illnesses which run in the family.

This can be worn in an identification tag or be kept with your diabetes record book.

Example Instruction Sheet 6b: Managing your diabetes when you are ill: patients with Type 2 diabetes

MANAGING YOUR DIABETES WHEN YOU ARE ILL

Illnesses (such as colds and flu) cause the body to make hormones which help the body fight the illness. These hormones usually also cause the blood glucose to go high. High blood glucose levels can lead to unpleasant symptoms like thirst, tiredness and passing a lot of urine.

By taking some simple precautions the minor illness can usually be treated at home.

What to Do

(1) Continue to take your diabetes tablets. This is very important, because as we have said the blood glucose usually goes high. In severe illnesses or during an operation insulin injections may be needed until you recover.

(2) Test your blood glucose every 2–4 hours. Write down the test results.

(3) Continue to drink fluids or eat if possible (see recommended food list).

(4) Read the labels on any medication you take to treat the illness because it may contain sugar, sugar substitutes or other ingredients which cause the blood glucose to go high.

(5) Rest.

(6) Keep the phone number of your doctor, diabetes clinic or diabetes nurse specialist/ diabetes educator beside the telephone.

When to Call the Doctor

(1) If you have diarrhoea and/or vomiting.

(2) If the blood glucose continues to rise.

(3) If you develop signs of dehydration (loss of skin tone, sunken eyes, dry mouth).

(4) If the illness does not get better in 2–3 days.

(5) If you feel you need advice.

Example Instruction Sheet 6b *cont'd*

What to Tell the Doctor When You Call

(1) How long you have been sick.

(2) What the blood glucose level is.

(3) How long the blood glucose has been high.

(4) How frequently you are passing urine and how much.

(5) If you are thirsty, tired or have a temperature.

(6) What medications you have taken to treat the illness.

(7) If you have vomiting or diarrhoea, how frequently and how much.

Food for Days When You are Sick

It is important to continue to eat and drink. Small frequent meals may be easier to digest.

Suggested foods

- sweetened jelly (not low cal)
- ice cream (1/2 cup)
- custard with sugar (1/2 cup)
- honey (3 teaspoons)
- sugar (1 tablespoon)
- sweetened ice block (one small or 90 ml)
- egg flip – sweetened (8 oz)
- tea or coffee + 4 teaspoons sugar
- milk (10 oz)
- Coke, lemonade or other sweetened soft drink (3/4 cup – not low cal)
- unsweetened tinned fruit (3/4 cup)
- orange juice (3/4 cup)
- apple juice (1/2 cup)
- pineapple juice (1/2 cup)
- orange (one medium)
- banana (one small)
- unflavoured yoghurt (100 g or 1/2 carton)
- flavoured (sweetened) yoghurt (200 g or one carton)
- broth or soup

Example Instruction Sheet 6b *cont'd*

Continuing Care

(1) If the doctor prescribes antibiotics to treat the illness it is important to complete the full course.

(2) Continue to test your blood glucose 2–4 hourly and record the results until you recover and then go back to your usual routine.

(3) Go back to your usual food plan when you recover.

(4) Consider writing down a medical history for quick reference in times of illness or in an emergency.

List:

- all the medications you are taking
- past illnesses
- blood group
- date of last tetanus and flu injection
- illnesses which run in the family.

This can be worn in an identification tag or be kept with your diabetes record book.

References

Anderson, R., Funnell, M. & Arnold, M. (1996) Using the empowerment approach to help patients change behaviour. In: *Practical Psychology for Clinicians* (eds B. Anderson & R. Rubin). American Diabetes Association, Alexandria, 163–172.

Coulter, A. (1997) Partnerships with patients: the pros and cons of shared clinical decision making. *Journal Health Service Policy*, **2**, 112–121.

Cox, D. & Gonder-Frederick, L. (1992) Major developments in behavioural diabetes research. *Journal of Consulting Clinical Psychologists*, **60**, 628–638.

Dunning, P. & Martin, M. (1997) Type 2 diabetes: is it serious? *Journal of Diabetes Nursing*, **2**, 70–76.

Ginsberg, B., Parkes, J. & Sparacina, C. (1994) The kinetics of insulin administration by insulin pens. *Hormone Metabolism Research*, **26**, 584–587.

Tope, R. (1998) The impact of interprofessional education in the south west region – a critical analysis. The literature review *www.doh.gov.uk/swrp/tope.htm*

Vaag, A., Handberg, M., Lauritzen, J., Pedersen, K. & Beck-Neilsen, H. (1990) Variation in absorption of NPH insulin due to intramuscular injection. *Diabetes Care*, **13** (1), 74–76.

Chapter 24
Discharge Planning

24.1 Key points

- Commence early (on admission).
- Arrange follow-up care.
- Give contact telephone number.
- Ensure self-care knowledge is adequate.
- Ensure insulin and monitoring equipment are available.
- Ensure patient understands how and when to take medication.
- Communicate with appropriate health professionals/carers.

A discharge plan must be established and conducted in a proactive manner. It is important to build discharge planning into the initial assessment and patient care plan, and to consider social and home needs, e.g. prevent falls. It should look beyond the current episode of care in order to prevent readmission and relevant health professionals, family and carers should be informed of admission and discharge.

(1) Inform allied health professionals of admission on day one or two of admission (diabetes nurse specialist/diabetes educator, dietitian, podiatrist, social worker).
(2) Ensure self-care status has been assessed so that the patient is capable of caring for their own diabetes and will be safe at home.
(3) Refer for home assessment early if indicated.

24.2 On day of discharge

(1) Ensure patient has necessary medications and supplies, insulin delivery device, blood glucose testing equipment, fingerprick device and diabetic record book and understands their use, and where to obtain future supplies.
(2) Ensure relevant follow-up appointments have been made, and a discharge letter has been written to the GP.
(3) If further diagnostic investigations are to be performed on an outpatient basis ensure patient has written instructions and understands what to do about medications and fasting and knows where to go for any investigations.
(4) Ensure the patient has a contact telephone number for assistance if necessary.
(5) Ensure the patient knows about the services offered by the diabetic association, and other relevant services, e.g. meals-on-wheels, low vision clinic, rehabilitation ser-

vices, community nurse for support especially when new to insulin and liaison with the diabetes nurse specialist/diabetes educator, counselling and council services, e.g. sharps disposal.

24.2.1 Transfer to another hospital or nursing home

In addition to the usual information provided relating to nursing and medical management the nursing letter accompanying the patient should contain information about:

- Diet.
- Progress of diabetes education.
- Skills assessment for performing blood glucose testing and insulin administration.

Ensure transport has been arranged and that the family is aware of the discharge. Some nursing homes and special accommodation facilities may not have cared for people with diabetes in the past, or have done so on an infrequent basis. Diabetes education for the staff of the facility in this situation is desirable.

Chapter 25
District Nursing and Home-based Care

25.1 Key points

- Establish communication link with referring agency or practitioner.
- Assess patient before seeking medical advice.
- Ascertain if hyperglycaemia is a new occurrence.
- Seek cause for hypoglycaemia.

25.2 Introduction

Domiciliary care allows the provision of technical and professional care to acutely and chronically ill patients at home. The provision of the service will be influenced by the home environment and the person's condition and capabilities, and available home support services. A nursing care plan should be prepared to complement the medical management plan.

Supporting people to enable them to remain at home is an important consideration of diabetic management. Visiting district and community and home-care nurses play an important role in this respect. They are often responsible for:

- Preparing insulin doses.
- Administering insulin.
- Performing blood glucose tests.
- Assessing the general condition of the patient.
- Supporting the continuing education of the patient and of family/carers.
- Attending to wound dressing.
- Attending to personal hygiene.
- Assisting with medication management, e.g. preloading dosette boxes.

Making clinical decisions about the patient in the home situation without advice and support can be stressful and difficult. In addition, the home situation must be carefully assessed to ascertain how to obtain access to the home, and the correct address and telephone number. The safety of the nurse is an important consideration and issues such as the surrounding environment and household composition should be assessed beforehand, if possible. The service base should have some idea of the route the nurse is likely to take. Other information (e.g. presence of dogs) should also be noted.

This chapter outlines the important diabetes-related information needed to gauge whether medical assessment is necessary.

25.3 How to obtain help

It is important for home care and domiciliary nursing bodies to establish open communication links with the referring agency or practitioner.

The referring agency should be the first point of contact for advice.

25.4 General points

(1) Ensure diabetes teaching is consistent with that of the diabetic unit.

(2) Before recommending equipment, e.g. meters, insulin delivery systems, ensure the person will be able to use it, can afford it and can obtain further supplies. This is particularly important if the person is visiting from another country or is travelling overseas where some brands of equipment may not be available. Assess:
- vision
- manual dexterity
- comprehension.

There may be costs associated with purchasing diabetes equipment and medications in some countries. It is important that the person understands the costs and any government initiatives to reduce/eliminate those costs.

(3) Ensure the patient is enrolled in the National Diabetes Services Scheme so that they can obtain syringes, lancets and test strips at the subsidised price (relevant only in Australia).

25.5 Diabetic problems nurses commonly encounter in the home

(1) Finding an elevated blood glucose level.
(2) Hypoglycaemia.
(3) The patient has not taken their insulin/diabetes tablets and it is 11 AM or later.
(4) The patient who does not follow the diabetes management plan.
(5) Management of diabetic wounds (foot ulcers).
(6) Disposal of sharps (needles, monolets) in the home situation.
(7) How and where to obtain help/advice about specific patient problems.

25.6 Nursing actions

(1) Assess general clinical state (see Chapter 2).

(2) If the patient appears unwell, record:
- temperature
- pulse
- respiration and presence of respiratory distress
- blood pressure
- colour.

(3) Assess presence, location, duration and severity of any pain.
(4) Note nausea, diarrhoea and/or vomiting.
(5) Note presence of any symptoms of urinary tract infection:
   - frequency
   - burning
   - scalding
   - itching.

(6) Assess state of hydration.
(7) Note time and dose of last diabetic medication.
(8) Note time and amount of last meal.
(9) Measure blood glucose level.

25.7 Interpreting the blood glucose level

To assess the diabetic status one must first ascertain whether the patient is in danger because of the blood glucose level. Ascertain:

- The present level.
- The usual blood glucose range.
- Why the blood glucose is outside the usual range. Whether the patient has suffered any illness, committed a dietary indiscretion, commenced on a new medication, missed a medication dose, or is using a complementary or self-prescribed medication.
- Whether it is likely to go up or down.

When ascertaining the blood glucose level check whether:

- The test was performed correctly.
- There was enough blood on the strip; if using a meter that the meter was calibrated and used correctly.
- The strips have exceeded the expiry date (see Chapter 4, Monitoring 1: blood glucose).
- The patient has commenced any new medication that could alter the blood glucose level (see Chapter 6).

The patient may require attention if the blood glucose level is:

- Low – hypoglycaemia <3 mmol/L.
- High – hyperglycaemia >17 mmol/L for a significant number of tests.

25.8 Hypoglycaemia

For more detailed information see Chapter 8.

(1) Treat according to the severity and time of occurrence of hypoglycaemia.
(2) Avoid overtreatment.
(3) Give rapidly absorbed glucose, i.e. high GI, if symptomatic, e.g.:
   - orange juice
   - tea/coffee with sugar
   - jelly beans.

(4) Give more slowly absorbed glucose, i.e. low GI, if the hypoglycaemia is asymptomatic and there is some time before the next meal is due.
(5) Suggest they have their meal if it is due in half an hour.
(6) Ensure patient has recovered before leaving the home. Check the blood glucose. Wash the person's hands before testing the blood glucose if they have been handling glucose to treat the hypoglycaemia.
(7) Record incident.

If severe follow the procedure for managing unconscious hypoglycaemia (Chapter 8). IM glucagon can be administered if it is available. If not manage the airway and seek medical or ambulance assistance.

Practice point

The next dose of medication is not usually withheld.

Discuss recognition and treatment of hypoglycaemia with patient and family. Ensure that the person and/or their family and carers know how to manage hypoglycaemia, that there is appropriate food/fluids to manage hypoglycaemia and they know who to call in an emergency.

25.9 Hyperglycaemia

For more detailed information see Chapter 10. Ascertain:

- How long the blood glucose level has been elevated.
- Whether the patient is unwell.
- Whether there are any symptoms of hyperglycaemia, e.g. polyuria, polydipsia, thirst or lethargy.
- Whether there are ketones present in the urine.

If moderate/heavy ketones are detected seek medical advice (this usually only occurs in Type 1 people).

Check for any obvious source of infection:

- Urinary
- Foot ulcer wound
- Cold or flu.

Practice point

Infection can be present without any overt signs and symptoms.

Counsel the patient about managing at home when unwell. (Patient information guidelines are shown in Chapter 23.) The important points are that the patient should:

- Continue to take insulin or OHAs.
- Maintain fluid and carbohydrate intake.
- Test and record blood glucose regularly, e.g. 2 to 4 hourly.

In addition:

(1) If the patient has Type 1 diabetes they should test their blood or urine for ketones every 4 hours.
(2) Maintain contact with the patient and liaise with the diabetes team.
(3) Advise them to seek medical advice if vomiting and/or diarrhoea occur, if the blood glucose continues to increase, if ketones develop in the urine or their conscious state changes.

25.10 The patient with chest pain

(1) Reassure the patient and family.
(2) Instruct the patient to stop current activity and to sit or lie down. Loosen tight clothing.
(3) Instruct patient to take anginine if prescribed by doctor.
(4) Assess the severity of the discomfort and the frequency of attacks.
(5) People with long-standing diabetes may have 'silent myocardial infarcts'. Complaints of vague chest discomfort should be investigated. The classic pain radiating into the jaw, arm and chest may be absent.
(6) Seek medical advice/ambulance service.
(7) Record BP.
(8) Discuss decreasing risk factors for cardiac disease (see Chapter 11).

25.11 The patient who has not taken their insulin or diabetes tablets and it is 11 AM or later

More than 80% of people miss medication doses (Morris *et al.* 2001; Gilbert *et al.* 2002). If medication is missed frequently, self-care capability, cognitive functioning and mental status (e.g. depression), beliefs about medications should be assessed. Often medications are missed or taken incorrectly because the person is given inaccurate, hurried or conflicting information or the information is presented in a format the person cannot read or does not understand.

Stopping medications without consulting a doctor and inappropriately altering doses is common (Kriev *et al.* 1999). Older people in particular make more mistakes including incorrect doses when drawing insulin up in a syringe (DeBrew *et al.* 1998). Home-based nursing services play a vital role in assisting elderly people to manage their medicines safely.

Medications that have long duration of action are less of a problem if a dose is missed than medications with short duration of action. Missing several consecutive doses of drugs with a narrow therapeutic index may lead to a loss of efficacy, e.g. the effect of aspirin on platelet stickiness might be diminished. Time will be required to re-establish therapeutic blood concentrations if consecutive doses of drugs with a long half-life are missed.

(1) Check blood glucose level.
(2) Ascertain why medication was omitted.
(3) Ascertain whether this is a regular occurrence.
(4) Ascertain whether they have eaten breakfast, and what they ate.

In general medication may need to be modified and the dose reduced. The amount will depend on the dose and types of insulin and the blood glucose level:

(1) Seek the advice of the referring agency.
(2) Document any medication adjustment.
(3) Have the order signed by the appropriate doctor within 24 hours.
(4) Plan strategies with the individual that set out what to do if a dose is missed in future and set up cues to minimise the number of missed doses, e.g. a reminder on the refrigerator door. Medical information leaflets are provided with medications when they are dispensed as part of the Quality Use of Medicines Program in Australia, but this may not be the case in other parts of the world, including the UK. These information leaflets often contain advice about what to do if a dose of the drug is missed.

Readings <6.0 mmol/L may indicate good control and the usual dose should be taken. If non-diabetic medications have been missed the person should take their normal dose at the usual time.

If it is before 11 AM counsel the patient to check their blood glucose; if it is 6 mmol/L or above the patient should:

- Take usual medication dose and eat breakfast.
- Eat lunch within 3 to 4 hours then tea 3 to 4 hours after that.
- Have medication and breakfast at normal time the next day.

25.11.1 Follow-up visit

Ascertain whether:

- The patient followed advice.
- The management strategy was effective.
- Hypo/hyperglycaemia occurred as a result of missed medication and modified dose.
- Further dietary counselling is necessary.

25.12 Managing diabetic foot ulcers at home

Diabetic foot ulcers are a common complication of diabetes and occur as a result of peripheral neuropathy and vascular changes (see Chapter 19).

25.12.1 On first visit

(1) Ascertain the extent to which the individual can be involved in their care, e.g. cleanliness, knowledge.
(2) Check treatment plan and medication prescriptions.
(3) Assess ulcer to obtain a baseline for future comparison:
    - dimensions: width × depth
    - type and quantity of discharge

- colour of surrounding tissue
- presence of oedema.

(4) Counsel patient to:
 (a) rest with foot elevated as much as possible.
 (b) protect foot:
  - bed cradle (stiff cardboard or polystyrene box)
  - appropriate footwear
  - regular inspection.
 (c) complete full course of antibiotics.

(5) Monitor blood glucose tests.

25.12.2 Further visits

(1) Perform the dressing according to the prescription. The dressing may be:
- dry
- occlusive
- or the wound may be cleaned and left open.

(2) Assess progress of the wound.
(3) If the wound deteriorates:
- note odour and amount and type of discharge
- take a swab for culture and sensitivity
- record TPR
- record blood glucose level
- refer for assessment.

Practice point

If bandages are used ensure they are correctly applied and do not constrict the blood supply. People with neuropathy may not be able to tell if the bandage is too tight.

(1) Bandage from the foot upwards, even if the ulcer is on the leg.
(2) Do not put bandages or tape in a circular fashion around the toes.
(3) Never prick the toes to obtain a blood glucose test.

25.13 The patient who does not follow the management plan ('non-compliant'; see Chapter 22)

'Non-compliant' is a derogatory and negative term. There may well be good reasons why people do not follow prescribed treatment, including:

- A complicated regime that the patient does not understand.
- Treatment goals are those of the management team and not the patient.
- Inability to comply (patient may not have a refrigerator, may suffer from low vision, or loss of fine motor skills).
- Cultural and language differences.
- Economic factors – cost of supplies.
- Non-acceptance of diabetes and constraints imposed on lifestyle.
- Other concerns may outweigh those about diabetes.

- 'Burnout'.
- Learned helplessness.

Counselling, education and appropriate modification of health professional expectations may help. Behavioural changes may take years; patient, supportive health professionals and family can assist the patient to eventually make some changes.

25.14 Disposal of sharps in the home situation

In the community the person with diabetes is responsible for the safe disposal of used needles and lancets. There are thousands of diabetes needles discarded every week, outside hospitals. All health professionals have a responsibility to promote the safe disposal of used sharps. The safe disposal of used needles, syringes and lancets should be an integral part of teaching injection technique and blood glucose monitoring.

Practice point

Ensure the patient understands what you mean by a 'sharp'.

25.14.1 Guidelines for handling and disposing of sharps at home

(1) Take care with sharps at all times.
(2) Store needles and monolets out of reach of children.
(3) Use a 'standards approved' container if possible (check with the local council about how to obtain one).
(4) Only recap your own syringe and lancet.
(5) Recapping of syringes and lancets is a good idea if an approved container is not available, e.g. at a restaurant.
(6) If testing blood glucose for family/friends always use a new lancet.
(7) Check arrangements for disposal of full containers with:
    - your local diabetes association
    - your local council.
(8) If an approved container is not available it is advisable to:
    - recap needles and lancets
    - place immediately into a puncture-proof, unbreakable container, clearly labelled 'used sharps'
    - keep the container out of the reach of children
    - keep the lid tightly closed (Diabetes Australia 1999).

In the UK people are advised to use a safe-clip device to remove needles and to dispose of lancets in an opaque container.

25.15 Storage of insulin

Insulin should be stored in the refrigerator if possible; *it should not be frozen*. The vial in use can be stored at room temperature if it is protected from heat and light and should be used within one month of opening. Any unused insulin stored at room temperature should be discarded after one month.

Practice point

If there is any change in appearance or consistency of the insulin, or if the expiry date is exceeded, discard the insulin.

25.16 Guidelines for premixing and storing insulin doses for home and district nursing services

25.16.1 General recommendations

Mixing and storage of insulin for periods of 24 hours or more may be necessary for the management of the diabetes of elderly people, of those with poor vision and of those with limited hand mobility who live alone and where no other assistance is available.

The correct method of mixing short- and long-acting insulins is included in the Example Instruction Sheets at the end of Chapter 23 and refer to UK RCN Guidelines 1999a and b.

The proportions to be mixed are prescribed by the doctor to suit individual patient requirements. In practice, biphasic insulin is frequently used in these situations.

25.16.2 Recommended guidelines

(1) Use insulin syringes only for drawing up insulin.
(2) The filled syringe should be stored:
   - in the refrigerator if possible or in a cool dark place
   - vertically or horizontally; they should not be stored with the needle pointing downwards which may cause clogging in the needle, preventing insulin being injected.
(3) Syringes should be rolled between the palms of the hands before administration to mix the contents.
(4) If the patient is on more than one injection per day the doses should be clearly understood by the patient. The doses should be clearly marked and stored separately from each other, e.g. in plastic food storage containers marked 'morning' and 'evening' or with the administration times.
(5) Injection technique should be assessed periodically to ensure insulin administration is accurate, especially in people with low vision and those with unexplained hyperglycaemia.
(6) One extra dose could be drawn up in case of emergencies provided the patient understands that it is not an additional dose of insulin.
(7) Monitor blood glucose when visiting the patient.
(8) Any concerns about control, mental state or accuracy of technique should be discussed with the relevant doctor.
(9) Signed and dated records of all advance doses of insulin (type, dose, frequency of administration) should be maintained. All blood glucose results and insulin doses should be recorded and accompany the patient to medical appointments.
(10) Ensure there are enough supplies to last until the next visit.

Practice point

If the patient has required a period in hospital, unused previously drawn up doses of insulin should be discarded. A new batch should be drawn up when the patient is discharged.

References

DeBrew, K., Barba, B. & Tesh, S. (1998) Assessing medication knowledge and practices of older adults. *Home Healthcare Nurse*, **16** (10), 688–691.

Gilbert, A., Roughead, L. & Sanson, L. (2002) I've missed a dose; what should I do? *Australian Prescriber*, **25** (1), 16–18.

Kriev, B., Parker, R., Grayson, D. & Byrd, G. (1999) Effect of diabetes education on glucose control. *Journal of the Louisiana State Medical Society*, **151**, (2), 86–92.

Morris, A., Brennan, G., Macdonald, T., Donnan, P. (2000) Population-based adherence to prescribed medication in Type 2 diabetes: A cause for concern. *Diabetes*, **40**, A76.

St Vincent's Hospital (2001) Drawing up insulin doses for patients who are unable to draw up their own doses. Department of Endocrinology and Diabetes Policy Manual, Melbourne.

United Kingdom Royal College of Nursing Guidelines (1999a) Guidelines on premixing and preloading of insulin for patients to give at a later date.

United Kingdom Royal College of Nursing Guidelines (1999b) Guidelines on preparing and preloading of insulin for patients to give at a later date.

Chapter 26
Complementary Therapies and Diabetes

26.1 Key points

- Complementary therapy use is increasing.
- People are entitled to unbiased information about complementary therapies.
- Complementary therapies can work synergistically with conventional medicine to improve diabetes balance and quality of life.
- Many herbs have hypoglycaemic effects.
- Herb/drug and herb/herb interactions and other adverse events do occur.
- Questions about complementary therapy use should be incorporated into routine history-taking and assessment.

Rationale

Complementary therapy use is increasing. If used appropriately within a quality management framework some complementary therapies (CTs) can help people with diabetes retain control over their disease and provide management congruent with their health beliefs. It is essential that conventional diabetes treatments be continued.

26.2 Introduction

The upsurge in the use of complementary therapies (CTs) is part of the evolution of a new health paradigm seeking to solve the health problems peculiar to today, i.e. chronic lifestyle diseases and depression. Complementary therapies are used by over 50% of the general population of most western countries particularly by people with chronic diseases, especially women with education to high school level or higher who are in poor health often with a chronics disease who are employed and interested in self-care (Lloyd *et al.* 1993; MacLennan *et al.* 1996; Eisenberg 1998; Egede *et al.* 2002). People choose to use CT by complex non-linear pathways. When people are considering their therapeutic options they are likely to choose therapies congruent with their life philosophy, knowledge, experience and culture and choose to be actively involved in their own care.

The prevalence of CT use by people with diabetes is largely unknown but two studies, Leese *et al.* 1997 and Ryan *et al.* 1999, found approximately 17% of people with diabetes in diabetic outpatient settings were using a range of complementary therapies, particularly herbs, massage and vitamin and mineral supplements such as zinc. The people using CT were satisfied with their chosen therapy even if it 'did not work'. Wellbeing improves when people are satisfied with their treatment (see Chapter 22). In addition, individuals may have had different goals for using the therapy from those assumed by conventional health professionals, and controlling blood glucose is not always their aim. The author's experience in a diabetes service indicates a similar rate and that, in many cases, people use complementary therapies for conditions other than diabetes, such as arthritis, stress and to manage the unpleasant symptoms of diabetes complications, e.g. nausea, pain, anxiety, stress and depression.

Egede *et al.* (2002) found people with diabetes were more likely to use CT than people without diabetes, as were people with other chronic conditions in a national study in the USA. In particular, people with diabetes over 65 years were the most likely group to use CT. The most commonly used CTs were nutritional advice, spiritual healing, herbal medicine, massage and meditation. The high usage rates in people with diabetes are hardly surprising and accord with the established demographics of CT users.

Many health professionals, especially nurses and general practitioners (GPs), are incorporating CT into their practice to enrich and extend their practice and provide holistic care. Many nurses and GPs who use CT in their practices do not have formal CT qualifications and do not effectively document or monitor the effects of CT usage. They often use CT in their own healthcare. Dunning (1998) found that just under 50% of a sample of 37 diabetes nurse specialists/diabetes educators were using CT in their practice and none had a CT qualification.

There are a great many CTs ranging from well-accepted therapies with a research basis to 'fringe' therapies with little or no scientific basis. Commonly used CTs are shown in Table 26.1. Defining CT can be difficult. The Cochrane collaboration defines them as:

> All health systems, modalities and practices and their accompanying theories and beliefs, other than those intrinsic to the politically dominant health system of a particular society or culture in a given historical period. They include all such practices and ideas self-defined by their users as preventing or treating illness or promoting

Table 26.1 Commonly used complementary therapies.

Acupuncture	Meditation
Aromatherapy	Music
Ayurveda (traditional Indian medicine system)	Naturopathy
Chiropractic	Nutritional therapies
Counselling (a range of techniques)	Pet therapy
Herbal medicine (from several traditions – Indian, Chinese, North American, Australian Aboriginal)	Reflexology Reiki Therapeutic Touch
Homeopathy	Traditional Chinese Medicine (complex system that uses several techniques, e.g. herbs, cupping, moxibustion and exercise)

Note: Many therapies are combined, e.g. aromatherapy and masssage.

> health and wellbeing. The boundaries within and between complementary therapies are not always sharp or fixed.
>
> (Cochrane Collaboration 2000)

Several terms are in common use to describe CT including complementary and alternative medicine (CAM), traditional medicine and non-scientific therapies. These terms are generally understood to mean therapies that are not part of conventional medicine. As the Cochrane definition indicates, the status of CT is not fixed and some CTs become part of conventional medicine as the evidence base for their safety and efficacy accumulates, e.g. acupuncture.

26.3 Complementary therapy philosophy

Complementary therapies have a common philosophy. This philosophy is consistent with current diabetes empowerment strategies and the focus is on effective professional–patient partnerships, good communication and preventative healthcare.

- The individual is unique.
- Balance is important.
- The body has the capacity to heal itself.
- A positive attitude is important to health and wellbeing.
- The client–therapist relationship is a therapeutic part of the healing process.
- The mind and body cannot be separated – what affects one affects the other (mind–body medicine).
- Illness is an opportunity for positive change.

Practice point

Healing does not mean curing. It refers to a process of bringing the physical, mental, emotional, spiritual and relationship aspects of an individual's self together to achieve an integrated balance where each part is of equal importance and value (Dossey *et al*. 1998).

Understanding this philosophy is important to understanding why people use CT. They seek answers to their health problems that match their existing beliefs and their health choices are part of their larger orientation on life and are not made in isolation from their beliefs and attitudes. They frequently mix and match CT with CT and CT with conventional therapies to suit their needs. Adverse events can arise when due consideration is not given to the potential effects of such combinations, e.g. drug/herb interactions. Alternatively, CT can enhance the effects of conventional medicines, allow lower doses of drugs to be used, decrease unwanted side effects and improve healing rates (Braun 2001).

26.4 Integrating complementary and conventional care

Many health institutions are concerned with regulatory and supply issues as well as benefits and risks as part of the safe use of CT. The degree of statutory and professional regulation varies from country to country and from therapy to therapy. Frequently there is no formal regulatory process in place but the professional associations of some CTs have stringent training and ongoing professional development requirements as part of self-regulation. Some require competence in first aid, e.g. the International Federation of Aromatherapists.

The safe, effective combination of the conventional and CT involves consideration of the following issues:

- The safety of the client, allowing for their personal choices.
- Facilitating people to make informed choices based on an understanding of the risks and benefits involved when using CTs, especially combining CT and conventional care. When the patient is not competent to consent, guardianship issues may arise.
- The knowledge and competence of health professionals to give advice about CT and the knowledge of how to refer to a suitable practitioner if necessary. CTs need to be appropriate to the individual's physical, mental and spiritual status and used based on a thorough assessment considering the potential interactions with conventional therapies. The suitability of CT should be reviewed regularly because diabetes is a progressive disease and continued use may be dangerous, e.g. in renal disease (see Chapter 16). Conventional drug doses should be monitored and may need to be changed.
- Guidelines should be followed where they exist and consent is required in some settings. Policies and guidelines need to include processes for communication between CT and conventional practitioners and for collaboration and referral mechanisms to prevent fragmented care (Dunning 2001). Where possible, guidelines should be evidence-based to support best practice. They should not be prescriptive and inflexible.
- Processes for monitoring outcomes and accurately documenting the effects of the therapy should be in place and allow objective data to be collected.
- Ensuring that safe quality products are used is important. Dose variations, contamination and/or adulteration with potentially toxic substances such as heavy metals and unsubstantiated claims made about the product can lead to serious adverse events including irreversible kidney failure (Ko 1998).
- Safety data information should be available where possible and could be included with research papers in a portfolio on the ward.
- It is important that an accurate diagnosis is made and a thorough health history and assessment have been carried out prior to using any therapy. These considerations are often overlooked, especially when the person with diabetes self-diagnoses and self-treats. Such practices can result both in delays in instituting appropriate management and in deterioration in diabetic status.

Practice point

These considerations apply equally to the selection and use of conventional therapies.

26.5 Can complementary therapies benefit people with diabetes?

Managing diabetes effectively is about achieving balance. To achieve balance a range of therapies used holistically, are needed. From a general perspective CTs can assist people to:

- Incorporate diabetes into the framework of their lives.
- Accept and manage their diabetes to achieve balance in their lives by reducing stress and depression, which facilitates the achievement of blood glucose control (balance) by decreasing insulin resistance.
- Develop strategies to recognise issues that cause stress and methods to prevent stress from occurring.
- Take part in decision-making and increase their self-esteem, self-efficacy and sense of being in control by improving their quality of life and allowing personal growth.
- Increase insulin production and decrease insulin resistance, either by the direct effects of the therapy, by reducing stress or by enhancing the effects of conventional medications.
- Manage the unpleasant symptoms of diabetic complications such as pain and nausea.
- Preventative health care, e.g. foot care to maintain skin integrity and prevent problems such as cracks that increase the potential for infection and its consequences.
- Teaching and learning, e.g. facilitating knowledge acquisition, retention and recall.

Some specific benefits for people with diabetes have also been reported. They include:

(1) A decrease in blood glucose levels in children being given regular massage by their parents. The parents reported reduced anxiety levels in themselves (Field *et al.* 1997).
(2) Some herbs have been shown to decrease blood glucose, HbA1c and lipids, e.g. American ginseng (*Panex quinquefolius*) (Vuksan *et al.* 2000); gymnema/gurmar (*Gymnema sylvestre*) (Baskaran *et al.* 1990) and fenugreek (*Trigonella foeum-graecum*) (Sharma *et al.* 1990, 1996). These herbs have primarily been used in Type 2 diabetes, but fenugreek has also been shown to lower blood glucose in Type 1 diabetes (Sharma *et al.* 1990).
(3) Many people with diabetes use chromium. There is some evidence to support the claim that it improves metabolic control but more clinical trials are needed (Finney *et al.* 1997).
(4) Acupuncture can improve the pain of diabetic peripheral neuropathy (Abuaisha *et al.* 1998).
(5) There is a range of biofeedback, relaxation and counselling therapies that can decrease stress by attenuating the effects of increased autonomic activity and catecholamine production. Improved mood and reduced blood glucose levels have been reported with biofeedback (McGrady *et al.* 1991).
(6) Antioxidant therapies receive significant press coverage. There is accumulating evidence that oxidation plays a role in the development of vascular disease and that antioxidants may delay the progression of retinopathy (O'Brien & Timmins 1999; Verdejo *et al.* 1999). Antioxidants such as vitamin E increase blood flow to eyes and kidneys, vitamin C replenishes vitamin E, and the B group vitamins are necessary for nerve function. However, consensus has not been reached about the benefits of using antioxidants, the dose needed and when in the course of diabetes they should be used.
(7) In 2000 the media reported that baths could help reduce blood glucose levels. The claims have not been substantiated and there could be risks such as postural hypotension, falls and burns to neuropathic feet if the water is too hot. Faster uptake of injected insulin or reduced stress levels could be methods whereby blood glucose is reduced.
(8) Aromatherapy can be used to enhance wellbeing and relaxation and to reduce stress

which benefits metabolic control. It can also be used for physical conditions such as alleviating pain, reducing hypertension, improving sleep and foot care. Aromatherapy may also alleviate stress during procedures such as CAT scans, and post-cardiac surgery (Buckle 1997). These things improve the individual's quality of life and psychological wellbeing. It is beneficial for environmental fragrancing to increase work performance, reduce absenteeism and reduce keyboard errors. In this respect the benefit is for the health professional and organisation rather than an individual. Aromatherapy is often combined with music and massage. There is a strong link between touch and aroma and wellbeing. In elderly care settings aromatherapy is used to reduce pain, improve sleep, maintain skin integrity and manage behavioural problems (Thompson 2001).

Clinical observation

There were several media reports in late 2001 of dogs being able to recognise that their owners with diabetes were hypoglycaemic and alert them early enough to enable the person to manage the episode themselves, or to alert another person. Guide dogs for visually impaired people are standard therapy and allow visually impaired people to lead independent lives. Are 'hypo dogs' the way of the future?

26.5.1 Adverse events

A number of adverse events associated with CT use by people with diabetes have been reported in the literature in the last few years. They include:

- Stopping insulin in a person with Type 1 diabetes leading to ketoacidosis (Gill *et al.* 1994).
- Trauma and burns to neuropathic feet and legs from cupping and moxibustion (Ewins *et al.* 1993)
- Allergies, drug/herb interactions and hospital admissions, largely from adulterated traditional Chinese medicine (Beigel & Schoenfeld 1998; Ko 1998).
- Hypoglycaemia following prolonged massage and using herbal therapies.
- Bleeding from herb/anticoagulant interactions see Table 26.2.
- Kidney damage, see Chapter 16.
- Heavy metal poisoning (Keen *et al.* 1994).

A number of initiatives have been taken to limit some of these problems, e.g. in 1991 the World Health Organisation developed guidelines for the safe use, manufacturing and labelling of plant medicines.

26.5.2 Herb/drug interactions

There are four main potential mechanisms for herb/drug interactions. Herbs can:

(1) Induce production of liver enzymes, especially cytochrome P450, which leads to reduced drug availability.
(2) Induce intestinal D-glycoprotein, which leads to reduced drug absorption and metabolism which can be clinically significant.
(3) Stimulate neurotransmitter production especially serotonin enhancing the effects of

Table 26.2 Commonly used herbs and supplements, their potential interactions, reported adverse events and some management strategies to use should an adverse event occur.

Herb	*Potential interactions*	*Reported adverse events*	*Management strategies*
Echinacea	Hepatoxic drugs, e.g. anabolic steroids, amiodarone, methotrexate, ketaconazole Immunosuppressants, e.g. corticosteroids, cyclosporin	Allergic reactions especially in atopic people Impairs the action of immunosuppressive drugs Can cause immunosuppression if taken long-term In acute surgery impairs wound healing	Do not use continuously for >8 weeks at a time
Garlic	Aspirin Warfarin Cholesterol lowering agents	Risk of bleeding especially when taken with anticoagulants Increased GIT activity Decreased effectiveness of antacids Inhibits platelet aggregation Additive effects	Discontinue 7 days before surgery Do not use concomitantly with antacids
Gingko biloba	Aspirin Warfarin SSRI MAO inhibitors	Bleeding risk if used with anticoagulants	Stop 36 hours before surgery Do not use concurrently
Fenugreek	Anticoagulants Oral hypoglycaemic agents	Bleeding Hypoglycaemia	Do not use concurrently Monitor Adjust dose of OHA or the herb
Ginseng *Note:* there are several species in common use	Corticosteroids Oral contraceptives Warfarin Digoxin Oral hypoglycaemic agents MAO inhibitors and tricyclic antidepressants	Increased risk of bleeding with anticoagulants Suppresses immune system – infections risk Hypoglycaemia Headache Additive effects	Stop 7 days before surgery Do not use concomitantly

Cont'd

Table 26.2 *Cont'd*

Herb	*Potential interactions*	*Reported adverse events*	*Management strategies*
Ginger	Antacids Warfarin	Decreased effectiveness of antacids	Do not use at the same time
Guar and bulking agents	Antibiotics	Decreased food absorption – hypoglycaemia risk	Do not administer at the same time
Glucosamine		GIT complaints Allergy if allergic to seafoods Nausea, vomiting abdominal pain Sleepiness Hyperglycaemia	Avoid with seafoods
Zinc	Increased HbA1c in Type 1 diabetes		
Valerian, hops	Anaesthetic agents Barbiturates Hypnotics Antidepressive drugs	Enhance/potentiate the effects of sedatives With long-term use the amount of anaesthetic needed is increased	Withdrawal – symptoms resemble valium addiction Taper dose preoperatively
St John's Wort	MAO inhibitors SSRI Decreases effect of HIV medications Warfarin Anticonvulsants Activates liver enzyme, hastening drug metabolism and reducing their effectiveness	Alters metabolism of some drugs, e.g. cyclosporin, warfarin, steroids Interacts with psychotrophic drugs and can increase their effect Skin allergies	Stop 5 days before operation Do not use concomitantly
Slippery elm		Decrease GIT absorption Hypoglycaemia	
Vitamin supplements C & E, B group; often as antioxidants	Vitamin toxicity Niacin	Decreases the beneficial effects of statins on HDL levels	
Feverfew	NSAIDS, warfarin, offset the herb's effect for migraine and might alter bleeding time	Changed bleeding time	

some drugs, i.e. they both do the same thing. Others decrease the effects of serotonin-inhibiting drugs (Braun 2001).

(4) Compete with drugs for binding sites on serum protein increasing the amount of free drug available. People with low serum albumin are especially at risk, e.g. the elderly and those with malnutrition.

Herb/drug interactions are a two-way street – alone neither the drug nor the herb might be a problem, but when used together, the *combination* can be potentially dangerous. It should also be noted that liver failure (20–30%) and kidney damage (30%) are recognised side effects of readily available conventional medicines, but the benefits are considered to outweigh the risks.

26.5.3 People most at risk of herb/drug interactions are those who

- are taking drugs with a narrow therapeutic window such as lithium, phenytoin, barbiturates, warfarin and digoxin
- are at risk of, or have, renal and/or liver damage and therefore, have altered ability to metabolise and excrete herbs and drugs
- have atopic conditions such as allergies, asthma or dermatitis
- are elderly
- are children
- are taking many drugs (polypharmacy)
- take alcohol or drugs of addiction
- lack knowledge or consult practitioners who lack knowledge about appropriate therapies to use. This includes CT and conventional practitioners
- self-diagnose, delay seeking medical advice, do not tell conventional or CT practitioners about the therapies/drugs they are using
- import products or use products when travelling that are not subject to regulations governing good manufacturing practices. The danger of contamination of products from some countries is significant.

People with diabetes are at increased risk because they usually have more than one risk factor present and risk factors may be additive.

26.6 How can complementary therapies be used safely?

Giving people appropriate advice so they can make informed decisions is an important aspect of nursing care. The following information could help nurses assist people with diabetes to use CT safely and choose therapies appropriate for the problem they want to treat. Patients need to know that there could be risks if they do not follow conventional evidence-based diabetes management practices. They should not be made to feel guilty or lacking in judgement if they choose to use a CT. People can be advised to:

- Develop a holistic health plan and decide what they hope to achieve by using a CT and use a therapy that is best suited to achieve these goals, e.g. to reduce stress: use massage, counselling or time-line therapy.
- Find out as much about the therapy as they can before using it. Seek information from unbiased sources and be wary of information they find in chat rooms on the Internet and advertising material.

- Consult a reputable practitioner, e.g. a member of the relevant professional association, and buy products from reputable sources that are approved and have relevant safety data available.
- Store and maintain products appropriately and consider safety issues if children and confused elderly people are part of the household. This also applies to storage of products in healthcare settings.
- Ensure the condition for which they want to use a CT is correctly diagnosed before they treat it, otherwise appropriate treatment could be delayed and the condition deteriorate.
- Be aware that there are risks if they do not follow conventional evidence-based diabetes management recommendations.
- Be aware that they should not stop or change recommended conventional treatments without the advice of their doctor.
- Inform all practitioners, conventional and complementary, about the therapies they are using so the health plan can be coordinated.
- Some CTs should not be used continuously for long periods.
- Take extra care if they are old, very young, pregnant, breastfeeding, have kidney or liver damage or are taking a lot of other treatments, because these cases are at increased risk of adverse events.
- Seek advice about how to manage the therapy if they need an operation or investigation, or starting any new conventional treatment.
- Seek advice quickly if any of the following occur:
  - hypo/hyperglycaemia
  - mental changes
  - abdominal pain
  - skin rashes
  - nausea, vomiting, diarrhoea
- Monitor the effects on their diabetes, e.g. blood glucose, lipids and HbA1c as well as their response with respect to the reason they chose the therapy, e.g. to manage pain.

26.7 Nursing responsibilities

Nurses have a responsibility to respect people's choices and not to be judgemental about the choices they make. They also have responsibilities to their employer, other patients, visitors and staff. Nurses can use CT as part of holistic nursing care but they have a duty of care to practise at the level of their education and competence and use safe therapies. The following general advice applies. Specific information about individual CTs should be sought before using it or giving advice about it.

- Be sensitive to the philosophical and cultural views of people with diabetes and be aware that they may perceive risks and benefits differently from health professionals.
- Follow guidelines for the use of CT where they exist, e.g. those of the NMC in the UK. In Australia the state nurse registering authorities, the Australian Nursing Federation and Royal College of Nursing, Australia, have all produced guidelines for nurses using CT (McCabe 2001).
- Ensure you are appropriately qualified and competent if you decide to use, recommend or offer advice about complementary therapies to a person with diabetes.
- Look for evidence of safety and efficiency but do not be too quick to accept or reject 'evidence'.
- Communicate the risks and benefits to people with diabetes and their families/carers.

If the person chooses not to follow advice, documentation should outline the information that was given.

- Develop a portfolio of evidence for reference on the ward.
- Use herbs and essential oils within the philosophy of the quality use of medicines and prescribe, administer, document and monitor within that philosophy. Nursing assessment should ask about CT. People are not always willing to disclose such information and skilful questioning is required. Questions should be asked in a framework of acceptance. The patient has a responsibility to disclose. Nurses can make it easier for them to do so.
- Value the nurse-client relationship as an essential aspect of the healing process.
- Consider staff reaction to environmental therapies, e.g. vaporising aromatherapy, playing music.
- Know how to contact the Poisons Advisory Service in the area.
- Have mechanisms in place to clean and maintain any equipment needed, e.g. aromatherapy vaporisers. Processes should be in place to deal with any CT products the patient brings with them.
- Document appropriately, in the same manner as conventional treatment, the type, dose and duration of the therapy, condition it is used for, advice given, expected outcome, actual outcome and report any adverse events.

Self-reflection

(1) How will you respond to a person who asks you about taking a traditional Chinese herbal medicine to control their blood glucose?
(2) What will you do when a person with diabetes and end stage renal failure elects to use herbal medicine?
(3) How would you advise a person with diabetes who asks you how she can use aromatherapy to help her sleep?

Clinical observation

A young Aboriginal man from Central Australia was studying research methods at the University. At the same time he was being educated about traditional tribal practices. He fractured his tibia and fibula playing football. It was a simple fracture but he became depressed and the bones were not mending as well as expected.

The young man's mother took him to consult with the Tribal Elders. On his return the doctor said to the mother, 'That won't cure him you know.' The mother replied, 'No – but it will put him in a frame of mind to accept your medicine. That will work now.'

References

Abuaisha, B., Boulton, A. & Costanz, J. (1998) Acupuncture for the treatment of chronic painful diabetic peripheral neuropathy: a long-term study. *Diabetes Research and Clinical Practice*, **39** (2), 115–121.

Baskaran, K., Kizar, A., Radha, K. & Shanmugasundaram, E. (1990) Antidiabetic effect of leaf extract from Gymnema sylvestre in non insulin-dependant diabetes mellitus patients. *Journal of Ethnopharmacology*, **30** (3), 295–300.

Biegel, Y. & Schoenfeld, N. (1998) A leading question. *New England Journal of Medicine*, **339**, 827–830.

Braun, L. (2001) Herb-drug interactions: a danger or an advantage? *Diversity*, **2** (6), 31–34.

Buckle, J. (1997) *Clinical Aromatherapy in Nursing*. Arnold, London.

Cochrane Collaboration (2001) *The Cochrane Library Complementary Medicine Field*. Oxford.

Dossey, B., Keegan, L., Guzzetta, C. & Kolkmeier, L. (1998) *Holistic Nursing: A Handbook for Practice*. Aspen Publications, Gaithersburg.

Dunning, T. (1998) Use of complementary therapies by diabetes educators. Unpublished data, St Vincent's Hospital, Melbourne.

Dunning, T. (2001) Developing clinical practice guidelines. In *Complementary Therapies in Nursing and Midwifery* (ed. P. McCabe). Ausmed Publications, Melbourne, 37–48.

Dunning, T., Chan, S.P., Hew, F.L., Pendek, R., Mohd, M. & Ward, G. (2001) A cautionary tale on the use of complementary therapies. *Diabetes in Primary Care*, **3** (2), 58–63.

Egede, L., Xiaobou, Y., Zheng, D. & Silverstein, M. (2002) The prevalence and pattern of complementary and alternative medicine use in individuals with diabetes. *Diabetes Care*, **25**, 324–329.

Eisenberg, D. (1998) Advising patients who seek alternative medical therapies. *American Journal of Health Medicine*, **127** (1), 61–69.

Ewins, D., Bakker, K., Youn, M. & Boulton, A. (1993) Alternative medicine: potential dangers for the diabetic foot. *Diabetic Medicine*, **10**, 980–982.

Fetrow, C. & Avila, J. (1999) *Professional's Handbook of Complementary and Alternative Medicines*. Springhouse Corporation, Pennsylvania.

Field, T., Hernandez-Reif, M., LaGreca, A., Shaw, K., Schanberg, S. & Kuhn, C. (1997) Massage lowers blood glucose levels in children with diabetes. *Diabetes Spectrum*, **10**, 237–239.

Finney, L. & Gonzalez-Campoy, J. (1997) Dietary chromium and diabetes: is there a relationship? *Clinical Diabetes*, **Jan/Feb**, 6–8.

Gill, G., Redmond, S., Garratt, F. & Paisley, R. (1994) Diabetes and alternative medicine: cause for concern. *Diabetic Medicine*, **11**, 210–213.

Keen, R., Deacon, A., Delves, H., Morton, J. & Frost, P. (1994) Indian herbal remedies for diabetes as a cause of lead poisoning. *Postgraduate Medicine Journal*, **70**, 113–114.

Ko, R. (1998) Adulterants in Asian patent medicines. *New England Journal of Medicine*, **339**, 847.

Leese, G., Gill, G. & Houghton, G. (1997) Prevalence of complementary medicine usage within a diabetic clinic. *Practical Diabetes International*, **14** (7), 207–208.

Lloyd, P., Lupton, D., Wiesner, D. & Hasleton, S. (1993) Choosing on alternative therapy: an exploratory study of sociodemographic characteristics and motives of patients resident in Sydney. *Australian Journal of Public Health*, **17** (2), 135–144.

McCabe, P. (ed.) (2001) *Complementary Therapies in Nursing and Midwifery*. Ausmed Publications, Melbourne.

McGrady, A., Bailey, B. & Good, M. (1991) Controlled study of biofeedback assisted relaxation in Type 1 diabetes. *Diabetes Care*, **14** (5), 360–365.

MacLennan, A., Wilson, D. & Taylor, A. (1996) Prevalence and cost of alternative medicine in Australia. *The Lancet*, **347**, 569–573.

O'Brien, R. & Timmins, K. (1999) Trends. *Endocrinology and Metabolism*, **5**, 329–334.

Ryan, E., Pick, M. & Marceau, C. (1999) *Use of Alternative Therapies in Diabetes Mellitus*. Proceedings of the American Diabetes Association Conference, San Diego, USA.

Sharma, R., Raghuram, T. & Rao, N. (1990) Effect of fenugreek seeds on blood glucose and serum lipids in Type 1 diabetes. *European Journal of Clinical Nutrition*, **44**, 301–306.

Sharma, R., Sarkar, A. & Hazra, D. (1996) Use of fenugreek seeds powder in the management of non insulin-dependent diabetes mellitus. *Nutritional Research*, **16**, 1331–1339.

Thomson, S. (2001) Complementary therapies in aged care. In *Complementary Therapies in Nursing and Midwifery* (ed. P. McCabe). Ausmed Publications, Melbourne, 257–275.

Verdejo, C., Marco, P., Renau-Piqueras, J. & Pinazo-Duran, M. (1999) Lipid peroxidation in proliferative vitreoretinopathies. *EYE*, **13** (part 2), 183–188.

Vuksan, V., Stavro, M., Seivenpiper, J. *et al.* (2000) Similar postprandial glycaemic reductions with escalation of dose and administration time of American ginseng in Type 2 diabetes. *Diabetes Care*, **23**, 1221–1226.

Chapter 27
Nursing Care in the Emergency and Outpatient Departments

Rationale

Diabetes accounts for a great many presentations to outpatient clinics and emergency departments every year. In addition, people present to community centres and general practitioners with potential emergency situations, e.g. silent myocardial infarction, see Chapter 11.

This chapter gives an outline of important issues. The other chapters in the book should be cross-referenced for specific presenting conditions. It is important that diabetes is identified as soon as the individual presents for treatment and their metabolic status is assessed to limit the morbidity and mortality associated with diabetic emergencies.

It is important to be aware that presentation of conditions such as myocardial infarction and urinary tract infections can be present with few of the classical signs and symptoms.

Other chapters can be consulted depending on the presenting condition.

27.1 The emergency department

Medical emergencies are a major source of morbidity and mortality for people with diabetes. The particular presenting problem may be unrelated to diabetes; however, the existence of diabetes will usually affect metabolic control. Extra vigilance will be needed to reverse or limit the abnormalities arising as a consequence of altered glucose metabolism, due to stress, illness or trauma.

Diabetes-related abnormalities frequently seen in the emergency department are:

- myocardial infarction
- cerebrovascular accident
- severe hypoglycaemia
- infected/gangrenous feet
- hyperglycaemia
- ketoacidosis
- hyperosmolar coma.

Rapid effective therapy and effective nursing care increase the chance of a good recovery.

Practice point

In emergency situations clear short-acting insulin is used, preferably as an IV infusion for ketoacidosis, hyperosmolar coma and myocardial infarction.

27.1.1 Nursing responsibilities

(1) Carry out assessment and observations appropriate to the presenting complaint.
(2) Note identification tags.
(3) Enquire if the patient has diabetes.
(4) Record blood glucose.
(5) Record blood urine glucose and ketones.
(6) Ascertain time and dose of last diabetes medication.
(7) Ascertain time and amounts of last meal, especially the amount of carbohydrate consumed.
(8) Assess usual day-to-day diabetic control and the period of deteriorating control.
(9) Record any other medication, those prescribed by a doctor and anything taken to relieve present complaint including complementary therapies.
(10) Seek evidence of any underlying infection.
(11) Assess pain, severity, site, cause, and relieve appropriately.
(12) Consider the psychological aspects of the illness. Give full explanation to the patient and family.
(13) Avoid long delays in assessment if possible, and be aware of the possibility of a hypoglycaemic episode in people with diabetes on medication.
(14) Have appropriate carbohydrate available to treat promptly if hypoglycaemia does occur.
(15) Assess diabetic knowledge and refer for further education if necessary.
(16) Ensure the patient knows when to take their next diabetes medication if discharged, especially if the dose has been adjusted, and that the patient understands the new dose.
(17) Arrange appropriate follow-up care.

Clinical observations

(1) Blood glucose can be elevated by infection, pain and anxiety.
(2) TPR and BP can also be affected by emotional stress.
(3) Reassure, rest the patient, repeat the TPR and BP.

Practice points

(1) Hypoglycaemia may be masked by coma from other causes, some medications, and autonomic neuropathy.
(2) UTI and myocardial infarction can be present with few, if any, of the usual presenting signs due to autonomic neuropathy (see Chapters 11 and 16 and Section 14c).
(3) Repeated visits to the emergency department for hypoglycaemia or ketoacidosis can indicate an underlying psychosocial problem (see Chapters 8, 10 and 22).

27.2 The outpatient department

People with diabetes may present to the outpatient department for routine appointments or for minor surgical or radiological procedures. They are usually basically well and mobile, although some may require a wheelchair, interpreter and/or guide dog assistance. Water should be provided for the guide dogs of visually impaired people especially in hot weather.

27.2.1 Nursing responsibilities

(1) Avoid long delays in seeing the doctor.
(2) Be aware of the possibility of hypoglycaemia and know how to recognise and treat it effectively. Know where glucagon and other hypoglycaemic treatments are kept and be sure to restock after use, e.g. hypostop, glucose gel. Have available at least one of the following:
- dry biscuits
- sandwiches
- tea/coffee, sugar
- orange juice
- glucose.

(3) Have blood glucose monitoring equipment available.
(4) Test urine or blood of Type 1 diabetics for ketones if blood glucose is elevated.
(5) Ensure test results are available with the medical record.
(6) Ensure appropriate examination equipment is available, including:
- tendon hammer
- sterile pins
- Semmens-weinstein filaments
- ophthalmoscope
- tuning fork
- biothesiometer
- stethoscope
- eye chart
- midriatic drops.

(7) Ensure patient knows the location of toilets, other clinics, pharmacy.

Nurses and other health professionals should ensure that they are up-to-date with emergency procedures such as cardiopulmonary resuscitation especially when they are working in community settings.

Appendix A
Associations Providing Services for People with Diabetes

A.1 Diabetic associations

Diabetic associations have been established in most countries, including the UK (British Diabetic Association) and Australia (Diabetes Australia). Membership of these associations consists of lay people and health professionals who work together to develop management policies and educational material/programmes for the care of people with diabetes.

A.1.1 Diabetes Australia

Diabetes Australia (DA) is the national diabetes organisation in Australia. It has branches in all states. A magazine, *Diabetes Conquest*, is produced quarterly. A national diabetes supply scheme (NDSS) is organised through Diabetes Australia and allows diabetic equipment (blood and urine test strips, syringes, meters) to be purchased at subsidised prices. People must enrol in the scheme, and a doctor's signature is required on the enrolment form. There is no cost to enrol. Supplies can be ordered and received by mail under this scheme. Insulin is not available through the NDSS scheme.

Diabetes Australia
1st Floor Churchill House
218 Northbourne Avenue
Braddon ACT 2612
Australia

A.1.2 British Diabetic Association

The British Diabetic Association (BDA) is the national diabetes organisation in the UK, with 400 branches and groups. The BDA provides education, develops educational material and trains volunteers. A magazine, *Balance*, is produced six times each year.

British Diabetic Association
10 Queen Anne Street
London W1M 0BD
UK

Both associations can provide information about specific services available and whom to contact for advice or additional information. Both are active in promoting research into diabetes and fund-raising activities to help finance diabetic research. Most of the reading material suitable for people with diabetes listed in Appendix C can be obtained from these associations.

A.1.3 USA

Similar services are provided in the USA by the American Diabetes Association. Enquiries can be directed to:

American Diabetes Association
1660 Duke Street
Alexandria VA 22314
USA

A.2 Professional diabetes associations

Health professional groups with a particular interest in diabetes also work to ensure uniformity of diabetic information, a high standard of care and the professional development of their members. Such associations include:

- American Association of Diabetes Educators
- Australian Diabetes Educators' Association
- Australian Diabetes Society
- British Diabetic Association
- Diabetes Educators International
- European Association for the Study of Diabetes
- Juvenile Diabetes Foundation

A.3 International Diabetes Federation (IDF)

The IDF is an international federation of the national diabetes associations. An International Diabetes Federation Congress is held every three years in a different part of the world.

International Diabetes Federation
International Association Centre
40 Rue Washington B-1050
Brussels, Belgium

A.4 Other professional associations

Other professional associations have diabetic interest groups within their membership. They include:

- National heart foundations
- Kidney foundations
- Dietetics associations
- Podiatry associations

A.5 Pharmaceutical companies

Many of the pharmaceutical companies produce diabetic products and supply patient information material. The major companies producing diabetic products are:

- Bayer Diagnostics
- Becton Dickinson
- Boehringer Mannheim
- Farmatalia Carlo Erba
- Hoechst Pharmaceuticals
- Novo Nordisk
- Roche
- Servier Laboratories
- Terumo Corporation
- Wyeth

Addresses and telephone numbers can be found in the telephone directory, or from the diabetic association in your country.

Appendix B
Diabetes Reference Material for Nursing Staff

B.1 Reference texts

Galloway, J.A., Porvin, J.H. & Shuman, C.R. (eds) (1988) *Diabetes Mellitus*. Eli Lilly, Indianapolis.
Kozak, G.P. (ed.) (1992) *Clinical Diabetes Mellitus*. W.B. Saunders, Philadelphia.
Pickup, J.C. & Williams, G. (eds) (1991) *Textbook of Diabetes*. Blackwell Scientific Publications, Oxford.
Rifkin, H. & Porte, D. (eds) (1990) *Diabetes Mellitus, Theory and Practice*. Elsevier, New York.
Wilson, J. & Foster, D. (eds) (1985) *Williams Textbook of Endocrinology*. W.B. Saunders, Philadelphia.

B.2 Practical texts

Galloway, J. (ed.) (1988) *Diabetes Mellitus*. Eli Lilly, Indianapolis.
Williams, G. & Pickup, J. (eds) (1992) *Handbook of Diabetes*. Blackwell Scientific Publications, Oxford.

B.3 Recommended journals

The following journals are easy to read, contain clinically relevant articles and are available in most hospital libraries.

Diabetes Care (USA)
Diabetic Medicine (UK)
Diabetologia (Europe)
Practical Diabetes (UK)
The Diabetes Educator (USA)

Note: It is desirable to ensure that texts and articles are as current as possible so that information is not outdated.

Appendix C

Reading Material for People with Diabetes

Court, J. (1998) *Modern Living with Diabetes for All Ages*. Diabetes Australia.

Davidson, B. (1986) *New Diabetic Cookery*. Octopus, London.

Day, J. (1998) *The Diabetes Handbook: Insulin Dependent Diabetes*. Thorsons Publishing, London.

Day, J., Brenchlay, S. & Redmond, S. (1998) *Living with Non-Insulin Dependent Diabetes*. Medikos, Sussex.

Horn, B. (1990) *Living with Diabetes*. Houghton, Australia.

Krall, L. & Beaser, R.J. (1989) *Joslin Diabetes Manual*. Lea & Febiger, Philadelphia.

Moffit, P., Phillips, P. & Ayers, B. (eds) (1991) *Diabetes and You, An Owner's Manual*. Diabetes Australia.

Roberts, C., McDonald, C. & Cox, M. (1990) *Eat and Enjoy*. Rene Gordon, Melbourne.

Sonksen, P., Fox, C. & Judd, S. (1998) *Diabetes at your Fingertips: The Comprehensive Diabetes Reference Book for the 1990s*. Class Publishing, London.

Stacy, P. & Borushek, A. (1986) *The Best Australian Cookbook for Diabetes and Weight Control*. Family Health Publications, Perth.

Diabetes Conquest, *Diabetes Forecast* and *Balance* are magazines for people with diabetes produced by the diabetic associations of Australia, the USA and the UK, respectively. They are available to people who become members of the relevant association.

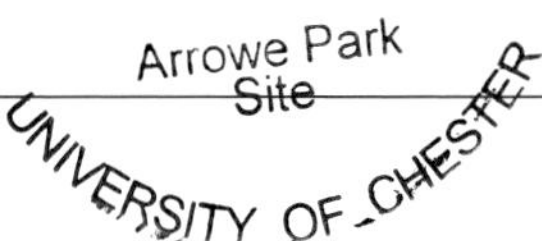

Index

Notes

As diabetes mellitus is the subject of this book, all references in the index concern diabetes mellitus unless otherwise specified: entries have been kept to a minimum under 'diabetes mellitus' (or 'diabetic') and readers are advised to seek more specific entries.

Page numbers in *italics* refer to figures; page numbers in **bold** refer to tables; *vs.* indicates a comparison or differential diagnosis.

acarbose **65**
acceptance, of diabetes 222
acetoacetate 42, 111
acetone 42
acromegaly 2
Actrapid® 73, *80*, *82*
acupuncture 265
acute hypoglycaemia 273
adolescents (diabetes mellitus in) 213–17
- attention-seeking 225
- eating disorders 214
- hypoglycaemia 225
- management compliance 215–16
- nursing responsibilities 216
- polycystic disease of ovary 214
- psychological issues 221–2, 224–5
- sexual problems 184
- *see also* children (diabetes mellitus in)

adrenaline, in hypoglycaemia **96**
adult respiratory distress syndrome (ARDS) 117
advanced glycation end products (AGE) 18
afternoon procedures 131, 133–4
age
- blood glucose levels 36
- children/adolescents *see* adolescents; children
- corticosteroid-related diabetes 157
- diabetes risk 11
- elderly *see* elderly (diabetes mellitus in)
- gestational diabetes 7
- hypoglycaemia 95
- obesity 53
- surgical complications 129
- type 2 diabetes development 4

age-related macular degeneration 167
albumin, nutritional support 146
alcohol consumption 52, 57
- blood glucose levels 36
- haemochromatosis 163
- hyperglycaemia 57
- hypoglycaemia 57, 199
- neuropathy management 205
- sulphonylurea interaction 66

alcoholic ketosis, ketoacidosis *vs.* 112
allergies
- corticosteroid therapy 156
- insulin 91–92
- surgery 130

alpha-glucoside inhibitors 63, **65**, 66
- adverse effects 66
- insulin combination 73
- mode of action 61, 63

American Diabetes Association (ADA) 277
- classification 1–2
- diagnosis 8–9

amputations 128, 203, 211
- physiotherapy 211

anaemia
- associated diseases/disorders 173
- fructosamine monitoring 49
- haemochromatosis 163
- renal disease 172–3

anaesthetists, blood glucose monitoring 131
analgesics
- hypoglycaemia masking 150
- neuropathy management 205
- oral glucose tolerance test 9

anaphylaxis 91
angiography 127
angioplasty 128
angiotensin-converting enzyme (ACE) inhibitors
- adverse effects 197
- cardiovascular disease therapy 124
- insulin sensitivity 192
- and lipid lowering therapy 68
- renal disease 172, 173
- retinopathy prevention 167

anorexia
- cancer 148
- lactic acidosis 62
- renal disease 173
- type 1 diabetes 2

antibiotics
- foot infections 204
- gastroparesis therapy 152
- post-surgery 132

anti-convulsant drugs, neuropathy management 205
anti-depressant drugs, adverse effects 185
antidiabetic agents *see* oral hypoglycaemic agents (OHAs)
anti-hypertensive drugs, oral glucose tolerance test 9
anti-inflammatory drugs, oral glucose tolerance test 9
anti-neoplastic drugs, oral glucose tolerance test 9
antioxidants 53
- complementary therapy 265

apligraft 210
aromatherapy 265–6
- renal disease 178

arthritis
- medication 138

sexual problems 181
aspartame 57
aspiration, enteral nutrition complications 143
aspirin
cerebrovascular disease management 127
cessation pre-colonoscopy 138
and lipid lowering therapy 68
neuropathy management 205
assessment 22–8
associations, for diabetes 276–7
atherosclerosis 121
at-risk groups (diabetes mellitus) 11
gestational diabetes 6–7
attention-seeking, children/ adolescents 225
Australian Diabetes Society Position Statements 12
Australian National Diabetes Strategy and Implementation Plan 225
autonomic neuropathy 18, 151–5, 205
aetiology 151–2
cardiovascular disease effects **122**
diagnosis 152
in elderly **191**
epidemiology 151–2
fall risk 201
hypoglycaemia masking 125, 199, 274
key points 151
management 152–4
myocardial infarction 274
non-diabetic causes 151
nursing care 154–5
organs affected 152, **153**, 154, 205
in pregnancy 219
sexual problems 183, 205
urinary tract infections 274
azathioprine 3

balanitis, thrush-induced 184
basal bolus regime 84, *85*
baseline information, nursing history 22
bed rest, foot disorder management 210
beta blockers
adverse effects 185
cardiovascular disease therapy 124
hypoglycaemia masking 66, 125
betahydroxybutyrate (B-OHB) 42, 111
monitoring 40
bicarbonate replacement
ketoacidosis treatment 115, 217
lactic acidosis therapy 119
biguanides 61–2, **65**
adverse effects 62, 119
in cancer 149
combination therapy 67
contraindications 62
mode of action 60, 61–2
in pregnancy 62
biofeedback techniques 265
biphasic insulin 74, 77
blood glucose levels
acceptable values 11–12, 20
affecting factors 36
children/adolescents 214
cognitive functioning 194
complementary therapies 36, 265
in elderly 194
foot disorders 208
herbal medicine effect 265
hypoglycaemia 94
ketoacidosis treatment 115
neuropathy management 205
nutritional support 143
outpatient stabilisation 105
pregnancy 219
preoperative care 130
sexual problems 183–4
surgery 128
targets 36
see also glucose meters
blood glucose monitoring 35–43, 48
anaesthetist role 131
brittle diabetes 35
cardiovascular disease 123
cardiovascular disease therapy 124
checklist 41
clinical observation 35–6
continuous ambulatory peritoneal dialysis 177
continuous subcutaneous insulin infusion 86
corticosteroids 157
dietary control 37
documentation 31
exercise 15–16
frequency 36–8
glycosylated haemoglobin 35
home-based care 253
hypoglycaemia diagnosis 35
inaccurate results 39, 151
insulin infusion 38
insulin therapy 35, 37, 87
investigative procedures 138
iron overload 164
key points 35
meters 38, 39
see also glucose meters
nephropathy 35
non-invasive testing 39
nutritional support 146
total parenteral nutrition 37, 38
oral hypoglycaemic agents 37, 61
outpatients 104, 275
patient demonstrable knowledge 231
pregnancy 35
protocol 37
purpose 34, 35–36
reverse iontophoreses 39
self-monitoring 34
stabilisation in hospital 104
steroid therapy 38
in surgery 131
visual impairment aids 169
see also glucose meters
blood ketone monitoring 40, 42–3
corticosteroids 157
disadvantages 43
hyperglycaemia 40
ketosis 40
levels and management **42**
outpatient departments 107, 275
polydipsia 41
polyuria 41
type 1 diabetes 41
see also ketoacidosis
blood pressure (BP)
cardiovascular disease therapy 124
documentation 31
emergency management 274
ketoacidosis treatment 115
stabilisation in hospital 104
blood urea nitrogen (BUN) 50
inadequate protein intake 53
blurred vision, hypoglycaemia 140
body mass index (BMI) 53
nutritional status 54
body weight
dietary management 55
monitoring 47
thiazolidinedione adverse effects 63
Boehringer Advantage 37
bowel preparations, colonoscopy 138
bradycardia, ketoacidosis 112
brain, autonomic neuropathy **153**
breakfasts 58–9
breast feeding 220
thiazolidinediones 63
British Diabetic Association 276–7
brittle diabetes mellitus 159–60
aetiology 159
blood glucose monitoring 35
management 159–60
nursing role 160
sliding scale insulin therapy 87
bypass surgery 128

cancer 148–50
care objectives 148–9
corticosteroid therapy 156
nursing responsibilities 149–50
signs/symptoms 148
therapy 148
candidiasis 17
oral 161

capsaicin, topical 205
captopril, adverse effects 43
carbohydrate modified foods 57
carbohydrates 52
  dietary management 55
  hypoglycaemia therapy 97
cardiac arrhythmias 89
cardiac disease 121
  corticosteroid-related diabetes 157
cardiac failure, thiazolidinedione adverse effects 63
cardiac insufficiency, in elderly **191**
cardiovascular disease 3, 18, 121–7
  aetiology 122, **122**
  clinical manifestations 121
  epidemiology 121–2
  investigation 125
  morbidity 123
  mortality 121, 123
  therapy 123–5
    lipid lowering therapy 68
  nursing responsibilities 123–5
  objectives 123
  rehabilitation 125
  risk factor modification 126
cardiovascular system, autonomic neuropathy therapy **153**, 154
care pathways 29
care plans 22
carotid bruits 127
carotid endarterectomy 127
carpal tunnel syndrome 174
cataracts 166, 167
caverject 185
central obesity 53
central parenteral nutrition 145
central venous pressure, ketoacidosis treatment 115
cerebral oedema 216–17
  post ketoacidosis 116
cerebrovascular accident 17, 273
cerebrovascular disease 126–7
Charcot deformity 203
Charcot's arthropathy 18
charting, patient care *see* documentation
cheiroarthropathy, mastopathy 163
chest pains, home-based care 255
children (diabetes mellitus in) 213–17
  assessment 213
  attention-seeking 225
  education 213
  epidemiology 213
  hypoglycaemia 225
  ketoacidosis 117, 215, 216–17
  management 215
  nursing responsibilities 216
  psychological issues 221–2, 224–5
  see also adolescents (diabetes mellitus in)
chlorpropamide 61, **64**
  pre-operative withdrawal 130
cholesterol monitoring 49
cholestyramine **69**
  gastroparesis therapy 152
cimetidine, sildenafil interactions 185
cirrhosis 119
cisapride 152
classification of diabetes 1–2
  see also type 1 diabetes mellitus; type 2 diabetes mellitus
Clinical Management Guidelines for Diabetes in General Practice 12
clofibrate, adverse effects 68
clonidine 205
codeine, neuropathy management 205
cognitive impairment
  blood glucose control 194
  in elderly **192**
  colestipol **69**
colonoscopy 138
communication
  brittle diabetes 159
  in elderly **191**
  outpatient stabilisation 106
comorbidities
  blood glucose levels 36
  surgery 130
  see also specific diseases/disorders
complementary therapies 261–72
  adverse effects 266
  blood glucose levels 36
  in cancer 149
  definition 262–3
  drug interactions 100
  epidemiology 261–2
  guidelines 270
  integration with conventional treatment 263–4
  nursing responsibilities 270–71
  quality of life 262
  renal disease 178
  safe use 269–70
  surgery 128
  types 262, **262**
    acupuncture 265
  antioxidant therapy 265
  aromatherapy 265–6
  biofeedback techniques 265
  cupping 266
  herbal medicine *see* herbal medicine
  moxibustion 266
  relaxation techniques 265
  traditional Chinese medicine *see* traditional Chinese medicine (TCM)
  vitamin supplementation **268**
compliance
  adolescents 215–16
  home-based care 255–6, 257–8
  hypoglycaemia 100
  psychological issues 226
complications (of diabetes mellitus) 3, 11, 17–18
  acute 17
  cardiovascular disease 18
  dietary therapy 54
  long term 17–18
  macrovascular disease 17, 204
  metabolic factors 19–20
  microvascular disease *see* microvascular disease
  patient demonstrable knowledge 231
  prevention 20
  risk factors 15
  screening 104
    see also specific diseases/disorders
confidentiality *see* patients
confusion 196
constipation 196
continuous ambulatory peritoneal dialysis (CAPD) 174–5
  commencement 176–7
  insulin administration 174, 177
  monitoring 50
  patient education 177–8
continuous subcutaneous insulin infusion (CSII) 84–6
control assessment, guidelines 13, **13**
control testing, glucose meters 37, *40*
coronary artery bypass grafting (CABG) 128
corticosteroids 156–8
  adverse effects 197
  blood glucose effects 156–7
  blood glucose monitoring 38
  cancer therapy 148
  diabetes predisposition 157–8
  oral glucose tolerance test 9
  treatment regimes 158
  uses 156
  withdrawal 157
cortisol, in hypoglycaemia **96**
cost (of diabetes mellitus) 18–19
counsellors 265
  sexual health 181, 186
C-peptide 50
  monitoring 49–50
creatinine
  clearance 50
  inadequate protein intake 53
crystal synovitis, in haemochromatosis 163
cupping 266
Cushing's disease 2

blood glucose levels 36
cyclamate 57
cyclosporin 3

daily injection regime 77, 84, *85*
Daonil **64**
'dawn phenomenon' 98
deep venous thrombosis
hyperosmotic non-ketotic coma 118
post ketoacidosis 117
dehydration
in elderly 196
investigative procedures 138
ketoacidosis 111
demographics 22
denial 222
depression 224
elderly 190
in elderly **191**
dermagraft 210
Diabetes Australia 276
Diabetes Control and Complications Trial (DCCT)
long term complications 17
outpatient stabilisation 107
quality of life 227
renal disease 171
diabetes mellitus
gestational *see* gestational diabetes mellitus
type 1 *see* type 1 diabetes mellitus
type 2 *see* type 2 diabetes mellitus
Diabetes Specific Quality of Life 227
'diabetic grief cycle' 222–3, *223*
diabetic ketoacidosis *see* ketoacidosis
Diabex **65**
Diabinese **64**
Diaformin **65**
diagnosis (of diabetes mellitus) 8–11
blood glucose monitoring *see* blood glucose monitoring
during cardiac surgery 122–3
see also screening (diabetes mellitus)
dialysis *see* renal dialysis
Diamicron **65**
diarrhoea
biguanide adverse effects 62
enteral nutrition complications 143
Diastix **45**
diazepam, neuropathy management 205
dietary characteristics
screening methods and problems 54–5
see also nutrition
dietary management, principles 55–6
see also nutrition
dietetic foods 57
differential diagnosis (diabetes mellitus) **6**, 50
DIGAMI protocol 124–5
digoxin, renal disease 173
discharge planning 249–50
district nursing *see* home-based care
dizziness, hypoglycaemia 95
documentation 29–33
clinical observation 31
diabetes specific 31–2, *32*
flow charts 29
medical record 29–32
nursing care plans 29, 31
nursing responsibilities 31, 33
parameters 31
by patient 33
patient confidentiality 31
preoperative care 130
dressings, foot disorders 204, 209
drug absorption, nutrition 56, **56**
drug addiction, brittle diabetes mellitus 159
drug-induced hypoglycaemia 199
drug interactions 66–7
blood glucose levels 36
complementary therapies 100
herbal medicine 197
hypoglycaemia **99**, 99–100
renal disease 173
drunkeness, hypoglycaemia *vs.* 57, 100
dual energy X-ray absorptiometry (DEXA) 53
duodenal tubes 144
dyslipidaemia 53

eating disorders, adolescents 214
echinacea **267**
ecograms 29
ecomaps 29
example *30*
education (diabetes) 13, 16–17, 230–48
affecting factors **236**
basic knowledge 230
cardiovascular disease rehabilitation 125
children/adolescents 213
continuous ambulatory peritoneal dialysis 177–8
dietary management 55
elderly 193–4
empowerment 234–5
instruction sheets 239–47
nursing role 235–7
ongoing 231, 233–4
outpatient stabilisation 104
record chart 232–3
renal disease therapy 174
sexual problem management 185
special issues 235
survival skills 230, 231
elderly (diabetes mellitus in) 189–202
blood glucose control 194
comorbidities 193
corticosteroid effects 157–8
dehydration 196
depression 190
epidemiology 189
falls 200–201
foot care 195
hyperglycaemia **190**, 195–6
hypoglycaemia 199–200
chronic 99
differential diagnosis 199
drug-induced 199
management 200
risk factors 199–200
infections 195
management 193–5, 196–7
access 194
affecting factors 194, **195**
aims 193
education 193–4
insulin 197
OHAs 196–7
polypharmacy 197
metabolic changes 192
nursing care 201
nutrition 198–9
dementia 199
enteral 198
malnourishment **190**, 198, **198**
status 193
obesity 192
post ketoacidosis 117
quality of life 195–6
renal disease **192**
safety issues 196
sexual problems 183, 184, 196
specific problems **190–92**
urinary tract infections 195
electrocardiography (ECG) 124
electrolyte balance
herbal medicine adverse effects 178
nutritional support 146
surgery 129
embolism, hyperosmotic non-ketotic coma 118
emergency departments 273–4
emergency surgery 134
empowerment 234–5
endocrine disorders
blood glucose levels 36
brittle diabetes 160
enteral nutrition 144
complications 143
elderly 198
see also parenteral nutrition; percutaneous endoscopic gastrostomy (PEG)
epidemiology (of diabetes mellitus) 2

erectile dysfunction *see* sexual problems
erythropoietin production, renal disease 173
ethnicity
gestational diabetes 7
as risk factor 11
Euglocon **64**
euglycaemic ketoacidosis 119
'exchanges' 58
exercise 15–16
blood glucose monitoring 15–16, 36
diabetes management 12
drug therapy modification 15
energy sources *15*
in hospital 16
nutrition 58
sexual problem management 185
eye diseases/disorders 166–70
detection 168
epidemiology 166–7
investigation 138–40, 168
see also retinopathy; visual impairment

falls
autonomic neuropathy 201
elderly 200–201
risk 201
family history, as risk factor 11
fasting
colonoscopy 138
hypoglycaemia 199
investigative procedures 137
ketones 42
pre-surgery 129
fasting blood glucose 8
fatigue
inadequate protein intake 52
sexual problems 181
fatty liver 53
fenugreek **267**
fever, ketoacidosis 113
feverfew **268**
fibrates **69**
fine needle aspiration biopsy 163
FlexPen® **76**, *81*, *82*, *83*
flow charts 29
fludrocortisone 154
fluid balance
cardiovascular disease therapy 124
emergency surgery 134
herbal medicine adverse effects 178
insulin infusion 89
ketoacidosis treatment 115
nutritional support 146
urine glucose testing 44
fluorescein angiography 168
patient care 139
food types *see* nutrition
foot disorders 203–12, 273
aetiology 204–7, **206**, *206*
assessment 207
autonomic neuropathy **153**
in elderly 195
examination 208
home-based care 252, 256–7
hospitalization 203, 204
infections 204–5
management 204
morbidity/mortality 203
nursing responsibilities 207–9
patient demonstrable knowledge 231
prevention 207
quality of life 203
risk factors **207**
therapy 209–11, **210**
amputations 211
care objectives 207
future work 210–11
hygiene 208
rehabilitation 211
ulcer classification 209
wound management 209–11
fructosamine monitoring 48–9

gabapentin 205
garlic **267**
gastrointestinal tract, autonomic neuropathy therapy 152, 153, **154**
gastroparesis 143, 152, **153**, 154, 205
brittle diabetes 159
therapy 155
gastroscopy tubes 144
genitals, autonomic neuropathy **153**
genograms 29
genomaps 29
example *30*
Geriatric Depression Scale 190
gestational diabetes mellitus 6–7, 219
classification 2
definition 6
diabetes risk 11
oral glucose tolerance test 219
at risk populations 6–7
screening 6
type 2 diabetes development 4
ginger **268**
gingko biloba **267**
ginseng **267**
glaucoma 167
glibenclamide 61, **64**
adverse effects 199
Glimel **64**
Glimepiride **65**
glipizide **64**
glitinides 63, **65**
in elderly 197
mode of action 60
glucagon administration **96,** 101–2
adverse reactions 102
contraindications 102
dosages 101
Glucophage **65**
glucosamine **268**
glucose
monitoring *see* blood glucose monitoring
transport into cell *5*
glucose meters 38, 39
control testing 37, *40*
light reflectance 38
inaccurate results 39
Glucowatch 39
glutamic acid decarboxylase (GAD) antibodies 50
gluten-free foods 152
glycaemic index 58
glycosuria 8
aetiology 44
ketoacidosis 111
glycosylated haemoglobin (HbA1c)
blood glucose monitoring 35
false results **49**
formation 48
hyperglycaemia 48
monitoring 48
outpatient stabilisation 105
granulocyte-stimulating factor 210
growth hormone, in hypoglycaemia **96**
Guillain–Barré syndrome 151

haemochromatosis 163
haemodialysis 176
haemoglobin, glycosylated *see* glycosylated haemoglobin (HbA1c)
haemoglobinopathies, fructosamine monitoring 49
halitosis 161
Hashimoto's thyroiditis 160
HbA1c *see* glycosylated haemoglobin (HbA1c)
Health-Related Quality of Life, Short Form 36 227
heparin 132
herbal medicine 262
adverse effects 178, 266
blood glucose level effect 265
common herbs **267–8**
drug interactions 197, 266, **267–8**, 269
high density lipoprotein (HDL) monitoring 49
HMG-CoA reductase inhibitors **69**
home-based care 251–60
advantages/disadvantages 251
blood glucose monitoring 253
chest pains 255
foot disorders 252, 256–7

hyperglycaemia 252, 254–5
hypoglycaemia 252, 253–4
insulin premixing 259–60
insulin storage 258–60
non-compliance 255–6, 257–8
nursing responsibilities 252–3
sharps disposal 252, 258
stabilisation 103
HONK *see* hyperosmolar non-ketotic coma (HONK)
HOPE studies 172
hops **268**
hormones
in hypoglycaemia 96, **96**
replacement therapy 156
surgery effects 129
hospitalization 19
foot disorders 203, 204
stabilisation 103–4
transfer 250
HUMA*PEN* **76**
Humulin® 73, 74, 77, *78–9*
types 73, *78*
Humulog® 72, 74, *78–9*
hydramnios 220
hypercholesterolaemia, thiazolidinedione adverse effects 63
hyperglycaemia 17, 110, 273
aetiology/causes
alcohol consumption 57
corticosteroids 156
drug interactions 66
enteral nutrition 143
exercise 16
during insulin therapy 74, 84, 86, 90
menstruation 184
polyuria 196
pregnancy 218
surgery 129, 132, 134
associated diseases/disorders
cancer 148, 149
cardiovascular disease 122
neuropathy 206
postural hypotension 196
pressure ulcers 196
renal disease 171
skin rashes 196
urinary tract infections 196
blood ketone monitoring 40
complications 196
blurred vision 140
documentation 31
in elderly **190**, 195–6
glycosylated haemoglobin 48
home-based care 252, 254–5
oral disease 196
overnight 84
prevention 119
rebound 160
therapy 113
see also ketoacidosis
hyperinsulinaemia 3–4
corticosteroids 156
hypernatraemia 143
hyperosmolar non-ketotic coma (HONK) 17, 117–18, 273
aetiology *118*
management 89, 274
mortality rate 117
precipitating factors 117
prevention 119
risk factors 19
surgical complications 129
treatment 117–18
see also hypoglycaemia
hypertension 122
cardiovascular disease effects **122**
retinopathy 167
hypoalbuminaemia 148
hypoglycaemia 17, 94–102
acute 273
aetiology/causes 97–8
drug-induced 61, 63, 66, **99**, 99–100, 150, 199
enteral nutrition 143
exercise 16
fasting 199
ketoacidosis 116
rapid-acting insulins 73
surgery 129, 131, 132
age 95
alcohol consumption *vs.* 57, 100, 199
associated diseases/disorders
autonomic neuropathy 154, 199, 274
brittle diabetes 160
in cancer 148, 149
cardiovascular disease 125
impaired cognitive function 199
liver disease 199
malnutrition 199
renal disease 199
sexual problems 181
chronic 89, 99
documentation 31
home-based care 252, 253–4
hormonal response 96, **96**
investigative procedures 138
masking 274
nocturnal 84, 98
outpatient departments 275
patient demonstrable knowledge 231
psychological effects 100–101
relative 99
repeated emergencies 274
at risk groups 100
children/adolescents 214, 225
in elderly *see* elderly (diabetes mellitus in)
gender 95
signs/symptoms 94–5, 95, **95**
blood glucose levels 94
blood glucose monitoring 35
blurred vision 140
therapy 96–8, 101–2
care objectives 96
conscious patient 96–7
impaired consciousness 97
insulin infusion 89
see also glucagon
see also hyperosmolar non-ketotic coma (HONK)
hypoglycaemic agents *see* oral hypoglycaemic agents (OHAs)
hypokalaemia
herbal medicine adverse effects 178
post ketoacidosis 116
thiazide diuretics adverse effects 124
hypotension
postprandial 201
postural
autonomic neuropathy 154
fall risk 201
hyperglycaemia/dehydration 196
therapy 154
renal dialysis 174
hypothermia, ketoacidosis 112
hypoxia, ketoacidosis 112
Hypurin 73
Hypurin neutral 73

idiopathic diabetes mellitus 2
immune-mediated diabetes mellitus 2
immunosuppression
corticosteroids 157
type 1 diabetes therapy 3
impaired cognitive function 19
hypoglycaemia 199
impaired fasting glucose 2
impaired glucose homeostasis 2
impaired glucose tolerance 2
corticosteroid-related diabetes 157
impaired insulin response 159
independence 20
infections 17
inflammatory diseases 156
influenza vaccinations 195
inhaled insulin 72, 91
InnoLet® **76**, *81*, *83*
Innovo® **75**, *81*, *83*
instruction sheets 239–47
type 1 diabetes 242–4
type 2 diabetes 245–7
insulin(s)
allergy 91–2
biphasic 74, 77
inhaled 72, 91
intermediate-acting 73, *79*

long-acting 73, 77, 91
mode of action *5*, 71–2
neutral *78*
oral 72
premixing *78*
home-based care 259–60
rapid-acting 72–3, *79*, *85*
hypoglycaemia 73
short-acting 73, 77, *85*
storage 74
home-based care 258–60
types 72–4, *78–80*
see also specific types
Insulin Aspart 72, 74
insulin-dependent diabetes mellitus (IDDM) *see* type 1 diabetes mellitus
Insulin Glargine 72
insulin infusions 87–90
affecting factors 90
associated risks 89
blood glucose monitoring 38
cardiovascular disease therapy 123
emergency situations 274
hyperosmolar non-ketotic coma management 274
infusion rate 88
ketoacidosis management 274
lactic acidosis therapy 119
mistakes 90, *91*
myocardial infarction management 274
neuropathy management 205
pump 89
solution preparation 88
insulin Lispro *78*
insulin resistance syndrome 3–4, *4*
corticosteroids 156
terminal patients 19
type 2 diabetes development 3
insulin therapy 71–93
administration 74–7
blood glucose monitoring 37
in cancer 149
combination therapy
alpha-glucoside inhibitors 73
biguanides 67
oral hypoglycaemic agents 67, 133
sulphonylureas 67
continuous ambulatory peritoneal dialysis 174, 177
devices **75–6**
jet injectors 76
'pens' **75–6**, *81–3*
syringes **75**
see also individual types
dose modification 157
education 237–8
elderly 197
instruction sheets 239–41
investigative procedures 138
ketoacidosis treatment 115
objectives 72
patient demonstrable knowledge 231
pre-surgery 130
pumps **76**
Quality Use of Medicines 71
regimes 72–4, 77, 84
basal bolus 84, *85*, 133
continuous subcutaneous insulin infusion 84–6
daily injection 77, 84, *85*
intravenous *see* insulin infusions
twice daily 84, *85*
renal disease 172
sliding scale 86–7
top-up (stat) doses 87
in type 2 diabetes 71–2
vision effects 87
visual impairment aids 169
see also management (of diabetes mellitus)
Insultard® 73, *82*
intensive care unit (ICU), insulin infusions 89
intermediate-acting insulin 73, *79*
intermittent claudication 17, 204
International Diabetes Federation (IDF) 277
intravenous lines 146
investigative procedures 137–44
blood glucose monitoring 138
care objectives 137–8
hypoglycaemia 138
instructions 137
insulin therapy 138
nursing management requirements 138
see also specific procedures
iron overload 163–4
iron supplements 138
islet cell antibodies 50
isomalt 57
isophane insulin *78*, *79*

jejunal tubes 144
jejunostomy 152
jet injectors **76**

ketaconazole, sildenafil interactions 185
ketoacidosis 3, 17, 110–17, 273
aetiology 110–11, *112*
pregnancy 219
surgery 129
assessment 112–13
children 215, 216–17
complications 116–17
consequences **113**
differential diagnosis 112
emergency surgery 134
euglycaemic 119
prevention 119
repeated emergencies 274
risk factors 19
signs/symptoms **111**, 111–12, *112*
treatment 113
bicarbonate replacement 217
insulin infusions 89, 274
nursing care 114, 115–16
observations 115–16
unit preparations 114
see also blood ketone monitoring; hyperglycaemia
Keto-diabur-Test 5000 **45**
Ketodiastix **45**
ketones 42, 111
blood, monitoring *see* blood ketone monitoring
urinary, monitoring 37
ketonuria 45
ketoacidosis 111
Ketostix **45**
kidney biopsy 174
kidney function, urine tests 346
Kussmauls respiration, ketoacidosis 111

lactic acidosis 119–20
biguanide adverse effects 62
drug-related 119
management 119–20
signs/symptoms 62
lactose intolerance, thiazolidinediones 63
left ventricular hypertrophy, anaemia 173
lente insulin *78*, *79*
leptin 53
lethargy
hypoglycaemia 95
ketoacidosis 111
type 1 diabetes 2
leukocyte function 19
libido decrease 183–4
lichen planus 161
lifestyle modifications
cardiovascular disease management 126
outpatient stabilisation 105
light reflectance meters *see* glucose meters
lignocaine, neuropathy management 205
limbs, lower *see* foot disorders
lipase inhibitors 53
lipid lowering agents 68–9, **69**
adverse effects 68–9
erectile dysfunction 185
cardiovascular status 68
lipids
dietary management 52, 55
outpatient stabilisation 105

serum, monitoring 49
lispro 72
liver damage
iron overload 163
sulphonylurea adverse effects 61
thiazolidinedione adverse effects 63
liver disease
blood glucose levels 36
hypoglycaemia 95, 199
long-acting insulin 73, 77, 91
low-density lipoproteins (LDLs) 68
monitoring 49

macroproteinuria 172
macrovascular disease 17, 204
maculopathy 166, 167
magnetic resonance imaging (MRI) 204
malnourishment 55
elderly **190**, 198, **198**
hypoglycaemia 199
nutritional support 143
malnutrition
anaemia 173
in cancer 148
hypoglycaemia 199
renal disease 173
malnutrition-related diabetes mellitus 7
mammograms 163
management (of diabetes mellitus) 11–16
aim 12–14
blood glucose monitoring 35
in cancer 148–9
clinical observation 13
control assessment **14**
dietary modification 55–6
education *see* education
exercise *see* exercise
investigative procedures 137–41
model *14*
during surgery 128–36
team 11–12
see also insulin therapy; oral hypoglycaemic agents (OHAs)
Mason-type diabetes *see* maturity onset diabetes of the young (MODY)
massage 262, 265
mastopathy 165
maturity onset diabetes of the young (MODY) 2, 7–8
type 1 diabetes *vs.* 7
medical records 29–32
Medisense PC 37
meditation 262
menstruation, hyperglycaemia 184
metabolic acidosis 111
metformin **65**
in elderly 196–7
pre-operative withdrawal 130
metoclopramide 152
Micral-test 46
microalbuminuria 172
monitoring 46
renal disease 171–2
renal failure 172
microangiopathy 162
Microbumin test 46
micronutrient deficiency 52
microvascular disease 18, 204
cardiovascular disease effects **122**
mastopathy 163
midrodrine 154
mineral deficiencies 53
Minidiab **64**
Mini Mental State Examination 194
misinformation
sexual problems 182
type 2 diabetes 17, 224
Mixtard® 74, 77, *80*, *82*
monitoring 34–51
betahydroxybuterate 40
cholesterol 49
continuous ambulatory peritoneal dialysis 50
C-peptide 49–50
creatinine clearance 50
education 47
fructosamines 48–9
glucose *see* blood glucose monitoring; urinary glucose testing
glycosylated haemoglobin 48
islet cell antibodies 50
ketones *see* blood ketone monitoring; urinary ketone monitoring
kidney function 46
lipids 49
lipoproteins 49
microalbuminuria 46
nursing responsibilities 47
nutritional status 54–5
oral glucose tolerance testing *see* oral glucose tolerance test (OGTT)
physical examination 47
renal function 50
total parenteral nutrition 50
triglycerides 49
weight 47
Monotard® 73, *80*
morning procedures 131, 133, 134
moxibustion 266
myocardial infarction 17, 122, 123, 273
autonomic neuropathy 154, 274
insulin infusions 89
management 274
post ketoacidosis 117

nasogastric tubes 144
nursing responsibilities 145–6
nataglitinide **65**
National Diabetes Services Scheme 252
National Diabetes Strategy 12
National Standards Framework, elderly care 194
nausea/vomiting
biguanide adverse effects 62
investigative procedures 138
lactic acidosis 62
sulphonylurea adverse effects 61
nephropathy 18
blood glucose monitoring 35
in haemochromatosis 163
see also renal disease
nerve blocks, neuropathy management 205
neuropathies 3, 18, 205–7
autonomic *see* autonomic neuropathy
in elderly **191**
in haemochromatosis 163
hyperglycaemia 206
management 205
motor nerves 205
peripheral 18
development 206–7
in elderly **190**
foot disorders 204
sensory nerves 205
sexual problems 181
neutral insulin *78*
nicotinic acid (low-dose) **69**
nocturnal hypoglycaemia 84, 98
non-alcoholic fatty liver disease (NASH) 163
non-insulin-dependent diabetes mellitus (NIDDM) *see* type 2 diabetes mellitus
non-insulin-dependent diabetes of the young (NIDDY) *see* maturity onset diabetes of the young (MODY)
non-invasive testing 39
non-mydriatic fundus photography 168
non-nutritive sweeteners 57
noradrenaline **96**
Novolet® **75**, *81*
NovoMix® **76**, *80*, *82*
Novo Nordisk Product Range *82–3*
NovoPen® **75**, *81*, *83*
NovoRapid® 72, *80*, *82*
nursing care 19–20
aims 20
ketoacidosis 114, 115–16
objectives 20
plans 20, 29, 31
visual impairment 169–70
nursing history 22–8
assessment chart 24–8
baseline information 22

care plans 22
characteristics 22–3
demographics 22
notes 31
patient confidentiality 22
patient independence 22
physical disability 23
nursing responsibilities 235–7
brittle diabetes 160
cancer 149–50
cardiovascular disease 123–5
children/adolescents 216
complementary therapies 270–71
documentation 33
emergency departments 274
foot disorders 207–9
home-based care 252–3
hospital stabilisation 104
intravenous lines 146
monitoring 47
nasogastric tubes 145–6
nutrition 52–3, 56
nutritional support 145–7
outpatient departments 275
percutaneous endoscopic gastrostomy 146
photocoagulation 139–40
renal disease 176
nutrition 12, 52–9
blood glucose monitoring 37
body weight 55
cardiovascular disease 126
deficiencies 54
dietary management, principles 55–6
drug absorption 56, **56**
education 55
elderly *see* elderly (diabetes mellitus in)
exchanges and portions 58
exercise 58
food types
carbohydrates 52, 55
dietetic foods 57
fat 52, 55
gluten-free foods 152
protein 55
salt 52
sugar 55
'sugar-free' foods 56–7
glycaemic index 58
key points 52
lipid lowering therapy 68
monitoring 54–5
neuropathy 205
nursing responsibilities 56
nursing role 52–3
in pregnancy 220
renal disease 173, 174
screening 54–5
sexual problems 185
nutritional support 143–7
administration routes 144–5
aims 143
blood glucose monitoring 143, 146
complications 143
fluid balance 146
formula choice 145
malnourishment 143
nursing responsibilities 145–7
recommencing oral feeding 147
see also enteral nutrition; parenteral nutrition

obesity 53–4
age 53
assessment 53
calculation 53
in elderly 192
gestational diabetes 7
inadequate protein intake 52
medication effects 54
therapy 53–4
type 2 diabetes development 3–4
ocular oedema 166
oliguria, ketoacidosis 112
open heart surgery 89
oral candidiasis 161
oral cavity disease 161–2
aetiology 162
hyperglycaemia/dehydration 196
management 162
signs/symptoms 161
oral glucose tolerance test (OGTT) 8, 9–11, 50
contraindications 9
drug interactions 9
gestational diabetes 6, 219
patient instructions 10
patient preparation 9
test protocol 9–11
oral hypoglycaemic agents (OHAs) 60–7
adverse effects **64–5**
hypoglycaemia 199
blood glucose monitoring 37, 61
combination therapy 61, 67
insulin 67, 133
dosage/frequency **64–5**
corticosteroid effect 157
drug interactions 66–7, **67**
elderly 196–7
enteral nutrition 144
gestational diabetes 7
investigative procedures 138
in pregnancy 220
renal disease 173
surgery 128
see also management (of diabetes mellitus); *individual agents*
oral insulin 72
osmotic diuresis 111
outpatient departments 275
overnight hyperglycaemia 84
oxygen therapy
ketoacidosis 115
lactic acidosis 119

pancreas transplants 92
pancreatic disease, blood glucose levels 36
parenteral nutrition 145
blood glucose levels 36
hyperosmotic non-ketotic coma 117
see also enteral nutrition
Parkinson's disease 151
patients
confidentiality 22
documentation 31
independence 22
instructions
oral glucose tolerance test 10
surgery 133
oral glucose tolerance test 9
responsibilities 33
PenMate 3 **76**
'pens' **75–6**, *81–3*
percutaneous endoscopic gastrostomy (PEG) 144
nursing responsibilities 146
see also enteral nutrition
periodontal disease 161
peripheral neuropathy *see* neuropathies
peripheral parenteral nutrition 145
peripheral vascular disease, in haemochromatosis 163
peritoneal dialysis 176
hyperosmotic non-ketotic coma 117
pharmaceutical companies 278
phenytoin 205
photocoagulation 139–40, 168
goals 139
nursing responsibilities 139–40
post-operative complications 140
physical disability 23
physical examination 47
physiotherapy
amputations 211
ketoacidosis treatment 116
neuropathy management 205
pioglitazone **65**
platelet-derived growth factor 210
PLISSIT model 187
polycystic disease of the ovary (PCOS)
adolescents 214
as risk factor 11
thiazolidinedione adverse effects 63
polydipsia
ketoacidosis 111
ketone monitoring 41
type 1 diabetes 2

polypharmacy
  elderly 197
  hypoglycaemia 199
polyuria
  hyperglycaemia/dehydration 196
  ketoacidosis 111
  ketone monitoring 41
  type 1 diabetes 2
'portions' 58
postprandial hypotension 201
postural hypotension *see* hypotension
preadmission clinics 130
Precision PCx 37
prednisolone, adverse effects 156
pre-eclampsia 220
pregnancy 218–20
  autonomic neuropathy 219
  blood glucose monitoring 35, 36, 219
  complications 18
  diabetes screening 218
  fructosamine monitoring 49
  hyperglycaemia predisposition 218
  ketoacidosis 42, 219
  management goals 219–20
  nutrition 220
  oral hypoglycaemic agents 220
    biguanides 62
    sulphonylureas 61
    thiazolidinediones 63
  retinopathy 167
premixed insulin *78*
pre-operative care 130
pressure ulcers 196
primary care settings 103
professional associations 277
protein
  dietary management 55
  inadequate intake 52
  intake inadequate 53
  urine testing 46
proteinuria 171–2
Protophane® 73, *80*
psychological illness
  repeated emergencies 274
  sexual problems 181
psychological issues 221–7
  children/adolescents 221–2, 224–5
  compliance 226
  'diabetic grief cycle' 222–3, *223*
  diagnosis 221–2
  patient requirements 226–7
  type 1 diabetes 221–2, 224–5
  type 2 diabetes 223, 225–6
  see also quality of life
pumps, insulin therapy **76**

quality of life 227–9
  complementary therapies 262
  determinants 227
  elderly 195–6
  foot disorders 203
  hypoglycaemia 100
  improvement 227–8
  measurement 227
  see also psychological issues
Quality Use of Medicines 71

radiocontrast media injection 140–41
rapid-acting insulins 72–3, *79*, *85*
  hypoglycaemia 73
Rastinon **65**
record chart 232–3
reflux 143
relaxation techniques 265
renal dialysis 174–5, 176–8
  continual ambulatory peritoneal dialysis *see* continuous ambulatory peritoneal dialysis (CAPD)
  haemodialysis 176
  peritoneal dialysis *see* peritoneal dialysis
  priorities 174
renal disease 171–9
  anaemia 172–3
  assessment 174
  blood glucose levels 36
  cardiovascular disease 125
  care objectives 175
  complementary medicine 178
  diet 173
  in elderly **192**
  erythropoietin production 173
  hypoglycaemia 199
  insulin therapy 172
  management 173–5, 176–8
  nursing responsibilities 176
  retinopathy 172
  risk factors 171–2
    see also nephropathy
renal failure 172
renal function monitoring 46, 50
repaglinide **65**
  in elderly 197
resins **69**
retinal photography 139, 168
retinopathy 3, 18, 166, 174
  aetiology 167
  cardiovascular disease therapy 125
  epidemiology 167
  investigation 139
  prevention 167
  renal disease 172
  risk factors 167
reverse iontophoresis 39
risk factors
  hyperosmolar non-ketotic coma 19
  ketoacidosis 19
  type 2 diabetes 3–4

rosiglitazone **65**
  contraindications 197
  in elderly 197
Royal National Institute for the Blind 168

saccharin 57
salt 52
screening (diabetes mellitus) 11, *12*
  gestational 6
  nutrition 54–5
  pregnancy 218
    see also diagnosis (of diabetes mellitus)
self-monitoring 34
serotonin reuptake inhibitors 53
serum albumin 146
serum creatinine 53
serum lipids 49
serum potassium 115
serum urea 146
sexual assault, ketoacidosis 116
sexual development 181
sexual health 180–88
  counsellors 181, 186
  sexual history 186
sexual problems 181–2
  adolescents 184
  arthritis 181
  autonomic neuropathy 183, 205
  blood glucose levels 183–4
  causes 182–3
  elderly 183, 184, 196
  erectile dysfunction 18, 183, 184–5
    age-associated 184–5
    drug-associated 185
    epidemiology 185
    non-diabetic causes 184
    therapy 154, 185
  fatigue 181
  hypoglycaemia 181
  infections 184
  investigation 185–6
  libido decrease 183–4
  management 185–8
    drug interactions 185
    nursing role 187–8
    PLISSIT model 187
  men 184–5
  misinformation 182
  neuropathy 181
  psychological illness 181
  vaginal lubrication 183–4
  vaginal thrush 184
  women 183–4
sharps disposal 238
  home-based care 252, 258
  patient demonstrable knowledge 231
shock, corticosteroid therapy 156
short-acting insulin 73, 77, *85*
sialosis 161

sibutamide 53
sildenafil 154, 185
  drug interactions 185
skin atrophy **191**
skin rashes 196
sliding scale, insulin therapy 86–7
slippery elm **268**
smoking cessation 154
  cardiovascular disease management 126
  lipid management 68
  neuropathy management 205
  oral glucose tolerance test 9
  pre-surgery 130
snacking 59
sodium restriction 173
Somoygi effect 98
sorbitol 57
stabilisation (of diabetes mellitus) 103–9
  definition 103
  home settings 103
  hospitalization 103–4
    nursing responsibilities 104
  outpatients 104–7
    objectives 105
    patient criteria 106
    protocol 106–7, 108–9
    rationale 106
  primary care settings 103
starvation ketosis 112
statins **69**
steatosis 163
Stevia 57
St John's Wort **268**
stress
  blood glucose levels 36
  in elderly **191**
  nocturnal hypoglycaemia 98
strokes 126–7
sugar
  dietary management 55
  hypoglycaemia therapy 97
'sugar-free' foods 56–7
sulphonylureas 61, **64–5**
  adverse effects 61
  in cancer 149
  combination therapy 67
  drug interactions 99, **99**
  introduction 60
  mode of action 60, 61
  in pregnancy 61
  pre-operative withdrawal 130
    see also specific drugs
surgery 128–36
  afternoon procedure 131, 133–4
  at-risk populations 129
  basal bolus regime 133
  comorbidities 130
  complementary therapies 128
  complications 129
  debridement
    foot disorders 209
    foot infections 204
  electrolyte imbalance 129
  emergency 134
  hormonal effects **129**
  hypoglycaemia 129, 131
  insulin infusions 88–9
  long-term effects **129**
  major procedures 131
  management aims 129–30
  metabolic effects **129**
  minor procedures 132–4
  morning procedure 131, 133, 134
  oral hypoglycaemic agents 128
  patient instructions 133
  post operative nursing care 132
  preoperative nursing care 130–31
see also specific procedures
sweeteners, non-nutritive 57
syncope 123
syringes **75**

takeaway foods 59
Taxus celebica, adverse effects 178
temperature, pulse and respiration (TPR)
  documentation 31
  emergency management 274
  ketoacidosis treatment 115
  nutritional support 146
  stabilisation in hospital 104
tetracycline 152
thalassaemia, haemochromatosis 163
thiazide diuretics
  adverse effects 124
    erectile dysfunction 185
  hyperosmotic non-ketotic coma 117
  oral glucose tolerance test 9
thiazolidinediones (TZIs) 63, **65**
  adverse effects 63
  contraindications 63
  in elderly 197
  mode of action 61
thrombolytic agents 124
thrush-induced balanitis 184
tolbutamide **65**
tolrestat 205
total parenteral nutrition (TPN) 145
  blood glucose monitoring 37, 38
  monitoring 50
traditional Chinese medicine (TCM)
  adverse effects 266
  renal disease 178
traditional medicine *see* complementary therapies
transient ischaemic attacks (TIAs) 126
tricyclic antidepressant drugs 205
triglycerides 68
  monitoring 49
trimethoprim 152
tropical diabetes mellitus 7
truncal obesity 53
twice daily regime 84, *85*
type 1 diabetes mellitus 1, 2–3
  characteristics **6**
  C-peptide 50
  differential diagnosis **6,** 50
    maturity onset diabetes of the young *vs.* 7
  idiopathic 2
  immune-mediated 2
  instruction sheets 242–4
  islet cell antibodies 50
  ketoacidosis 3
  ketone monitoring 37, 41
  ketonuria 45
  management *see* management (of diabetes mellitus)
  progression *3*
  psychological issues 221–2, 224–5
  sexual problems in women 183
type 2 diabetes mellitus 1, 2, 3–6
  characteristics **6**
  complications 3
    see also individual complications
  C-peptide 50
  development 3
  differential diagnosis **6**
  hyperosmolar non-ketotic coma 117
  instruction sheets 245–7
  insulin therapy 71–2
  ketonuria 45
  management
    oral hypoglycaemic agents *see* oral hypoglycaemic agents (OHAs)
      see management (of diabetes mellitus)
  misinformation 17, 224
  psychological issues 223, 225–6
  risk factors 3–4
  sexual problems in women 183
  urinary ketone monitoring 37

ultralente insulin *78*, *79*
ultrasound 163
Ultratard® 73, *80*
United Kingdom Prospective Diabetes Study (UKPDS)
  cardiovascular disease findings 122
  insulin and oral hypoglycaemic agent combinations 67
  long term complications 17
  outpatient stabilisation 107
urea, nutrition 146
urinalysis
  documentation 31
  protein 46
  protocol 37

urinary glucose testing 44–6
  controls 44
  indications 45
  limitations 44–5
  stabilisation in hospital 104
  test strips **45**
urinary ketone monitoring 37, 45
urinary tract, autonomic neuropathy **153**
urinary tract infections (UTIs) 17
  autonomic neuropathy 274
  in autonomic neuropathy 154
  in elderly 195
  hyperglycaemia/dehydration 196

vaginal lubrication 183–4
vaginal thrush 4
valerian **268**
Valsalva manoeuvre 152
vascular changes 204
venesection 163
venous thrombosis, post-surgery 132
very-low density lipoproteins (VLDL) 49
vision, blurred 140
Vision Australia 168
visual impairment
  aids/resources 168–9
  in elderly **191**
  fall risk 201
  insulin therapy commencement 140
  nursing care 169–70
    see also eye diseases/disorders
vitamin A 53
vitamin B_{12} absorption 62
vitamin C 53
vitamin deficiencies 53
vitamin E 53
vitamin supplementation **268**
  renal disease therapy 173

white cell count 19
World Health Organization (WHO)
  diabetes diagnosis 8, **8**
  sexuality definition 180–81
wound healing 196

xenical 53
xerostomia 161

zinc supplements **268**